Interactions between microbes and metals have a huge economic importance. Metallic structures and apparatus can be corroded leading to reduced efficiency of operation and even danger to users. However, microorganisms have enormous potential for the removal of economically important metals from their ores. There has been intense research in this field of biotechnology in recent years, and this is reviewed here. Specialists cover the different aspects of the subject in separate chapters, which include marine corrosion and the prospects and management of biomining bacteria. The chemical and electrochemical aspects and the prospects for controlling the positive and negative effects of these microorganisms are covered in detail.

Mining and oil industries engineers and researchers will find the contents of this book extremely pertinent. Researchers in biotechnology, metallurgy and microbiology will also find much of interest here.

Bioextraction and biodeterioration of metals

The Biology of World Resources Series

The impact of organisms on the world's materials, foodstuffs, structures and environments

Series Editors

DR DENNIS ALLSOPP

Head of Genetic Resources and External Services, International Mycological Institute

DR BRIAN FLANNIGAN

Reader, Department of Biological Sciences, Heriot-Watt University

DR RITA COLWELL

President, University of Maryland Biotechnology Institute and Professor of Microbiology

The Biology of World Resources is an international research series that examines the influence of living organisms (both micro and macro) on the world's manufactured, built and natural resources. The important role played by organisms in the world-wide economy requires a greater understanding if resources of all kinds are to be used responsibly and to the best effect.

Initial volumes will be concerned with biodeterioration of materials such as the microbial deterioration of metals, hydrocarbons and plastics materials. More traditional materials of organic origin such as lignocellulosic materials and foodstuffs will also be covered.

The negative aspect of biodeterioration of materials will be balanced by chapters and volumes concerned with the biodegradation of wastes and their bioconversion into less harmful or useful products. Biological extraction and concentration of materials will also be covered.

These materials-centred works will be complemented by volumes covering the broader problems presented by composite structures and systems such as buildings (domestic and commercial), transport systems, utilities and natural environments utilized for production or environmental purposes.

The Biology of World Resources Series 1

Series Editors
Dennis Allsopp
Brian Flannigan
Rita Colwell

Bioextraction and biodeterioration of metals

Edited by

CHRISTINE C. GAYLARDE

Departamento de Solos, Universidade Federal do Rio Grande do Sul, Brazil

HÉCTOR A. VIDELA

Sección de Electroquímica, INIFTA, Universidad Nacional de la Plata,
Argentina

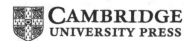

CAMBRIDGE
UNIVERSITY PRESS

CAMBRIDGE UNIVERSITY PRESS
Cambridge, New York, Melbourne, Madrid, Cape Town, Singapore,
São Paulo, Delhi, Dubai, Tokyo

Cambridge University Press
The Edinburgh Building, Cambridge CB2 8RU, UK

Published in the United States of America by Cambridge University Press, New York

www.cambridge.org
Information on this title: www.cambridge.org/9780521122351

First published 1995
This digitally printed version 2009

A catalogue record for this publication is available from the British Library

Library of Congress Cataloguing in Publication data

Bioextraction and biodeteriodarion of metals / edited by Christine C.
  Gaylarde and Héctor A. Videla.
     p.   cm. – (The Biology of world resources : series 1)
   ISBN 0 521 41757 0
   1. Metals – Biodegradation.   2. Bacterial leaching.   I. Gaylarde,
Christine C.   II. Videla, Héctor A.   III. Series.
QR135.5.M37B54   1995
620.1.′623 – dc20   94–26747 CIP

ISBN 978-0-521-41757-0 Hardback
ISBN 978-0-521-12235-1 Paperback

Contents

Contributors

PROFESSOR S. C. DEXTER

College of Marine Studies, University of Delaware, Lewes, DE 19958-1298, USA

DR R. G. J. EDYVEAN

Department of Chemical Engineering, University of Leeds, Leeds IS2 9JT, UK

PROFESSOR T. FORD

Harvard School of Public Health, Department of Environmental Health, 665 Huntington Avenue, Boston, MA 02115, USA

PROFESSOR C. C. GAYLARDE

Departamento de Solos, Universidade Federal do Rio Grande do Sul, Avenida Bento Gonçalves 7712, 91540-000 Porto Alegre, RS, Brazil

DR R. A. KING

Corrosion Services, 34 Cecil Road, Manchester M9 2RQ, UK

DR J. S. MAKI

Department of Biology, Marquette University, Wehr Life Sciences Building, Milwaukee, WI 53233, USA

PROFESSOR R. MITCHELL

Laboratory of Microbial Ecology, Division of Applied Sciences, Harvard University, 40 Oxford Street, Cambridge, MA 02138, USA

DR D. MORIN

Direction de Recherches, Département Géomatériaux et Géoprocédés, Avenue de Concyr, Orléans-La Source, BP 6009, 45060 Orléans cedex 2, France

PROFESSOR H. H. PARADIES

Biotechnology and Physical Chemistry, Markische Fachhochschule, Frauenstuhlweg 31, D-58644 Iserlohn, Germany

PROFESSOR D. E. RAWLINGS

Microbiology Department, University of Cape Town, 22 University Avenue, Private Bag, Rondebosch 7700, South Africa

PROFESSOR C. A. C. SEQUEIRA

Laboratorio de Electroquímica, Instituto Superior Técnico, Avenida Rovisco Pais, 1096 Lisboa, Portugal

PROFESSOR H. A. VIDELA

Sección de Electroquímica, INIFTA, Universidad Nacional de La Plata, Sucursal 4, Casilla de Correo 16, (1900) La Plata, Argentina

DR D. R. WOODS

Microbiology Department, University of Cape Town, 22 University Avenue, Private Bag, Rondebosch 7700, South Africa

Series Editors' Foreword

The natural, manufactured or environmental resources of the world constitute a vast range of substrates and habitats, which to a lesser or greater degree may be influenced or modified by the activities of living organisms. In the case of materials such as metals, plastics, cellulosics and stored food the response to organisms is only passive, but where a resource is a complex environmental one such as a lake or agricultural land there is an extra dynamic element, provided by its living components, that will respond to changes in an active manner.

The material and environmental resources of the world are under increasing pressure, both from the increasing demands of growing populations and also from increasing standards and aspirations of consumers. The demand for 'more and better' in all things places us in a doubly difficult situation. Imbalance in economic activities also can create difficulties; higher crop yields in one area may be at the expense of harmful eutrophication in another. Sustainability is a term now well recognized in agriculture and in certain areas of manufacturing that have planned recycling programmes, but the universal acceptance and implementation of such concepts is still some way off. Current and future innovations in materials manufacture, use and disposal may bring their own particular problems. These problems will be difficult to forecast, with no long experience to draw on.

This series of books aims to address the involvement of biological factors in material and environmental resources. The concept grew from a proposed series on the biodeterioration of materials and the biodegradation of wastes, to one which also encompassed complex environmental resources, as all these topics are interlinked.

It is the biological factors, which are so central and infringe on all human activity and yet are often overlooked, that will be examined. A building constructed with only engineering or aesthetic considerations in mind may be rendered uninhabitable if a large microbial load builds up in its atmosphere. For example, the creation of energy-economical 'tight buildings' has led to problems of condensation and attendant mould growth that have implications for both the fabric of the buildings and the health of the occupants. Again, an electrical component designed with regard only for its physical, chemical and electrical properties may be rendered useless by attack by organisms. Conformal coatings, designed to protect delicate electrical components against water, corrosion and vibration may be broken down by fungi, which can also cause direct electrical malfunctions by bridging circuits on small components.

A better understanding of how materials and organisms interact is therefore vital to the sensible and most economic choice and use of such resources both long and short term, and is the starting point for studies on the use of complex natural and artificial environments as resources. It is the intention of both the Series Editors and the Volume Editors to reflect the need for this understanding, and to present the complexities of important areas and issues in which living organisms have a profound influence.

Dennis Allsopp
Brian Flannigan
Rita Colwell

Preface

This volume links together two important aspects of the biology of metals: the extraction of metals from their ores using bacteria and the corrosion of artificial metallic objects by biological activity. The bioextraction of metals is a centuries old process, but the role of living organisms in metal leaching was only recognized some years after the discovery that microorganisms were involved in metal corrosion. Both topics are currently commanding much interest from both research and industrial sectors of society because of their great economic importance. The contributors to this volume have produced up-to-date reviews of progress in their areas of expertise. This introduction provides some basic and historical background information.

Bioextraction of metals

Leaching methods for the extraction of copper from ores were used in combination with the cementation process as early as the fifteenth century in northern Hungary. Dump leaching has been employed in many countries since this time, although the pioneer is generally regarded to be the Rio Tinto mine in Spain in 1725. The Russians and North Americans were active in the field from an early stage and by the mid-1970s the world production of copper using the dump leaching technique was estimated to be 280 000 tons, of which the USA produced 230 000 tons.

Bacteria of the genus *Thiobacillus* were first isolated by Beijerinck in 1902 and *Thiobacillus thiooxidans* was identified by Waksman in 1922. Until the 1960s, the leaching process was generally considered to be purely chemical, even though it had been shown that sulfur-oxidizing microorganisms could oxidize pyrite and sulfide ores of zinc. Even after the isolation of a pure culture of *T. ferrooxidans* from acid mine waters in 1947, it was some years before real attention was paid to the importance of these organisms in metal leaching. The first patent utilizing *Thiobacillus* was granted in the USA in 1958 and the method was used commercially in dump leaching of copper in Bingham Canyon, Utah.

The introduction of leaching technology for other metals may be considered to be the extraction of uranium from its sulfide ores in the 1960s. The commercial recovery of uranium from acid mine drainage at Eliot Lake, Canada, was begun in 1960, although it was not until 1964 that *T. ferrooxidans* was shown to be present in the drainage waters. The Agnew Lake Mines, in Northern Ontario, Canada, began full-scale leaching of uranium in 1977. The direct bioleaching of other metals has still not been shown to be economically competitive with existing methods.

In addition to direct extraction of metal, bioleaching may also be used to remove unwanted components from ores such as gold or lead prior to refining. Tank leaching of ores, leading to the modern methods used for gold extraction, did not begin even on a laboratory scale until the 1960s. Initial results were unpromising, with low oxidation rates produced by bacteria on sulfide ores (some mg/l per h). Later improvements in technology had allowed this to be increased to over 1 g/l per h by 1971, but maximum rates reported since this time seem to imply that a plateau has been reached and future increases will have to come from improvements in the microorganisms. Genetic engineering techniques applied to the leaching bacteria may offer the answer and the genetic systems of *Thiobacillus* are currently the subject of intensive research. The economics of optimum use of the world's mineral resources means that this will be an interesting and highly active research and development area in future years.

Adhesion of microorganisms to surfaces and biofilm formation

The bacteria utilized in bioleaching have been found to adsorb to the surface of the ore particles and this physical contact is believed to be important in the industrial process. Similarly, contact between microbial cells and metal has been shown to be necessary for some biocorrosion phenomena. Hence research into the adsorption of microbial cells to metal-containing surfaces is essential for an understanding of both processes.

The importance of surfaces on microbial activity was first noted in the literature by Sohngen in 1913 and, in 1918, the adsorption of bacteria on to solid particles was studied by Eisenberg. He noted that Gram-positive bacteria of high lipid content adsorbed more strongly than did Gram-negative bacteria. In the 1920s, Mudd & Mudd showed in an elegant series of experiments that bacterial adsorption to an oil/water interface depended on the degree of hydrophobicity of the cell surface. Put simply, the greater the cell surface hydrophobicity, the greater the tendency to collect at the aqueous/non-aqueous interface and also the greater the tendency to pass into the non-aqueous phase.

Following the initial adhesion of cells to an interface, further build-up of the biofilm will depend on factors such as ability of cells to form aggregates and the possible synthesis of extracellular polymeric materials, which may act as gums. Biofilms cause fouling of industrial equipment such as heat exchangers, pipelines and ship hulls, resulting in reduced heat transfer, increased corrosion and increased frictional resistance. Fouling is also of commercial concern in the microelectronics industry and in the production of paper and rolled steel. In the medical field, biofilms are of importance for their ability to harbour and protect pathogenic microorganisms. Research into biofilm formation and activity is currently changing many of the traditional views on microbially influenced metal corrosion.

Biodeterioration of metals

The first suggestion that bacteria might be involved in metal corrosion was made in relation to lead pipes by Garrett in 1891, whilst the role of bacteria in the corrosion of ferrous metals was first recognized by Gaines in 1910. A landmark in the history of microbially induced corrosion was the proposal, by the Dutch workers von Wolzogen Kühr and van der Vlugt in 1934, of an electrochemical explanation for the anaerobic corrosion of pipes in soil induced by sulfate-reducing bacteria (SRB). Their Cathodic Depolarization Theory implicated the activity of the bacterial enzyme hydrogenase in the corrosion process. They concluded that only active sulfate reduction could effect the anaerobic corrosion of cast iron. Although the role of hydrogenase in corrosion has since been questioned, notably by Booth & Tiller in 1968, there is no doubt that the process of sulfate reduction is essential. Following the Dutch publication, a number of alternative theories to explain SRB-mediated corrosion were proposed by workers such as King & Miller in 1971, Costello in 1974, and Iverson & Olson in 1983 and it is now generally accepted that the phenomenon is multifactorial.

The relatively recent recognition of the importance of sessile (attached) microbial cells and biofilms in corrosion has led to the elaboration of a number of new monitoring techniques and has shown that the traditional electrochemical view of corrosion, which has held sway since the early pioneer work of Booth, Tiller and Iverson, among others, is in need of radical rethinking. In addition, the need for improved control methods, both by cathodic protection and coatings and by the use of biocides, has become obvious. Future research in this subject will include the development of more sensitive and more rapid detection techniques, together with the elaboration of control agents and processes designed to combat sessile, as well as planktonic, organisms. Economic losses caused by biologically mediated corrosion have been estimated to be above 1% of the gross national product in the UK and hence investment into the understanding and control of these processes should have a high priority.

It is intended that this volume should indicate the economic importance of the bioextraction and biocorrosion of metals, in addition to reviewing the current research in progress. We hope that we have achieved these aims and should like to thank all the authors for their excellent contributions.

Christine C. Gaylarde
Héctor A. Videla

1

Metal–microbe interactions

TIM FORD, JAMES MAKI
and RALPH MITCHELL

Introduction

The interaction between microorganisms and metals in any environment is one of balance. Microorganisms require metals in trace quantities for metabolism and growth (Table 1.1), but higher concentrations can be toxic. Metals can be categorized in terms of their toxicity and availability (Duxbury, 1985): type 1, non-critical (Table 1.1); type 2, potentially toxic and relatively available (in addition to the metals in Table 1.1, these include Ag, Sb, Cd, Bi, Pt, Cr, Au, Sn, Hg, Pd, Pb and Tl); type 3, potentially toxic but relatively unavailable due to their rarity or insolubility (includes Hf, Ta, Os, Zr, Re, Rh, W, Ga, Ir, Nb, La and Ru). The toxicity of metals is caused primarily by their ability to denature proteins (Gadd & Griffiths, 1978). This denaturing can be caused by blocking of functional groups, displacing an essential metal or modifying the active conformation of the molecule (Collins & Stotzky, 1989). Biotic and abiotic influences on the toxicity of metals to microbes have been reviewed in detail (Collins & Stotzky, 1989).

Microbial cells require mechanisms for the acquisition of the essential metals to metabolize, grow and reproduce. However, in order to survive in environments containing high concentrations of available metals, they need mechanisms for dealing with their inherent toxicity. Both types of mechanism are exploited in bioextraction (Hutchins et al., 1986; Brierley et al.,

Table 1.1. *Physiological functions of metals and their relative availability and toxicity*

Metal	Biological function[a]	Accessibility and toxicity[b]
Fe	Present in cytochromes and an enzyme cofactor	Type 1
Mg	Enzyme cofactor	Type 2
Mn	Enzyme cofactor	Type 2
Mo	Present in special enzymes	Type 2
Co	Present in vitamin B_{12} and coenzyme derivatives	Type 2
Cu	Present in special enzymes	Type 2
Zn	Present in special enzymes	Type 2
Ni	Present in special enzymes	Type 2
Va	Present in special enzymes	—

Note: [a]Modified from Stanier *et al.* (1986), Wackett *et al.* (1989) and Neidhardt *et al.* (1990).
[b]Adapted from Duxbury (1985). Type 1, non-critical; type 2, relatively available and potentially toxic.

1989) and can contribute to biodeterioration (Houghton *et al.*, 1988; Ford & Mitchell, 1990).

There is a considerable volume of work on metal–microbe interactions. This chapter attempts to provide a broad overview of these processes, using some recent examples. We focus primarily on bacteria, although all microbes will interact with metals during their life cycles.

Iron and manganese

Iron and manganese oxidizing/depositing or reducing bacteria deserve special mention for two reasons: (a) interactions between microorganisms and iron and manganese are central to many bioextraction processes, due to the ability to coprecipitate other metals; and (b) iron and manganese oxide formation creates serious fouling and corrosion problems. Excellent reviews have been written on the mechanisms of iron and manganese oxidation and reduction (e.g. Ghiorse, 1984; Jones, 1986; Nealson *et al.*, 1988, 1989). There is evidence that mechanisms exist for iron deposition both intracellularly and extracellularly. Extracellularly, iron may have a structural role in colony morphology, or in the coprecipitation of toxic ions. In addition, it may also protect the cell from oxygen. Intracellularly, iron deposition may prevent accumulation of toxic levels of iron and, in some bacteria, a high intracellular concentration of magnetite ensures migration of the bacterium toward the sediments and away from high oxygen concentrations (Frankel & Blakemore, 1984).

Microorganisms are the major catalysts of manganese cycling in the environment (Nealson *et al.*, 1989). Depending on growth conditions, some organisms are capable of both oxidation of Mn(II) and reduction of Mn(III) or Mn(IV). These mechanisms were fully discussed by Nealson *et al.* (1989). There is no direct evidence for a biochemical function for manganese oxidation, although manganese-oxidizing proteins have been isolated. In contrast, direct biochemical proof has recently been obtained that a specific bacterium can use MnO_2 and Fe(III) as terminal electron acceptors for anaerobic respiration (Myers & Nealson, 1988; Lovley & Phillips, 1988).

Summary of interactions

Microbe–metal interactions can be conveniently divided into three types:

1. *Extracellular interactions.* These cover a wide range involving extracellular polymers, proteins, acid metabolites and changes in the localized environment due to biochemical processes.
2. *Cell-surface interactions.* Many metals readily bind to microbial cell surfaces as a result of specific functional groups.
3. *Intracellular interactions.* Metals may accumulate in microbial cells due to specific transport processes. This may result in detoxification through transformation to insoluble or more volatile forms, or incorporation of specific metals into enzymes.

Extracellular interactions

Microorganisms do not have to be in direct contact with metals in order to interact. Many interactions between microorganisms and metals occur indirectly due to the production of metabolites or as the indirect consequence of a biochemical reaction. A number of processes are important in biodeterioration and bioextraction: (a) leaching of metals from alloys or natural ores by production of acidic metabolites; (b) release of metals bound to iron and manganese oxides as the result of microbial reduction; (c) immobilization of metals in the form of insoluble metal salts or exopolymer/ metal complexes; (d) production of siderophores to concentrate specific metals in deficient environments.

Acids

Research into industrial uses for microbe–metal interactions, particularly mining practices, has provided insights into mechanisms of metal solubiliz-ation and transport. Organic or inorganic acids produced by microorganisms including *Thiobacillus* spp., *Serratia* spp., *Pseudomonas* spp., *Bacillus* spp., *Penicillium* spp. and *Aspergillus* spp. can be used to extract metals from solid substrates (Schinner & Burgstaller, 1989). For example, Schinner & Burgstaller (1989) used citric acid production by a *Penicillium* sp. to extract zinc selectively from industrial waste.

Coprecipitates

Francis & Dodge (1990) have shown that toxic metals can be mobilized under anaerobic conditions as coprecipitates with iron oxides. They used highly defined pure culture systems with a N_2-fixing *Clostridium* sp. and concluded that metals closely associated with iron (i.e. Cd and Zn) were solubilized by enzymic reduction of Fe(III), whereas others (particularly Pb) were solubilized by the indirect action of bacterial metabolites. This could be an important process in industry because coprecipitation of toxic metals with ferric iron is a widely used treatment for waste streams that have a high metal content (DeCarlo & Thomas, 1985).

Insoluble complexes

Many metal salts are insoluble and their formation results in immobilization of metals by sequestering to sediments or adsorption to soil particles. Fre-quently, metals form insoluble complexes with, for example, hydroxides, carbonates, phosphates and sulfides. Probably the best-known microbial immobilization process results from sulfide production by the sulfate-reducing bacteria, characteristic of anoxic sediments. As a result, these sediments often contain high concentrations of lead and mercuric sulfides.

Extracellular materials

Many microorganisms produce extracellular polysaccharides (EPS) and/or proteins that strongly bind metals. They may be important in biogeochemical cycling of metals (Black *et al.*, 1986; Ford & Mitchell, 1992) and have been strongly implicated in corrosion reactions (Geesey *et al.*, 1986; Ford & Mitchell, 1990).

Most research on EPS–metal interactions stems from the importance of biological flocculation of metals in waste water treatment processes (Brown & Lester, 1979, 1982*a,b*). As a result of extensive chemical studies of EPS (Sutherland, 1972, 1982, 1985) and EPS–metal binding studies (Mittelman & Geesey, 1985; Geesey *et al.*, 1986, 1987; Ford *et al.*, 1987, 1988, 1990; Geesey & Jang, 1989; Ford & Mitchell, 1990) a clearer picture of the interactions now exists. The structure and complexity of a typical EPS molecule is shown in Fig. 1.1. Interaction between EPS and metal ions is generally considered to be a direct consequence of negatively charged functional groups on the exopolymer, for example pyruvate, succinate, uronate, hydroxyl and phosphate. A pH-dependent binding of positively charged cations can rapidly occur with stability constants in excess of those generally measured for humic substances and other naturally occurring ligands (Mittelman & Geesey, 1985). Table 1.2 shows some of the binding characteristics of bacterial EPS and different metal ions. In metal corrosion, EPS–metal ion interactions are thought to change surface equilibrium conditions. Binding of metals to EPS molecules results in release of protons, providing an electron sink to promote the cathodic reaction. Binding also results in reduction of free metal ion concentration in the biofilm. This in turn promotes ionization of the metal from a corroding surface, promoting the anodic reaction. The overall effect is stimulation of the corrosion cell (Geesey *et al.*, 1988; Ford *et al.*, 1991).

Along with EPS, bacteria also secrete extracellular proteins that bind metals. Two examples of these types of protein come from recent characterizations of a manganese-binding and -oxidizing protein (Adams & Ghiorse, 1987; Boogerd & de Vrind, 1987) and copper-binding proteins (Harwood-Sears & Gordon, 1990; Schreiber *et al.*, 1990). The manganese

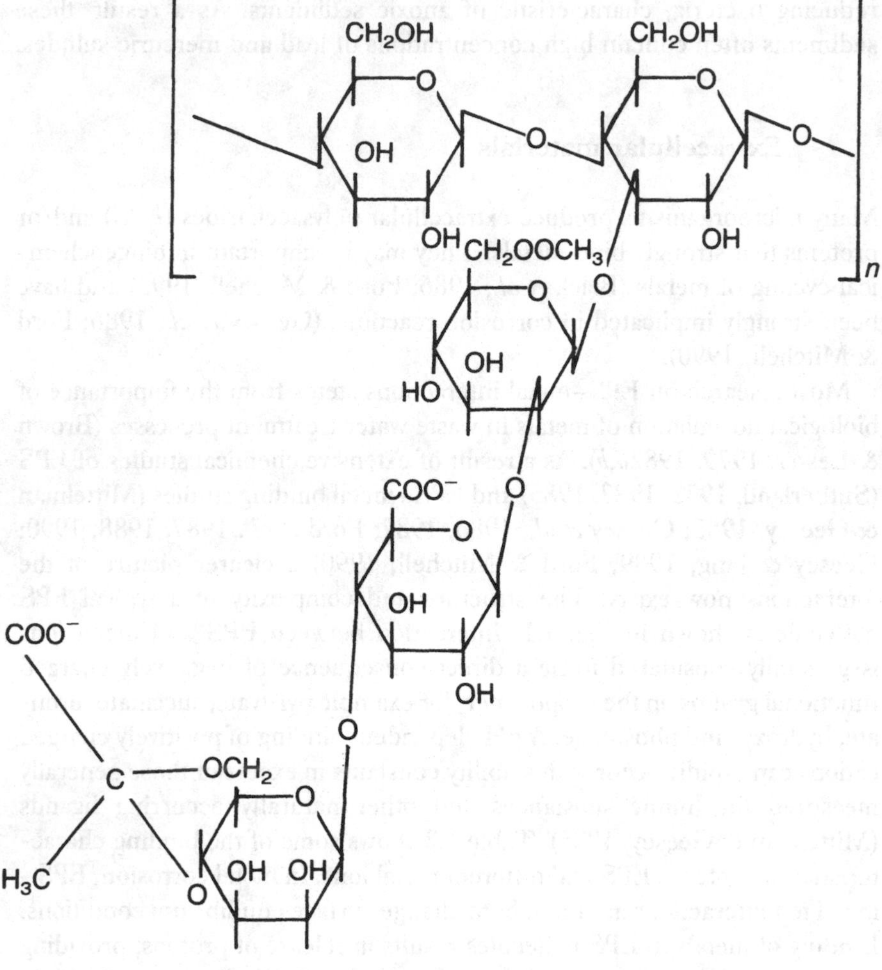

Fig. 1.1 Structure of extracellular polysaccharide from *Xanthomonas campestris* (redrawn from Sutherland, 1982).

(Mn(II))-binding protein $(110\,000\,M_r)$ is secreted by a sheathless mutant of *Leptothrix discophora*. It appears to be associated with high relative molecular mass polysaccharides (Adams & Ghiorse, 1987) and thus may be a component in the sheath of the wild-type parent (Nealson *et al.*, 1989). This protein may be an oxidase that catalyses the oxidation of Mn(II) (Adam & Ghiorse, 1987; Boogerd & de Vrind, 1987). Adam & Ghiorse (1987) have suggested that this protein acts to detoxify Mn(II) by converting it to

Table 1.2. *Maximum binding abilities (MBA) and conditional stability constants* (K_c) of bacterial EPS–metal complexes

Bacterium	Growth conditions	Metal	nmol/mg	K_c ($\times 10^8$)
Thermus sp.	Batch culture	Cu	9	0.7
Thermus sp.	Surface attached	Cu	85	0.09
Deleya marina	Batch culture	Cu	263	24.0
D. marina	Batch culture	Mn	556	9.0
D. marina	Batch culture	Fe	39	1.0
D. marina	Batch culture	Ni	435	14.0
Pedomicrobium *manganicum*	Batch culture	Fe	13	750.0
P. manganicum	Batch culture	Mn	184	19.0
P. ferrugineum	Batch culture	Mn	409	2.9

Note: Compiled from Ford *et al.* (1986, 1987), and Black *et al.* (1986).

MnO_x because the growth of the *L. discophora* mutant is inhibited by Mn(II). The copper-binding proteins (*ca* 19 000–21 000 M_r) are produced by *Vibrio alginolyticus* when it is exposed to copper (Harwood-Sears & Gordon, 1990; Schreiber *et al.*, 1990). These proteins, induced by exposure to copper, act to detoxify the metal by complexation (Harwood-Sears & Gordon, 1990; Schreiber *et al.*, 1990).

Siderophores

Many microorganisms excrete specific chelating agents to facilitate the uptake of ferric ions. These agents, known as siderophores (iron loving), have extremely strong binding affinities for ferric ions. Their function depends on their ability to concentrate iron in iron-deficient environments, and facilitate transport into the cell. Siderophores are low relative molecular mass organic compounds (*ca* 500–1000; Neilands, 1989) containing functional groups such as hydroxamate or catecholate. Binding ability is a function of the size and charge of the ion, hence analogues to ferric iron may also be strongly bound by these siderophores; for example, aluminium, gallium and chromium form trivalent metal ions of similar size (Raymond *et al.*, 1984). Aluminium may be a particular competitor for catecholate siderophores. In a review, Hider (1984) reported stability constants of Fe(III) and Al(III) for catechol of 10^{44} and 10^{46}, respectively. In addition, molybdenum and copper have been shown to form strong complexes with siderophores. Hider (1984) reported that a number of nitrogen-fixing bacteria secreted dicatecholate siderophores under molybdenum-deficient conditions. Dicatecholate siderophore–molybdenum complexes may provide an important uptake mechanism for intracellular molybdenum accumulation, required for nitrogenases. Cu(II) complexation with both hydroxamate and catecholate siderophores has been reported and may be important in sequestering copper for production of tyrosinase enzyme (Davis & Byers, 1971). In addition, McKnight & Morel (1980) suggested that hydroxamate siderophores may play an important role in the reduction of copper toxicity to cyanobacteria. They speculated that the geometry of the copper siderophore complex made it unlikely that it would be assimilated by cyanobacterial cells. It would not be recognized by the iron transport system.

Cell-surface interactions

Binding of metals to cell surfaces is an important factor in the distribution of metals in natural waters (Sigg, 1987; Xue *et al.*, 1988). Both bacterial (Beveridge, 1989) and algal (Xue *et al.*, 1988) surfaces are well suited to binding metals. This sorption of metals to living or dead cells is considered to be a practical solution to many metal contamination problems (Sigg, 1987). Algal surfaces contain functional groups (e.g. carboxylic, amino, thio, hydroxo and hydroxy-carboxylic groups) that can interact with metal ions (Xue *et al.*, 1988).

Lipopolysaccharides

Gram-negative bacteria possess lipopolysaccharides (LPS) in their outer membranes (Fig. 1.2). The LPS are complex, consisting of a hydrophobic, phosphorylated section known as lipid A, a core oligosaccharide section, and variable O-specific side-chains consisting of a number of unusual sugars. The O-specific side-chains project out from the cell membrane and contain different functional groups capable of binding metals.

Phosphoryl groups of LPS and phospholipids are the most abundant electronegative sites available for metal binding (Coughlin *et al.*, 1983;

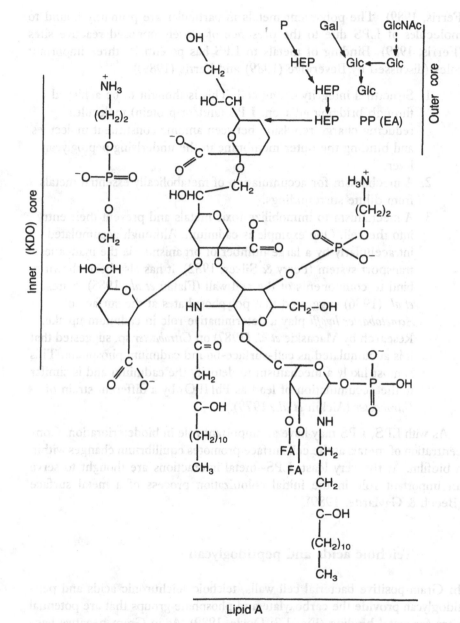

Lipid A

Fig. 1.2 Structure of lipopolysaccharide from *Escherichia coli* K12 (redrawn from Ferris, 1989). FA, fatty acid; EA, ethanolamine; HEP, L-glycero-D-mannoheptose; PP, pyrophosphate; KDO, 2-keto-3-deoxyoctonate.

Ferris, 1989). The polyvalent metals in particular are primarily bound to molecules of LPS due to the presence of closely opposed reactive sites (Ferris, 1989). Binding of metals to LPS has potentially three important roles (discussed by Beveridge (1989) and Ferris (1989)):

1. Structural integrity of the cell. This is thought to be achieved through bridging adjacent LPS (and/or protein) molecules, reducing charge repulsion between anionic constituent molecules and binding the outer membrane to the underlying peptoglycan layer.
2. A mechanism for accumulation of metabolically essential metals from dilute surroundings.
3. A mechanism to immobilize toxic metals and prevent their entry into the cell. One example is cadmium. Although accumulated intracellularly by a large number of organisms via the manganese transport system (Perry & Silver, 1982), it has also been shown to bind to components of the cell wall (Flatau *et al.*, 1985). Suresh *et al.* (1986) suggested that polyphosphates at the surface of *Acinetobacter lwoffi* play a determinative role in cadmium uptake. Research by Macaskie *et al.* (1987) on *Citrobacter* sp. suggested that it is accumulated as cell-surface-bound cadmium phosphate. This is most likely a mechanism to detoxify the cadmium and is similar to the accumulation of lead as $PbHPO_4$ by a different strain of *Citrobacter* (Aickin *et al.*, 1979).

As with EPS, LPS may have an important role in biodeterioration. Concentration of metals at the cell surface promotes equilibrium changes within a biofilm. At the very least, LPS–metal interactions are thought to serve an important role in the initial colonization process of a metal surface (Beech & Gaylarde, 1989).

Teichoic acids and peptidoglycan

In Gram-positive bacterial cell walls, teichoic/teichuronic acids and peptidoglycan provide the carboxylate and phosphate groups that are potential sites for metal binding (Fig. 1.3; Doyle, 1989). As in Gram-negative bacteria, binding of metals to functional groups on the surface of Gram-positive bacteria is thought to be an important step to intracellular accumulation. The importance of cation binding to the morphology of Gram-positive

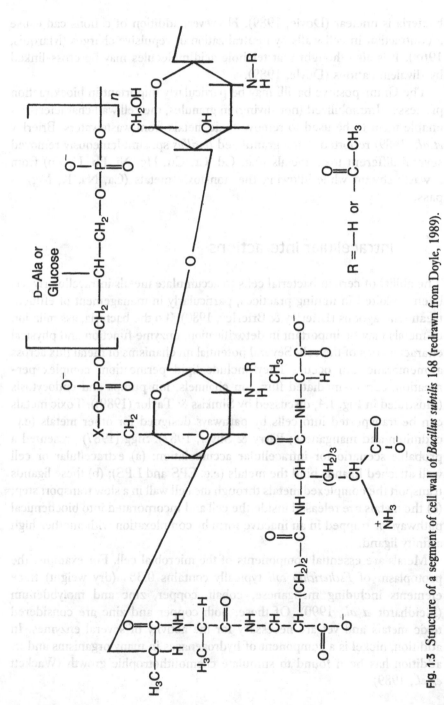

Fig. 1.3 Structure of a segment of cell wall of *Bacillus subtilis* 168 (redrawn from Doyle, 1989).

bacteria is unclear (Doyle, 1989). However, addition of cations can cause a contraction in cell walls by neutralization of repulsive charges (Marquis, 1968). It is also thought that teichoic acid molecules may be cross-linked by divalent cations (Doyle, 1989).

The Gram-positive bacilli may be particularly important in bioextraction processes. Immobilized (non-living) in granules, the cell wall characteristics enable them to be used to remove toxic metals from wastewaters. Brierley *et al.* (1989) reported that a granulated *Bacillus* sp. simultaneously removed several different toxic metals (e.g. Cd, Cr, Cu, Hg, Ni, Pb, U, Zn) from a waste stream while allowing the non-toxic metals (Ca, Na, K, Mg) to pass.

Intracellular interactions

The ability of certain bacterial cells to accumulate metals intracellularly has been exploited in mining practices, particularly in management of effluent treatment lagoons (Brierley & Brierley, 1980). To the bacteria, assimilation of metals may be important in detoxification, enzyme function and physical characteristics of the cell. Several potential mechanisms of metal flux across a membrane can occur. They include lipid permeation, complex permeation, carrier-mediated flux, ion channels, ion pumps and endocytosis (illustrated in Fig. 1.4, discussed by Simkiss & Taylor (1989)). Toxic metals can be transported into cells by pathways designed for other metals (e.g. cadmium and manganese; Perry & Silver, 1982). Sigg (1987) presented a probable scenario for intracellular accumulation: (a) extracellular or cell wall attached ligands bind the metals (e.g. EPS and LPS); (b) these ligands transport the complexed metals through the cell wall in a slow transport step; (c) the metals are released inside the cell and incorporated into biochemical pathways or trapped in an inactive form by complexation with another high affinity ligand.

Metals are essential components of the microbial cell. For example, the protoplasm of *Escherichia coli* typically contains 0.3% (dry weight) trace elements including manganese, cobalt, copper, zinc and molybdenum (Neidhardt *et al.*, 1990). Of these, both copper and zinc are considered toxic metals and yet are necessary for the activity of several enzymes. In addition, nickel is a component of hydrogenases in many organisms and its addition has been found to stimulate chemolithotrophic growth (Wackett *et al.*, 1989).

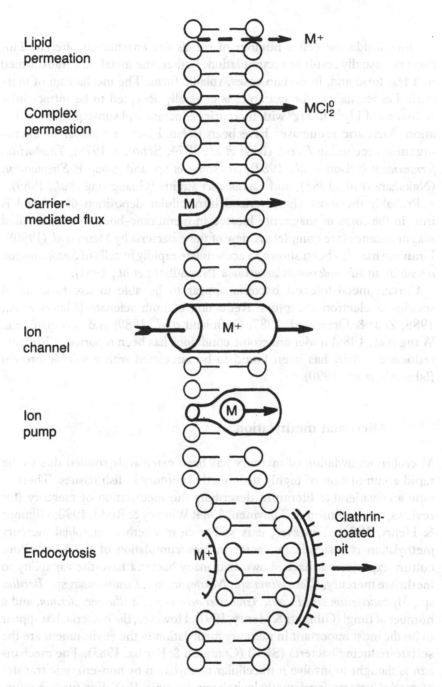

Fig. 1.4 Potential mechanisms of metal (M) flux across a membrane (redrawn from Simkiss & Taylor, 1989).

Once inside the cell a number of metals are enzymically altered. This does not usually result in accumulation. Rather, the metals are transformed to a less toxic and, in certain cases, volatile form. The mechanism of mercuric ion resistance, for example, is generally accepted to be intracellular reduction of Hg^{2+} to Hg^0 with mercuric reductase and subsequent volatilization. Mercuric reductases have been isolated from a number of microorganisms including *E. coli* (Izaki *et al.*, 1974; Schottel, 1978), *Thiobacillus ferrooxidans* (Olson *et al.*, 1982), *Streptomyces* sp. and group B *Streptococcus* (Nakahara *et al.*, 1985), and *Caulobacter* strains (Guangyong *et al.*, 1989).

Probably the most characterized intracellular deposition of a metal is iron in the form of magnetite located in membrane-bound vesicles called magnetosomes (see complete review of these bacteria by Mann *et al.* (1990)). Uranium has also been shown to accumulate rapidly in cells of *Saccharomyces cerevisiae* and *Pseudomonas aeruginosa* (Strandberg *et al.*, 1981).

Certain metal-tolerant bacteria appear to be able to use toxic metal species as electron acceptors. Reduction of both selenate (Maiers *et al.*, 1988; Zehr & Oremland, 1987; Oremland *et al.*, 1989) and chromate (e.g. Wang *et al.*, 1989) under anaerobic conditions has been reported. Chromate reductase activity has been found to be associated with a soluble protein (Ishibashi *et al.*, 1990).

Microbial methylation

Microbial methylation of mercury has been extensively studied due to the rapid accumulation of highly toxic methylmercury in fish tissues. There is now a considerable literature describing the methylation of mercury (for reviews, see Robinson & Tuovinen, 1984; Winfrey & Rudd, 1990; Gilmour & Henry, 1991). However, it is still unclear whether microbial mercury methylation is a significant factor in bioaccumulation of the metal. Pure culture experiments have shown that many bacteria have the capability to methylate mercury, *Clostridium* sp., *Neurospora* sp., *Pseudomonas* sp., *Bacillus* sp., *Mycobacterium* sp., *E. coli*, *Aerobacter aerogenes*, *Bacillus megaterium*, and a number of fungi (Gilmour & Henry, 1991). However, the bacteria that appear to be the most important in mercury methylation in the environment are the sulfate-reducing bacteria (SRB) (Compeau & Bartha, 1985). The mechanism is thought to involve intracellular methylation by non-enzymic transfer of methyl groups from methylcobalamin (vitamin B_{12}). For further information on this mechanism, see the review by Robinson & Tuovinen (1984).

The volatilization of other metals by microbial methylation and other forms of transformation have received less attention than mercury. These processes have been reviewed by Thayer & Brinckman (1982). These authors suggested that rates of other transformations, e.g. ethylation and phenylation, are unlikely to be significant due to the large size of these organic groups. Methylation of other metals, however, has been shown for arsenic, lead, selenium, tellurium, tin, thallium and antimony. For example, Gilmour *et al.* (1985, 1987) correlated production of monomethyl tin in whole sediment samples with numbers of sulfate-reducing and sulfide-oxidizing bacteria. In addition, these authors were able to show that *Desulfovibrio* spp. isolated from the sediments were able to methylate tin in culture medium at rates similar to those of sediment methylation. Methylation of arsenic by fungi was studied extensively as a result of poisoning from fungal transformations of arsenic in paints (for an early review, see Challenger, 1945). More recent work has been concerned with transformation and mobilization in sediments and soils (e.g. Brannon & Patrick, 1987). However, there is little information on the microbial role in these processes.

Genetic considerations

Bacterial metal resistance occurs widely in nature and is often mediated by plasmids. As a result, genetic manipulation may be used to enhance specific microbe–metal interactions. This may play an important role in bioextraction and biodeterioration in the future.

Metal resistance in bacteria can be induced in the laboratory by chromosomal mutation, usually involving changes in membrane transport systems (Silver & Misra, 1988). However, in the environment, metal resistance is generally coded for on plasmids or on transposons (Silver & Misra, 1988; Silver *et al.*, 1989). Some of the better-defined genetically determined metal resistances are presented in Table 1.3. In addition, other less well-defined genetic determinants for resistance to metals include those for bismuth, cobalt, nickel, lead, antimony, thallium, zinc and most probably others (Silver & Misra, 1988). A variety of mechanisms for metal resistance exists (Table 1.3). One of these involves an energy-dependent efflux of the metal. Because many of the toxic metals enter the cell via transport systems for other nutrients, these efflux systems must have a high specificity for the toxic metal in order to avoid the loss of any nutrients (Silver & Misra, 1988). Many of the advances in understanding these genetically determined

Table 1.3. *Some defined genetically determined resistances to heavy metals*

Compound	Location	Mechanism of resistance
Arsenic	Plasmid	Reduced metal uptake due to energy-dependent efflux system
Tellurium	Plasmid	Unknown
Chromate	Plasmid	Uptake of metal blocked
Cadmium	(a) Plasmid	Energy-dependent efflux system (also works for Zn)
	(b) Plasmid	Increased binding of metal
	(c) Plasmid	Energy-dependent efflux system (specific for Cd)
	(d) Chromosomal	Membrane transport system changed so metal no longer accumulated
	(e) Chromosomal	Synthesis of polythiol Cd^{2+} binding protein
	(f) Plasmid	Unknown (also confers resistance to Zn and Co)
Mercury	Plasmid and chromosome	Selective transport system catches Hg outside cell and passes it to mercuric reductase
Copper	Plasmid	Possible cellular metal isolation
Silver	Plasmid	Dependent upon presence of silver complexing components (halide ions)

Note: Compiled from Silver & Misra (1988) and Silver *et al.* (1989).

resistance systems have come through the use of molecular and genetic techniques. The methods of cloning and sequencing the resistance genes have led investigators to develop an understanding of both the quantity and structure of the proteins involved in the actual resistance mechanism and in the regulation of the genes themselves. However, as pointed out by Silver & Misra (1988), sometimes the use of these sophisticated techniques does not necessarily lead to a basic understanding of how the system works.

Eventually, use of molecular and genetic techniques as tools will enable microbiologists to elucidate the detailed mechanisms for most of the microbe–metal interactions we have briefly described above. Understanding how these systems work will provide a greater potential for the use of microorganisms in bioextraction (e.g. Hutchins *et al.*, 1986; Brierley *et al.*, 1989) and hopefully provide humankind with ways to decrease the effects of microorganisms involved in biodeterioration (e.g. Ford & Mitchell, 1990). One method that will be employed will be to use genetically engineered microorganisms (GEMs) as biotechnological solutions to solve problems. Concern has arisen about the release of GEMs into the environment, partly due to the ready exchange of genetic information that is possible between microorganisms in the environment (for a review, see DeFlaun & Levy, 1989). However, it is believed that these effects can be decreased with careful planning with an end result of minimizing the ecological effect of GEMs while maximizing their ability to perform the desired task for which they were engineered (Miller & Levy, 1989). However, release of GEMs in the environment is only one way they can be used. For example, the bacteria used for metal extraction could be immobilized (e.g. Brierley *et al.*, 1989) and/or kept in enclosed reactors to prevent release. Alternative technologies for GEMs can be devised so that environmental release is not a problem.

Conclusions

It should be evident from the above discussion that microbe—metal interactions are varied and numerous. Greater understanding of the various mechanisms involved in these interactions should lead to better use of microorganisms in bioextraction and possibly methods to avoid the effects of microbially based biodeterioration. The complete understanding of the mechanisms requires not only a combination of morphological, physiological and genetic information about the microorganisms involved but also information about the chemistry of the metals themselves.

References

Adams, L. F. & Ghiorse, W. C. (1987). Characterization of extracellular Mn^{2+}-oxidizing activity and isolation of an Mn^{2+}-oxidizing protein from *Leptothrix discophora* SS-1. *Journal of Bacteriology*, 169, 1279–85.

Aickin, R. M., Dean, A. C. R., Cheetham, A. K. & Skarnulis, A. J. (1979). Electron microscope studies on the uptake of lead by a *Citrobacter* sp. *Microbios Letters*, 9, 7–16.

Beech, I. B. & Gaylarde, C. C. (1989). Adhesion of *Desulfovibrio desulfuricans* and

Pseudomonas fluorescens to mild steel surfaces. *Journal of Applied Bacteriology*, 67, 201–7.

Beveridge, T. J. (1989). Role of cellular design in bacterial metal accumulation and mineralization. *Annual Review of Microbiology*, 43, 147–71.

Black, J. P., Ford, T. E. & Mitchell, R. (1986). The role of bacterial polymers in metal release into water. In *International Symposium on Biofouled Aquifers: Prevention and Restoration*, ed. R. Cullimore, pp. 37–42. American Water Resources Association, Bethesda, MD.

Boogerd, F. C. & de Vrind, J. P. M. (1987). Manganese oxidation by *Leptothrix discophora*. *Journal of Bacteriology*, 169, 489–94.

Brannon, J. M. & Patrick, W. H. (1987) Fixation, transformation, and mobilization of arsenic in sediments. *Environmental Science and Technology*, 21, 450–9.

Brierley, J. A. & Brierley, C. L. (1980). Biological methods to remove selected inorganic pollutants from uranium mine wastewater. In *Biogeochemistry of Ancient and Modern Environments*, ed. P. A. Trudinger, M. R. Walter & B. J. Ralph, pp. 661–7. Australian Academy of Science, Canberra.

Brierley, C. L., Brierley, J. A. & Davidson, M. S. (1989). Applied microbial processes for metals recovery and removal from wastewater. In *Metal Ions and Bacteria*, ed. T. J. Beveridge & R. J. Doyle, pp. 359–82. John Wiley & Sons, New York.

Brown, M. J. & Lester, J. N. (1989). Metal removal in activated sludge: the role of bacterial extracellular polymers. *Water Resources*, 13, 817–37.

Brown, M. J. & Lester, J. N. (1982*a*). Role of bacterial extracellular polymers in metal uptake in pure bacterial culture in activated sludge. I. Effects of metal concentration. *Water Resources*, 16, 1539–48.

Brown, M. J. & Lester, J. N. (1982*b*). Role of bacterial extracellular polymers in metal uptake in pure bacterial culture in activated sludge. II. Effects of mean cell retention time. *Water Resources*, 16, 1549–60.

Challenger, F. (1945). Biological methylation. *Chemical Reviews*, 36, 315–61.

Collins, Y. E. & Stotzky, G. (1989). Factors affecting the toxicity of heavy metals to microbes. In *Metal Ions and Bacteria*, ed. T. J. Beveridge & R. J. Doyle, pp. 31–90. John Wiley & Sons, New York.

Compeau, G. C. & Bartha, R. (1985). Sulfate-reducing bacteria: principal methylators of mercury in anoxic sediments. *Applied and Environmental Microbiology*, 50, 498–502.

Coughlin, R. T., Tonsager, S. & McGroarty, E. J. (1983). Quantitation of metal cations bound to membranes and extracted lipopolysaccharide from *Escherichia coli*. *Biochemistry*, 22, 2002–7.

Davis, W. B. & Byers, R. R. (1971). Active transport of iron in *Bacillus megaterium*: role of secondary hydroxamic acids. *Journal of Bacteriology*, 107, 491–8.

DeCarlo, E. H. & Thomas, D. M. (1985). Removal of arsenic from geothermal fluids by adsorptive bubble flotation with colloidal ferric hydroxide. *Environmental Science and Technology*, 19, 538–44.

DeFlaun, M. F. & Levy, S. B. (1989). Genes and their varied hosts. In *Gene Transfer in the Environment*, ed. S. B. Levy & R. V. Miller, pp. 1–32. McGraw-Hill, New York.

Doyle, R. J. (1989). How cell walls of Gram-positive bacteria interact with metal ions. In *Metal Ions and Bacteria*, ed. T. J. Beveridge & R. J. Doyle, pp. 275–93. John Wiley & Sons, New York.

Duxbury, T. (1985). Ecological aspects of heavy metal responses in microorganisms. *Advances in Microbial Ecology*, 8, 185–235.

Ferris, F. G. (1989). Metallic ion interactions with the outer membrane of Gram-negative bacteria. In *Metal Ions and Bacteria*, ed. T. J. Beveridge & R. J. Doyle, pp. 295–323. John Wiley & Sons, New York.

Flatau, G. N., Clemant, R. L. & Gauthier, M. J. (1985). Cadmium binding sites on cells of a marine pseudomonad. *Chemosphere*, 14, 1409–12.

Ford, T. E., Black, J. P. & Mitchell, R. (1990). Relationship between bacterial exopolymers and corroding metal surfaces. *Corrosion 90*. Paper no. 110. NACE, Houston, TX.

Ford, T. E., Maki, J. S., Black, J. P. & Mitchell, R. (1986). Interaction of *Thermus* with metal surfaces. Abstracts of the 86th Annual Meeting of the American Society for Microbiology, Abstract I.33, p. 170.

Ford, T. E., Maki, J. S. & Mitchell, R. (1987). The role of metal-binding bacterial exopolymers in corrosion processes. *Corrosion 87*, Paper no. 380. NACE, Houston, TX.

Ford, T. E., Maki, J. S. & Mitchell, R. (1988). Involvement of bacterial exopolymers in biodeterioration of metals. In *Biodeterioration 7*, ed. D. R. Houghton, R. N. Smith & H. O. W. Eggins, pp. 378–84. Elsevier Applied Science, London, New York.

Ford, T. & Mitchell, R. (1990). The ecology of microbial corrosion. *Advances in Microbial Ecology*, 11, 231–62.

Ford, T. E. & Mitchell, R. (1992). Microbial transport of toxic metals. In *Environmental Microbiology*, ed. R. Mitchell, pp. 83–101. John Wiley & Sons, New York.

Ford, T. E., Mitchell, R. & Geesey, G. G. (1991). Mechanisms of metal deterioration by bacterial exopolymers. In *Biocorrosion Mechanisms*, Proceedings of the Research in Progress Symposium. *Corrosion 91*. NACE, Houston, TX.

Francis, A. J. & Dodge, C. J. (1990). Anaerobic microbial remobilization of toxic metals co-precipitated with iron oxide. *Environmental Science and Technology*, 24, 373–8.

Frankel, R. B. & Blakemore, R. P. (1984). Precipitation of Fe_3O_4 in magnetotactic bacteria. *Philosophical Transactions of the Royal Society, London, Series B*, 304, 567–74.

Gadd, G. M. & Griffiths, A. J. (1978). Microorganisms and heavy metal toxicity. *Microbial Ecology*, 4, 303–17.

Geesey, G. G., Iwaoka, T. & Griffiths, P. R. (1987). The characterization of interfacial phenomena occurring during exposure of a thin copper film to an aqueous suspension of an acidic polysaccharide. *Journal of Colloid and Interface Science*, 120, 370–6.

Geesey, G. G., Jang, J., Jolley, J. G., Hankins, M. R., Iwaoka, T. & Griffiths, P. R. (1988). Binding of metal ions by extracellular polymers of biofilm bacteria. *Water Science Technology*, 20, 161–5.

Geesey, G. G. & Jang, L. (1989). Interactions between metal ions and capsular polymers. In *Metal Ions and Bacteria*, ed. T. J. Beveridge & R. J. Doyle, pp. 325–57. John Wiley & Sons, New York.

Geesey, G. G., Mittelman, M. W., Iwaoka, T. & Griffiths, P. R. (1986). The role of bacterial exopolymers in the deterioration of metallic copper surfaces. *Materials Performance*, **25**, 37–40.

Ghiorse, W. C. (1984). Biology of iron- and manganese-depositing bacteria. *Annual Review of Microbiology*, **38**, 515–50.

Gilmour, C. C. & Henry, E. A. (1991). Mercury methylation in aquatic systems affected by acid deposition. *Environmental Pollution*, **71**, 131–69.

Gilmour, C. C., Tuttle, J. H. & Means, J. C. (1985). Tin methylation in sulfide bearing sediments. In *Marine and Estuarine Geochemistry*, ed. A. C. Sigleo & A. Hattori, pp. 239–58. Lewis, Chelsea, MI.

Gilmour, C. C., Tuttle, J. H. & Means, J. C. (1987). Anaerobic microbial methylation of inorganic tin estuarine sediment slurries. *Microbial Ecology*, **14**, 233–42.

Guangyong, J. I., Salzberg, S. P. & Silver, S. (1989). Cell-free mercury volatilization activity from three marine *Caulobacter* strains. *Applied and Environmental Microbiology*, **55**, 523–5.

Harwood-Sears, V. & Gordon, A. S. (1990). Copper-induced production of copper-binding supernatant proteins by the marine bacterium *Vibrio alginolyticus*. *Applied and Environmental Microbiology*, **56**, 1327–32.

Hider, R. C. (1984). Siderophore mediated absorption of iron. *Structure and Bonding*, **58**, 26–87.

Houghton, D. R., Smith, R. N. & Eggins, H. O. W. (eds) (1988). *Biodeterioration 7*. Elsevier Applied Science, London, New York.

Hutchins, S. R., Davidson, M. S., Brierley, J. A. & Brierley, C. L. (1986). Microorganisms in reclamation of metals. *Annual Review of Microbiology*, **40**, 311–36.

Ishibashi, Y., Cervantes, C. & Silver, S. (1990). Chromium reduction in *Pseudomonas putida*. *Applied and Environmental Microbiology*, **56**, 2268–70.

Izaki, K., Tashiro, Y. & Funaba, T. (1974). Mechanisms of mercuric chloride resistance in microorganisms. III. Purification and properties of a mercuric ion reducing enzyme from *Escherichia coli* bearing R factor. *Journal of Biochemistry* (Tokyo), **75**, 591–9.

Jones, J. G. (1986). Iron transformations by freshwater bacteria. *Advances in Microbial Ecology*, **9**, 149–85.

Lovley, D. R. & Phillips, E. J. P. (1988). Novel mode of microbial energy metabolism: organic carbon oxidation coupled to dissimilatory reduction of iron or manganese. *Applied and Environmental Microbiology*, **54**, 1472–80.

Macaskie, L. E., Dean, A. C. R., Cheetham, A. K., Jakeman, R. J. B. & Skarnulis, A. J. (1987). Cadmium accumulation by a *Citrobacter* sp.: the chemical nature of the accumulated metal precipitate and its location on the bacterial cells. *Journal of General Microbiology*, **133**, 539–44.

Maiers, D. T., Wichlacz, P. L., Thompson, D. L. & Bruhn, D. F. (1988). Selenate reduction by bacteria from a selenium-rich environment. *Applied and Environmental Microbiology*, **54**, 2591–3.

Mann, S., Sparks, N. H. C. & Board, R. G. (1990). Magnetotactic bacteria:

microbiology, biomineralization, paleomagnetism and biotechnology. *Advances in Microbial Physiology*, **31**, 125–81.

Marquis, R. E. (1968). Salt-induced contraction of bacterial cell walls. *Journal of Bacteriology*, **95**, 775–81.

McKnight, D. M. & Morel, F. M. M. (1980). Copper complexation by siderophores from filamentous blue-green algae. *Limnology and Oceanography*, **25**, 62–71.

Miller, R. V. & Levy, S. B. (1989). Horizontal gene transfer in relation to environmental release of genetically engineered microorganisms. In *Gene Transfer in the Environment*, ed. S. B. Levy & R. V. Miller, pp. 405–20. McGraw-Hill, New York.

Mittelman, M. W. & Geesey, G. G. (1985). Copper binding characteristics of exopolymers from a freshwater sediment bacterium. *Applied and Environmental Microbiology*, **49**, 846–51.

Myers, C. R. & Nealson, K. H. (1988). Bacterial manganese reduction and growth with manganese oxide as the sole electron acceptor. *Science*, **240**, 1319–21.

Nakahara, H., Schottel, J. L., Yamada, T., Miyakawa, Y., Asakawa, M., Harville, J. & Silver, S. (1985). Mercuric reductase enzymes from *Streptomyces* species and group B *Streptococcus*. *Journal of General Microbiology*, **131**, 1053–9.

Nealson, K. H., Rosson, R. A. & Myers, C. A. (1989). Mechanisms of oxidation and reduction of manganese. In *Metal Ions & Bacteria*, ed. T. J. Beveridge & R. J. Doyle, pp. 383–411. John Wiley & Sons, New York.

Nealson, K. H., Tebo, B. M. & Rosson, R. A. (1988). Occurrence and mechanisms of microbial oxidation of manganese. *Advances in Applied Microbiology*, **33**, 279–318.

Neidhardt, F. C., Ingraham, J. L. & Schaechter, M. (1990). *Physiology of the Bacterial Cell*. Sineaur Associates, Sunderland, NY.

Neilands, J. B. (1989). Siderophore systems of bacteria and fungi. In *Metal Ions & Bacteria*, ed. T. J. Beveridge & R. J. Doyle, pp. 141–63. John Wiley & Sons, New York.

Olson, G. J., Porter, F. D., Rubinstein, J. & Silver, S. (1982). Mercuric reductase enzyme from a mercury-volatilizing strain of *Thiobacillus ferrooxidans*. *Journal of Bacteriology*, **15**, 1230–6.

Oremland, R. S., Hollibaugh, J. T., Maest, A. S., Presser, T. S., Miller, L. G. & Culbertson, C. W. (1989). Selenate reduction to elemental selenium by anaerobic bacteria in sediments and culture: biogeochemical significance of a novel, sulfate-independent respiration. *Applied and Environmental Microbiology*, **55**, 2333–43.

Perry, R. D. & Silver, S. (1982) Cadmium and manganese transport in *Staphylococcus aureus* membrane vesicles. *Journal of Bacteriology*, **150**, 973–6.

Raymond, K. N., Muller, G. & Matzanke, B. F. (1984). Complexation of iron by siderophores. *Trends in Current Chemistry*, **123**, 49–102.

Robinson, J. B. & Tuovinen, O. H. (1984). Mechanisms of microbial resistance and detoxification of mercury and organomercury compounds: physiological, biochemical, and genetic analyses. *Microbiological Reviews*, **48**, 95–124.

Schinner, F. & Burgstaller, W. (1989). Extraction of zinc from industrial waste by a *Penicillium* sp. *Applied and Environmental Microbiology*, **55**, 1153–6.

Schottel, J. L. (1978). The mercuric and organomercurial detoxifying enzymes from a plasmid-bearing strain of *Escherichia coli*. *Journal of Biological Chemistry*, 253, 4341–9.

Schreiber, D. R., Millero, F. J. & Gordon, A. S. (1990). Production of an extracellular copper-binding compound by the heterotrophic marine bacterium *Vibrio alginolyticus*. *Marine Chemistry*, 28, 275–84.

Sigg, L. (1987). Surface chemical aspects of the distribution and fate of metal ions in lakes. In *Aquatic Surface Chemistry. Chemical Processes at the Particle–Water Interface*, ed. W. Stumm, pp. 319–49. John Wiley & Sons, New York.

Silver, S. & Misra, T. K. (1988). Plasmid-mediated heavy metal resistances. *Annual Review of Microbiology*, 42, 717–43.

Silver, S., Misra, T. K. & Laddaga, R. A. (1989). Bacterial resistance to toxic heavy metals. In *Metal Ions & Bacteria*, ed. T. J. Beveridge & R. J. Doyle, pp. 121–39. John Wiley & Sons, New York.

Simkiss, K. & Taylor, M. G. (1989). Metal fluxes across the membranes of aquatic organisms. *Review of Aquatic Science*, 1, 173–88.

Stanier, R. Y., Ingraham, J. L., Wheelis, M. L. & Painter, P. R. (1986). *The Microbial World*, 5th edn. Prentice-Hall, Englewood Cliffs, NJ.

Strandberg, G. W., Shumate, S. E. & Parrott, J. R. (1981). Microbial cells as biosorbents for heavy metals: accumulation of uranium by *Saccharomyces cerevisiae* and *Pseudomonas aeruginosa*. *Applied and Environmental Microbiology*, 41, 237–45.

Suresh, N., Roberts, M. F., Coccia, M., Chikarmane, H. M. & Halvorson, H. O. (1986). Cadmium-induced loss of surface polyphosphate in *Acinetobacter lwoffi*. *FEMS Microbiological Letters*, 36, 91–4.

Sutherland, I. W. (1972). Bacterial exopolysaccharides. *Advances in Microbiology and Physiology*, 8, 143–213.

Sutherland, I. W. (1982). Biosynthesis of microbial exopolysaccharides. *Advances in Microbiology and Physiology*, 23, 79–150.

Sutherland, I. W. (1985). Biosynthesis and composition of Gram negative bacterial extracellular and wall polysaccharides. *Annual Review of Microbiology*, 39, 243–70.

Thayer, J. S. & Brinckman, F. E. (1982). The biological methylation of metals and metalloids. *Advances in Organometallic Chemistry*, 20, 313–56.

Wackett, L. P., Orme-Johnson, W. H. & Walsh, C. T. (1989). Transition metal enzymes in bacterial metabolism. In *Metal Ions & Bacteria*, ed. T. J. Beveridge & R. J. Doyle, pp. 165–206. John Wiley & Sons, New York.

Wang, P. C., Mori, T., Komori, K., Sasatsu, M., Toda, K. & Ohtake, H. (1989). Isolation and characterization of an *Enterobacter cloacae* strain that reduces hexovalent chromium under anaerobic conditions. *Applied and Environmental Microbiology*, 55, 1665–9.

Winfrey, M. R. & Rudd, J. W. M. (1990). Environmental factors affecting the formation of methylmercury in low pH lakes. *Environmental Toxicology and Chemistry*, 9, 853–69.

Xue, H.-B., Stumm, W. & Sigg, L. (1988). The binding of heavy metals to algal surfaces. *Water Resources*, 22, 917–26.

Zehr, J. P. & Oremland, R. S. (1987). Reduction of selenate to selenide by sulfate-respiring bacteria: experiments with cell suspensions and estuarine sediments. *Applied and Environmental Microbiology*, **53**, 1365–9.

2

Bacterial leaching of refractory gold sulfide ores

DOMINIQUE MORIN

Introduction

The use of biotechnology in relation to precious metals is essentially in the bioleaching of gold-bearing sulfide ores as the pretreatment of ores difficult to process by direct cyanidation.

For a long time gold was recovered only by physical methods, namely gravity separation followed by melting. Then came amalgamation of gold with mercury. For the last 100 years, however, cyanidation has been the main process for extracting gold from ores.

The attraction of the cyanidation process lies in its simplicity. The principle of the process is the oxidation and dissolution of gold in a cyanide solution at ambient temperature, an enhancement effect being provided by the very high stability of the chemical gold cyanide complex. Generally a 1 g/l solution of sodium or potassium cyanide in a reactor suitably agitated and aerated is able, selectively, to bring gold from ores into solution in a few hours. The gold is then extracted from solution by adsorption on activated carbon, cementation on zinc dust or ion exchange on synthetic resins. Finally it is recovered as a coarse product, known as doré, to be ultimately refined.

By comparison with the physical processes, where only relatively coarse particles (>100 μm) of gold can be recovered, cyanidation can deal with finely disseminated gold ores. To make gold accessible to the cyanide solution the ores have to be ground. Where the costly operation of grinding can be economically applied and make the ore amenable to efficient gold recovery by direct cyanidation the material is named a 'free-milling ore'. However, many ores do not respond well to cyanidation, even after fine grinding. Such ores are said to be refractory.

Until recently, only free-milling ores were treated by the processing companies. The refractory facies in a deposit of an otherwise cyanidable ore were simply discarded with the tailings of the milling circuit. However, concurrently with the oil crisis, gold has been subjected to strong demand and reserves of free-milling ores are being depleted. Consequently, the interest in refractory ores has considerably increased. Jha (1987) pointed out that during the last 10 to 15 years, many major gold projects have focused on the processing of refractory ores.

Gold occurs commonly in association with base metals, where the ore is frequently refractory because gold is trapped in the matrix of metallic sulfides, mainly pyrite (FeS_2) and arsenopyrite (FeAsS). In such cases the standard process for liberating gold is to roast the sulfides. The residual calcine is then treated by cyanidation. However, roasting of sulfides is becoming less and less environmentally acceptable because of the pollution of the atmosphere by sulfur dioxide. Only five pyrometallurgical facilities in the Western world continue to accept gold-bearing pyrite–arsenopyrite materials for roasting (Chryssoulis & Cabri, 1990). Alternative hydrometallurgical processes have been developed to replace roasting and have been implemented to varying degrees. Bioleaching is one of these processes and is now recognized as technically and economically viable.

The pretreatment of a refractory gold-bearing sulfide ore by bioleaching leads to the destruction of the sulfide matrix in order to liberate the gold physically and to make the ore amenable to cyanidation. The microorganisms used in the process are mainly the autotrophic thiobacilli. The process is operated in aerated reactors, with the thermostat set at 35–45 °C on a pulp of finely ground ore. This chapter describes the various aspects of this technique, the conditions in which it can be applied and its potential for industrial development.

Mineralogical definition of refractory gold ores

The main mineralogical factors causing the refractoriness of a gold ore are the following (Hausen, 1989; Komnitsas & Pooley, 1989; Petruk, 1989; McDonald *et al.*, 1990):

Physical lock-up. Gold is only locked if it can be economically liberated by grinding. Otherwise it is said to be encapsulated. In this case the gold is usually disseminated as fine grains or submicrometre-size particles in various gangue phases, such as cherty quartz. Gold present in host minerals such as pyrite or arsenopyrite may be of submicroscopic size, and even methods such as scanning electron microscopy fail to show how finely and in what chemical state it is dispersed (Wagner *et al.*, 1988). This type of trapping generally occurs with pyritic or arsenopyritic ores. A study using Mössbauer spectroscopy to determine the nature of the invisible gold has recently been made on the ore of Fairview Mine, Eastern Transvaal, South Africa (Wagner *et al.*, 1989). The results show that the refractory character of the ore is caused by the chemical bonding of the gold rather than by the physical inclusion of small, discrete metallic particles in the matrix of FeAsS and FeS$_2$. In the same way, this technique, employed on a pyrite concentrate from the Olympias mine in Greece, has confirmed results obtained by laser ablation and ion microprobe indicating that the major part of the gold identified is chemically combined with arsenic in arsenic-rich mineral sites encountered in both arsenopyrite and pyrite matrices (Adam *et al.*, 1990). The chemical combination of gold and arsenic in both arsenopyrite and pyrite was previously postulated by Swash (1988) for a South African ore.

Overconsumption of cyanide. Certain sulfide minerals react in water to form cyanicides, which combine with and deplete the cyanide necessary to dissolve the gold.

Oxygen depletion. Some reducing ions such as ferrous, sulfide, thiosulfate and arsenite, consume oxygen when released in water.

Carbonaceous material. Such substances can have an adsorbing effect (pregnant solution robbing) on gold dissolved by cyanidation.

Coating. Certain sulfides, of antimony for instance, and iron
    hydroxides (tarnishing effect) can create a coating on gold
    particles during leaching, thus impeding dissolution.

Insoluble gold alloys. Gold may be associated with tellurium,
    arsenic, antimony or bismuth as more or less refractory alloys.

An ore is pretreated by bioleaching when it contains encapsulated gold
in pyrite and/or arsenopyrite. Bacteria decompose the sulfides by oxidation,
liberating gold so that during the cyanidation the leachant can penetrate
into the interior of the residual solid to reach the gold.

Microorganisms and chemical reactions

Microorganisms

*Most of the work on the biological treatment of refractory gold ores and
their general operating conditions described here is related to thiobacilli:
Thiobacillus ferrooxidans alone or in mixed culture with Thiobacillus thiooxidans and/or Leptospirillum ferrooxidans.* Since the chemical reactions of
oxidation of the sulfides are exothermic it is generally necessary to cool the
system, according to the local climate and unit size, in order to maintain
the temperature optimal for these mesophilic microorganisms. Moderate
thermophilic thiobacillus-like strains and thermophilic *Sulfolobus* are therefore also taken into consideration.

Helle & Onken (1988) have observed that the presence of leptospirillum-
like bacteria in a mixed culture of thiobacilli can significantly accelerate leaching. Budden & Spencer (1990) reported pilot tests with a moderately
thermophilic culture, but they did not describe the different strains used.
Hutchins *et al.* (1988) compared the treatment of various refractory sulfide
and carbonaceous ores by *T. ferrooxidans*, a facultative thiobacillus-like
thermophilic strain, and an extremely thermophilic *Sulfolobus* sp. They concluded that the thermophiles are more efficient in terms of the kinetics of iron
extraction and can have the advantage of less cooling requirement. However,
they also observed that in some instances gold recovery does not correlate
directly with iron extraction when different microorganisms (and different
temperatures) are used. A comparison carried out by Coastech Research Inc.
(Lawrence & Marchant, 1988) between *T. ferrooxidans* and *Sulfolobus* has
shown no significant metallurgical or economic advantage in using a thermophilic strain.

Chemistry of solution

Many different reactions are involved in the oxidation of pyrite and arseno-pyrite, forming a complex system that is not yet understood in detail. The decomposition reactions of pyrite on which the bacterial activity plays an accelerating role are successively: (a) the direct oxidation of the pyrite, (b) the oxidation of the ferrous ions in solution, and (c) the oxidation of sulfur yielded by the ferric ion of the pyrite. The main chemical reactions are:

$$4FeS_2 + 14O_2 + 4H_2O \rightarrow 4FeSO_4 + 4H_2SO_4 \qquad (2.1)$$

$$4FeSO_4 + O_2 + 2H_2SO_4 \rightarrow 2Fe_2(SO_4)_3 + 2H_2O \qquad (2.2)$$

$$FeS_2 + Fe_2(SO_4)_3 \rightarrow 3FeSO_4 + 2S^\circ \qquad (2.3)$$

$$2S^\circ + 2H_2O + 3O_2 \rightarrow 2H_2SO_4 \qquad (2.4)$$

Arsenic contained in arsenopyrite is solubilized in the form of arsenite, As(III), and arsenate, As(V) (Panin $et\ al.$, 1985), and iron in ferrous and ferric forms. The specific main reactions enhanced by bacterial metabolism are:

$$4FeAsS + 11O_2 + 6H_2O \rightarrow 4H_3AsO_3 + 4FeSO_4 \qquad (2.5)$$

$$4FeAsS + 13O_2 + 6H_2O \rightarrow 4H_3AsO_4 + 4FeSO_4 \qquad (2.6)$$

Arsenious acid, H_3AsO_3, produced by reaction (2.5) is partly oxidized into arsenic acid, H_3AsO_4. Arsenopyrite, like pyrite, is also chemically attacked by ferric iron.

Furthermore a large proportion of reaction products precipitate as follows (Livesey-Goldblatt $et\ al.$, 1983):

$$Fe_2(SO_4)_3 + 2H_3AsO_4 \rightarrow 2FeAsO_4 + 3H_2SO_4 \qquad (2.7)$$

$$Fe_2(SO_4)_3 + 6H_2O \rightarrow 2Fe(OH)_3 + 3H_2SO_4 \qquad (2.8)$$

$$Fe(OH)_3 + H_2SO_4 \rightarrow Fe(OH)(SO_4) + 2H_2O \qquad (2.9)$$

According to Panin $et\ al.$ (1985) the ratio $As^{3+} : As^{5+}$ of arsenic brought into solution is 5.1 : 1. However, Lawrence & Marchant (1987) considered that, although trivalent arsenic may predominate in the early stages of batch leaching when oxidation potentials are low (e.g. <620 mV (standard hydrogen electrode (SHE)), pentavalent arsenic will be formed in continuous leach conditions and in well-established batch leaches. Nevertheless,

Morin & Ollivier (1990) have reported that monitoring both forms of arsenic during a pilot test on an arsenopyrite concentrate has shown that arsenic in solution can be in major part arsenite. It must be emphasized that, in high concentrated mineral species, the precipitation of arsenate as ferric arsenate probably removes it from solution as fast as it is produced. Incidentally, the precipitation of iron salts in the medium is not reported to disturb bacterial growth in the bioleaching of pyrite and arsenopyrite in agitated bioreactors.

Mineralogical transformation of sulfide during bioleaching

The biological degradation of sulfides proceeds selectively. Each metal sulfide has its proper reactivity and the physical contact of different sulfides amplifies their differences in reactivity. This amplification, related to the

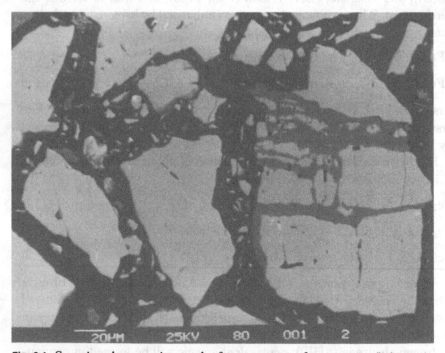

Fig. 2.1 Scanning electron micrograph of a concentrate of arsenopyrite (light grey) and pyrite (dark grey).

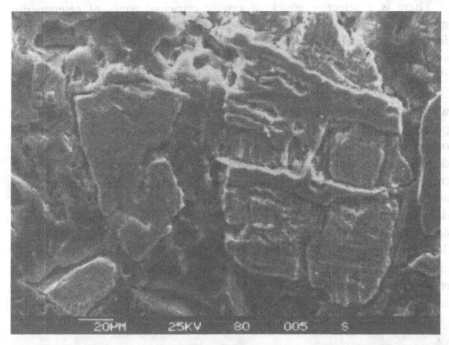

Fig. 2.2 View of the same polished section as in Fig. 2.1 after bioleaching, showing selectivity of attack between arsenopyrite and pyrite, and the galvanic effect on a mixed grain arsenopyrite–pyrite.

semiconducting property of the sulfides, is called the 'galvanic effect' (Berry & Murr, 1978). Thus, in the case of a substrate containing a mixture of pyrite and arsenopyrite, the preferential decomposition of arsenopyrite is generally observed (Karavaiko *et al.*, 1986; Marchant, 1986). In the case of mixed grains of both sulfides the decomposition of arsenopyrite is still accelerated (Morin *et al.*, 1989; Figs. 2.1 and 2.2).

Selectivity of attack can be an advantage when refractory gold is contained only in the soluble sulfide, but it can also be a drawback when refractory gold is distributed in compounds of different reactivity. The selectivity, in the restrictive meaning, i.e. the degradation of one sulfide and the passivation of the other, appears when the two sulfides have similar contents and when they are physically in intimate contact. If necessary the complete decomposition of the sulfides can then be achieved by lengthening the bioleach time in order to attack each of the sulfides successively (Shrestha, 1988; Adam *et al.*, 1989).

There is a selective attack of arsenic-enriched zones of arsenopyrite grains (Marion *et al.*, 1991). The attack rate may be faster or slower than for zones containing lower amounts of arsenic (Classen *et al.*, 1993). The surfaces of attacked sulfides show grooves, pits, holes and jagged edges. Pits of the same size and shape as the bacilli suggested to Norman & Snyman (1988) that direct mineral attack took place at the point of contact with bacterial cells. According to Southwood & Southwood (1986) the pores in pyrite are frequently oriented parallel to the crystallographic axes of the cubic lattice. They also, like previous authors, observed that pore development occurs in regions of structural disturbance. The fact that gold trapped within pyrite must occupy lattice defects and that the same sites are also preferentially attacked by bacteria implies that only a limited decomposition of pyrite can be sufficient to liberate gold. Hansford & Drossou (1988) have thus obtained 90% gold liberation for only 30% pyrite oxidation, showing that bioleaching is selective in the gold-rich regions. Figures 2.3 and 2.4 illustrate this phenomenon (Morin *et al.*, 1989).

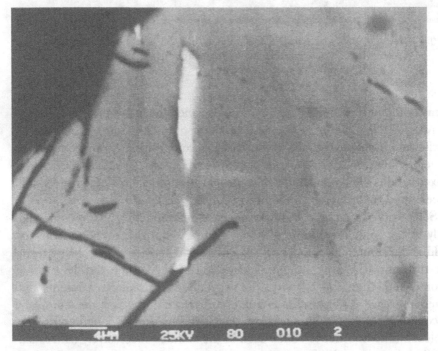

Fig. 2.3 Scanning electron micrograph of a gold grain trapped in arsenopyrite.

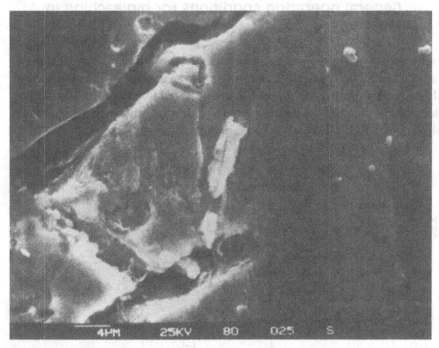

Fig. 2.4 Micrograph of the same arsenopyrite particle as in Fig. 2.3 after bioleaching, showing the selectivity of the attack along fractures and liberation of the gold grain.

Another situation occurs when refractory gold is uniformly and finely distributed within the sulfide(s). In this case, complete degradation is required. It sometimes happens that gold is even found partly in the bioleach solution. Lawrence & Gunn (1985) have found 4.9% of the gold of a pyrite concentrate in the bioleach situation. In the same experiment 18.3% of the silver was dissolved. It is not known whether the precious metals are associated in some way with bacteria or are in colloidal form.

Silver is frequently associated with gold and metal sulfides. It takes a greater variety of forms, however, than does gold, occurring as simple or complex sulfides, and it may be reactive or remain inert during both bioleaching and subsequent cyanidation, which is not fully explained.

Generally speaking, for bioleaching more than for other techniques, each ore is a specific case and needs to be tested before any conclusion is drawn. The reactivity, the degradation required and the conditions suitable for a given ore are largely unpredictable.

General operating conditions for bioleaching in reactors

A schematic flowsheet of the treatment is shown in Fig. 2.5. The treatment is applied either directly to the ore or to a concentrate by flotation of the gold-bearing sulfide compounds. Flotation is used to recover metal sulfides selectively in the froth of a pulp of a given ore through which air has been bubbled, exploiting the hydrophobic nature of the sulfides.

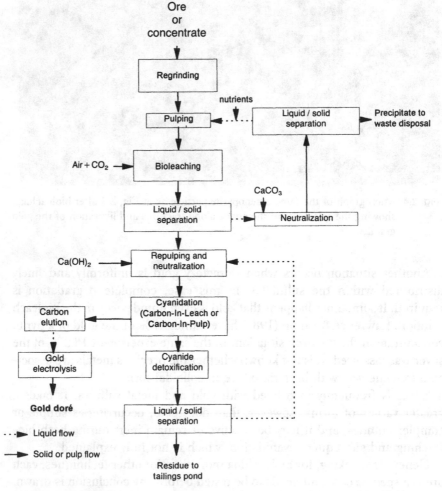

Fig. 2.5 Conceptual block diagram for the treatment of a refractory gold sulfide ore by bioleaching and cyanidation.

The selection depends upon several factors including:

The potential cost economy on the size of the equipment by feeding a concentrate and then a reduced flow rate of solid.

The gold grade of the ore and the gold balance of the flotation.

The sulfur content in the ore, which may be too low to enable bacterial growth.

Certain flotation reagents can affect the biological reaction on concentrates (Hackl *et al.*, 1990). Inhibition or toxicity can be eliminated or alleviated by acid washing, regrinding to create fresh surfaces and by bacterial adaptation.

Particle size

The ore must be ground very finely, to a particle size of less than approximately 40 to 100 μm, depending on the kinetics of biodegradation of the sulfides. The finer the particle size, the larger will be the surface available for bacterial attack and consequently the faster will be the reaction.

Pulp density

'Pulp density' as used in the mining industry means the weight percentage of solids in a slurry. It is obviously economically desirable to maximize pulp density consistent with satisfactory process performance (Gormely & Branion, 1990). The higher the pulp density, the smaller will be the size of bioreactors required to process a given feed rate for a selected residence time.

It is a general experimental observation that the kinetics of bioleaching deteriorate seriously at pulp densities higher than 20% (w/w) for reasons that have not yet been adequately determined. Among the explanations that have been suggested are disruption of cells adhering to surfaces through the effects of attrition (Miller *et al.*, 1986), interference with the mass transfer of oxygen and carbon dioxide into the leach medium (Sakagushi & Silver, 1976), nutrient limitation and insufficient biological adaptation (Marchant, 1986). Moore (1989) observed that bacteria can become gradually acclimatized to solid concentrations as high as 35% (w/w), with oxidation rates similar to those at 10%. Finally, the optimal pulp density is a compromise between the degradation of sulfides necessary to liberate gold and the acceptable time of retention in the unit.

Generally speaking, all measurements of the influence of solids content on sulfide degradation kinetics in bioleaching show that the kinetics slow down once the solids content increases above an optimum value that falls between 10% and 15% (solids weight/pulp weight). The reasons for this limitation are not precisely known, but the most commonly cited arguments (without any order of importance) are:

> *Attrition caused by grains on microorganisms* and which increases with the solids concentration. However, like other workers, we at BRGM have demonstrated that an increase of the proportion of *inert* materials, such as quartz, will have no influence in an environment with a constant quantity of sulfide grains (unpublished data).

> *Decrease in surface for exchange between gas and liquids*, for oxygen and carbon dioxide transfer, necessary for oxidation reactions and for the metabolism of the microorganisms. An increase in solids concentration leads to an increase in overall viscosity and thus to larger gas bubbles, but small solids particles can decrease coalescence through an adherence effect. Interpretation of this is difficult, the more so as agitation specialists do not agree on the effect of solids concentration, which also varies according to the size and type of the solid particles.

> *Sulfides can be inhibitors.* Sulfidic sulfur becomes an inhibitor above a certain concentration, like ferrous iron, which, although an energy substratum, inhibits growth above a certain concentration in the environment.

> *Excess bacterial population.* Some authors have observed a decrease of activity in terms of oxidation yield, when the seeded bacterial population becomes large. At BRGM, we have not observed this effect.

> *Excess number of microorganisms on solids surface compared to a deficit in solution*, which causes disequilibrium between the two modes of oxidation: direct (attack of sulfides through adherence of the bacteria) and indirect (oxidation of ferrous iron).

Disequilibrium in the proportions of species populations in a mixed culture. This explanation is part of the preceding one, the idea being that a culture will be optimum if the various species within it function satisfactorily together. Certain species are linked to solids, e.g. *T. thiooxidans* and *T. ferrooxidans*. Others, like *Leptospirillum ferrooxidans*, exist only in a liquid environment. The complementary effects of individual growth may be dependent upon a specific concentration field in the substratum.

Inhibition by organic excrement of microorganisms: in particular, organic acids or their derivatives in the environment.

In addition to this, it can be said that the solutions that are most accessible to the main two potential reasons to be retained, i.e. a mechanical reason (the availability of dissolved gas) and a biological reason, are:

1. Optimization of agitation efficiency. It is essential to provide sufficient quantities of O_2 and CO_2 when the solids concentration is increased.
2. Adaptation of the mixed culture to other than the initially determined optimum conditions. A culture can be adapted to a higher solids concentration than initially optimized, especially through continuous conditions of growth.

The operators who have worked at industrial or pilot scales have been using solids contents that varied from 14% to 35%. They are:

Genmin's BIOX at Fairview, Sao Bento and Wiluna, operating at 20% solids.

Shamrock's pilot plant, working at 14% solids.

The Salmita pilot plant, using 23–25% solids.

The Equity Silver pilot plant, using a feed of 10 to 25% solids.

The Asamera Minerals pilot plant, using 10 to 35% solids.

Use of more than 10% solids thus is current practice.

Temperature

The temperature used for bioleaching with thiobacilli in most studies is 35 °C. Although *T. ferrooxidans* grows most rapidly at 30 °C, it oxidizes iron faster at 35 °C (Homes, 1988), but since the oxidation of sulfides is exothermic, cooling must be considered to maintain the steady and satisfactory action of the system. In hot climates it may be permissible to operate at temperatures up to 40 °C, but with little margin for error at the upper limit (Gormely & Branion, 1990). It also seems possible to acclimatize mesophilic bacteria to grow as moderate thermophilic strains, namely at 40–45 °C (P. C. van Aswegen, personal communication). Spencer *et al.* (1990) also used a moderately thermophilic culture that is able to maintain an optimum oxidation rate over the range 30–49 °C.

Nutrients

Generally the 9K medium determined by Silverman & Lundgren (1959) is the reference, but the concentrations of the four mineral components ammonium, phosphorus, magnesium and potassium must be adapted according to the ore and to the bacterial culture. Nitrogen is the most essential, as shown by Marchant (1986), who has also found that a fertilizer grade (21-0-0) was acceptable. McCready (1988) has reported that, according to recent studies, a 9K medium would contain excessive concentrations of phosphate, magnesium and ammonium.

Oxygen and carbon dioxide

With a saturation concentration in water assumed to be 7.5 mg/l at 30 °C, Bos *et al.* (1986) estimated that a P_{O_2} at 10% is required to prevent oxygen limitation, which gives a minimal value of 0.75 mg/l for O_2 concentration. Pinches *et al.* (1988) obtained experimental results that suggest that the critical concentration is as low as 0.5 mg/l. However, Liu *et al.* (1988) showed that dissolved oxygen is not rate limiting for the oxidation of ferrous iron if its concentration is higher than 1.0 mg/l. These authors measure oxygen uptake rates close to 200 mg/l per h. In the case of pyrite oxidation the biological activity is generally more intense and the need for oxygen is greater, consequently the oxygen uptake rate can be higher. Chapman *et al.*

(1990) measured oxygen uptake rates up to $0.995 \, \text{kg/m}^3$ per h in the first stage of the continuous bioleaching of pyrite at pilot scale, and Griffin & Luinstra (1989) reported oxygen demand as high as 1500 mg/l slurry per h.

Oolman *et al.* (1990) observed that a sharp drop in O_2 and in CO_2 uptake occurs at dissolved oxygen levels below 10% saturation with air. Moreover, there is a correlation between the uptake rates of the gases.

Frequently, the addition of CO_2 is considered desirable to avoid limitation in an industrial process (Norris, 1990). Norris also considered that adequate growth of a moderate thermophile would require a higher concentration of CO_2 than would either *T. ferrooxidans* or *Sulfolobus*. CO_2-enriched air (1%) is used in the bioleach test procedure applied to Olympias ore (Adam *et al.*, 1989). The hydrodynamic aspects of aeration are considered on pp. 43–4, below.

Tolerance versus solution composition

Marchant (1986) has seen in a first estimation that chlorinated, fresh and process water sources were deleterious to biooxidation compared to distilled water. However, after adaptation of the bacteria, the water source was shown not to be a significant factor. Furthermore, if process water can be recycled, great care must be taken to eliminate residual cyanide and above all thiocyanate, which have been recognized as being seriously detrimental to bacterial growth (Marchant, 1986). Hackl & Wright (1989) noted an inhibiting effect with thiocyanate at levels as low as 5 p.p.m.

Concentrations of iron and arsenic in the solution used for continuous bioleaching of pyrite–arsenopyrite concentrates can reach 10–20 g/l and 20–40 g/l respectively, as obtained by Karavaiko *et al.* (1986). The ionic species derived from the decomposition of pyrite and arsenopyrite that have the most detrimental effect on the growth of *T. ferrooxidans* and *T. thiooxidans* are ferric and arsenite (Collinet & Morin, 1990). Arsenite (As(III)) at 5 g/l would be sufficient to inhibit growth, whereas for arsenate (As(V)) 40 g/l would be necessary. Barrett *et al.* (1989) detected the production of substantial concentrations of As(III) during the biooxidation of an arsenopyrite concentrate by a moderately thermophilic mixed culture, and concluded that, because of the risk of toxicity, the arsenite concentration must be monitored on a regular basis.

The acidity produced from the oxidation of the sulfides is also a source of inhibition. It is generally accepted that the optimum pH for *T. ferrooxidans* is around 2–3, but when the substrate is in large part pyritic the pH can reach extremely low values, considerably less than 1, owing to the availability of abundant sulfur and the precipitation of ferric hydroxide when the solution reaches saturation. It may also happen that neutralizing substances in the substrate, such as calcite, tend to impede the beginning of growth. Optimum acidity can be regulated by maintaining an adequate residence time in the first stage of bioleaching. Otherwise the conditions can be adjusted by addition of an appropriate reagent.

Retention time

The mean time of residence in the continuous bioleaching unit is highly variable, depending on the biodegradability of the ore, the grade of the sulfides to be decomposed or the degradation of the sulfides needed to achieve adequate subsequent gold recovery, and of course the capacity of the bacterial culture employed. The range is wide but generally between 2 and 5 days; for instance 40 h, for selective degradation of the gold-bearing sulfide contained in the Equity Silver Mine ore (Canada; Lawrence & Marchant, 1987), 115 h for the Arthur White Mine concentrate (USA; Chapman et al., 1990).

Biomass

Bacterial growth in the bioreactor obviously is the key parameter of the bioleaching kinetics. Nevertheless, there is no absolute method for controlling this. According to Karavaiko et al. (1966) the normal concentration of cells in solution of the T. ferrooxidans strain used in their pilot study should be at least $10^9/ml$ and the biomass concentration in the pulp maintained at 1–5 g/l. Another factor is that the greater part of the bacterial population is associated with solid particles.

The general approach to culture in a continuous bioleaching reactor is the application of the principle of the chemostat. The retention time is thus minimized to reach the highest rate of growth with the weakest inhibition by the products of reaction and also limited to avoid washout of the population. However, as the degree of sulfide transformation depends on the bacterial biomass concentration of bacteria, the addition of extra biomass is also frequently considered in two different ways. The first and more usual procedure is recycling of a part of the solution with or without partial neutralization to eliminate ferric iron in solution. The second, particularly suitable for arsenopyrite concentrate, is to feed the bioreactor with a solution with high concentrations in biomass and ferric iron (Grishin et al., 1985; Shrestha, 1988; Sutill, 1989). This is the separate generator concept (Pooley et al., 1987).

Cyanidation

Gold is recovered by cyanidation from bioleach solid residue after liquid/solid separation by settling or filtration. Generally, no specific unsolvable technical difficulty is encountered during these operations. However, Marchant (1986) recommended that attention be paid to the washing to remove dissolved cyanicides such as copper and ferrous iron in order to minimize cyanide consumption.

The equation for gold dissolution by cyanidation is as follows (Adamson, 1973):

$$2Au + 4NaCN + O_2 + 2H_2O \rightarrow 2NaAu(CN)_2 + 2NaOH + H_2O_2$$
$$(2.10)$$

The pH must be kept alkaline in order to avoid release of cyanhydric acid gas into the atmosphere. As the liberated gold is very fine, the cyanidation kinetic is rather fast and a few hours are sufficient to dissolve the gold.

Cyanidation on bioresidue is carried out in the usual manner and gold can be recovered from solution by selective adsorption on activated carbon or by zinc dust cementation. If carbonaceous matter is contained in the ore, adsorbing gold during cyanidation, the Carbon-In-Leach method is used (Hutchins et al., 1988; Moore, 1989).

Excessive cyanide consumption can happen, in particular when arsenopyritic concentrate rather than pyritic is being treated. In this case bioleaching can produce significant amounts of elemental sulfur, which is known to react with cyanide (Hackl, 1989). Komnitsas & Pooley (1990) cited consumptions above 100 kg cyanide/ton of the product of Olympias pyrite concentrate bioleaching, which is considerable as the usual cyanide consumption is at most a few kilograms per ton. Several procedures are available to circumvent this problem and can be tested so as to improve the efficiency of bioleaching up to complete sulfur decomposition and to optimize the duration of cyanidation.

Abundant troublesome foam can appear after neutralization, owing to the destruction of the biomass. Antifoaming agents are generally inefficient and other solutions proposed are a clearance for foams above the cyanidation pulp, a limited flow rate of air and mechanical breakers (Hackl, 1989).

The fraction of the precious metals that may be in the bioleach solution can be recovered by neutralizing the solution at the same time as the solid before cyanidation.

Another route to recovering gold from bioresidue is leaching with thiourea. Thiourea reacts on gold as follows (Torma, 1988):

$$Au + Fe^{3+} + 2CS(NH_2)_2 \rightarrow Au[CS(NH_2)_2]^{2+} + Fe^{2+} \tag{2.11}$$

The advantage of using thiourea is that the process does not need the neutralization required by cyanidation, since the reaction proceeds in acidic medium. Ferric iron necessary to the reaction is produced by bioleaching. However, the fact that the final objective of the neutralization is to eliminate the sulfate produced by bioleaching has to be kept in mind. The final consumption of neutralizing agent for each technique must thus be quite similar.

As suggested by Murthy (1990), gold recovery with thiourea would be very attractive if thiourea and bacterial leaching could be carried out simultaneously. However, Warburg respirometry experiments have shown the bacteria are inhibited at relatively low thiourea concentrations. Existing pilot and semicommercial plants employing bioleaching use only the conventional cyanidation process.

Bioreactors and the static method

Continuous leaching in reactors

Bioleaching in reactors is carried out continuously. The kinetics of bioleaching would be much longer batchwise owing to the fact that inhibitors are accumulated in the medium.

As the working pulp density is relatively low and the residence time is rather long, the reactors used for bioleaching at full scale have very large volumes. Additionally, oxygen must be as continuously available as possible and the solid suspension must be as homogeneous as possible. Consequently, the type of reactor and the system for agitation are fundamental to both the efficiency of the technique and its cost.

Oxygen is required as a terminal electron acceptor to satisfy the oxidation reactions of the sulfide compounds and also to accommodate the respiratory functions of bacterial growth. Air is quite suitable for providing oxygen. Since chemical reactions of oxidation in bioleaching are exothermic and the temperature must be regulated to maintain an optimal growth, heat transfer has also to be considered.

Two types of reactor have been seriously taken into consideration up to now, the airlift Pachuca-type reactor and mechanically agitated reactors. On the laboratory scale a very convenient system that has been extensively tested uses the airlift principle. This is the injection of air to obtain mixing by lifting pulp through a central core. The attraction of this method is that oxygen transfer and mixing of pulp are achieved by the same means. This type of reactor, called a Pachuca tank, has been extensively employed in the mineral-processing field and in particular in the gold mining industry.

Although used up to pilot scale (Karavaiko et al., 1986), such a device is inadequate for large volumes for several reasons. Simultaneously mixing and supplying oxygen leads to an overconsumption of air and difficulty of predicting performance for large pulp volumes. It is particularly difficult to restart such a system after a prolonged stoppage. If oxygen availability is high, the large volumes of air injected could lead to excessive cooling (Hardwick et al., 1988).

According to Acevedo et al. (1988) a comparison of performance on an equal total energy consumption basis (for aeration and agitation) shows that a stirred tank is superior to a Pachuca tank in terms of leaching efficiency per unit energy expenditure. Only stirred reactors are in use for large tanks at present. Generally, agitation and aeration are produced by the means of a combination of impellers and injection of air at the bottom of the tank. The configuration of impellers involves an axial flow impeller, as a propeller, on the upper part of the agitation shaft and a radial effect turbine, Rushton-like or vertical flat blade turbine, on the lower part. Radial flow impellers have a strong shear effect, which is used to split bubbles of air injected at the bottom and thus disperse the gas. This type of impeller is energy intensive. Axial flow impellers are good at maintaining solids in suspension as they have a high pumping capacity. They consume less energy, but generate much less shear.

The shear generated by radial flow impellers must be given consideration. Excessive shear stress could rupture the bacterial cell walls, or impede the attachment of microorganisms to the sulfide mineral. Hackl et al. (1990) have reported a detrimental effect due to excessive shear when using Rushton turbines at high rotational speeds. Oolman (1993) observed that the microbial activity is decreased at turbine tip speeds around 2 m/s. However, Dew & Godfrey reported that industrial scale tanks at Fairview Mine (South Africa) have been operated at impeller tip speeds of greater than 4.5 m/s and no adverse effects have been noted. Alternatives to the radial flow impeller *sensu stricto* are diffusers (Griffin & Luinstra, 1990) or impellers with more sophisticated shapes, such as hydrofoil blade impellers (Greenhalgh *et al.*, 1990). In both cases, lack of operator experience in the application of such systems to bioleaching is a difficulty. The A315 mobile of Lightnin, which is designed to have a mixed radial and axial effect, seems to have given satisfactory proofs of efficiency on an industrial scale.

Another approach, when the attachment of the bacteria to the mineral surface is not essential to the efficiency of bioleaching, is the application of the separate generator concept (Miller & Errington, 1989; Sutill, 1989). In this case the important phase of the bacterial activity is the regeneration of ferric iron as the oxidizing agent (the indirect mechanism of bioleaching). This is operated in a separate vessel where temperature, agitation and concentration of metal species can be closely controlled to optimize biomass growth, while leaching takes place in subsequent tanks where close control of conditions is not necessary.

The reaction heat produced by the oxidation of the sulfides must be removed, taking into account the extra heat generated by mechanical mixing, the heat lost through the tank walls and the heat lost by evaporation of water into the sparged air. Dew & Godfrey (1991) reported an installed length of internal cooling tube of 1.77 km for the cooling of the Sao Bento (Brazil) BIOX® 580 m^3 tank.

A typical bioleaching unit is made up of a series of cascade reactors with pulp transfer by means of overflow gravity and has the following general characteristics:

> For the first stage of leaching, two or more equal-sized tanks in parallel. This configuration ensures a longer residence time in this stage in order to avoid washout, to generate enough acid to neutralize natural alkalinity of the ore if it exists and to provide protection against a mechanical failure during this essential stage.

> The reactor height should not be more than 9 m (Gormely & Branion, 1990) because the air supply for higher tanks requires the use of compressors of significant greater cost than the blowers that can be employed otherwise.

The height/diameter ratio of the tanks is less than or close to 1.0 for reasons of efficiency and power cost.

The reactors are baffled to increase turbulence.

An internal cooling coil removes the heat produced by the oxidation of the sulfides.

The construction material commonly recommended is 316L stainless steel. Care should be taken to avoid using materials that may repress the culture (Griffin & Luinstra, 1990); in particular rubber-lining the vessels can cause problems of toxicity to the bacteria (Gormely & Branion, 1989).

Static bioleaching

The pretreatment of lean ores or residues from metallurgical plants by means of heap (or dump) leaching has also been envisaged. This technique has been applied for a long time to copper, uranium and gold ores, and has the great advantage of being much cheaper than treatment by leaching in reactors. In heap leaching the material, suitably fragmented, is piled up on impervious surfaces, so as to form heaps. The tops of the heaps are irrigated with solutions containing microorganisms and nutrients. After percolation the pregnant solutions are collected and treated before recycling. After the bioleaching treatment, alkaline neutralization is necessary to recover the gold by cyanidation.

Predicting the efficiency of the treatment is difficult as uniformity of attack through the heap cannot be ensured. Moreover, cyanidation by heap leaching after bioleaching in an acidic medium would lead to an environmental risk that cannot be neglected. Livesey-Goldblatt (1986) and Lawson et al. (1990) have reported a stepwise study of the optimization of the procedure to be applied in situ to slimes dams. Several laboratory-scale studies using columns have been carried out to simulate the heap bioleaching technique (Brierley & Luinstra, 1993; Mihaylov & Hendrix, 1993; Monroy et al., 1993).

When long-term biooxidation is acceptable and when a partial degradation of the trapping sulfide is sufficient to release gold, static bioleaching can be considered to improve further cyanide heap leaching recoveries. Burbank et al. (1990) have described such a situation justifying a campaign of tests carried out on low refractory gold ores.

Kinetic models and typical testwork programme

The need for predicting the performances of bioleaching from laboratory testwork to full-scale application has been an incentive to build quantitative models for the kinetics of the process. As pointed out previously, bacterial bioleaching has been observed to proceed selectively according to the nature of the mineral surface. Southwood & Southwood (1986) have examined the development of cylindrical pores and have proposed a model taking this into account. The model presented by Hansford & Drossou (1988) has been shown to fit the data of bioleaching of a refractory gold-bearing pyrite concentrate, supporting a propagating-pore mechanism. In contrast, Blancarte-Zurita & Branion (1988) have applied a shrinking-core model to simulate bioleaching in continuous reactors. These physical models based on the transformation of the attacked mineral require much more testing before they can be applied in reactor design.

Pinches *et al.* (1988) have developed a logistic growth model based on the following equation:

$$r = dF/dt = k_M F[1 - F/F_M] \tag{2.12}$$

where t is time, F the fraction of pyrite oxidized, F_M the maximum fraction of pyrite that can be oxidized, and k_M a rate constant.

After numerical determination of F_M and k_M by means of a first series of data, the model has been tested for different reactor arrangements and shown to be a helpful tool for performance prediction and decision making.

The comparison of laboratory-scale and pilot-scale results tends to indicate that scale does not affect the results of biohydrometallurgy or precious metals hydrometallurgy (Marchant, 1986; Hackl *et al.*, 1990; Morin & Ollivier, 1990).

In any case, testwork following rigorously a procedure of progressively increasing volume capacity is highly recommended to provide the required data for an adequate scale-up of the process in general and in order to size the equipment. This procedure will include the following items and related information:

Batch testing (a few grams to several hundred grams)

Bacterial selection and adaptation to the ore.

Kinetics and maximum degree of sulfide oxidation.

Gold recovery versus sulfide oxidation.

Typical medium composition, pH, Eh (electrochemical potential of solution), etc.

Optimization of the particle size.

Comparison between concentrate and ore treatment.

Effect of recycle.

Tracking of gold dissolved in the bioleachate.

First estimate of the consumption of reagents (cyanide and lime) for final gold recovery and neutralization of pregnant solution.

First tests of stability of the waste solids.

Optimized inoculum for the next step.

Continuous laboratory testing (one or several kilograms per day)

Determination of the residence time.

Gold recovery versus residence time.

Response to the variations in composition of the initial material.

Biomass resistance and stability.

Oxygen uptake rate.

Optimization of consumption of reagents.

Mineralogical transformation.

Optimized inoculum for the next step.

Economic balance and basic engineering.

Pilot plant testing (from 100 kg to several tons per day)

Power and heat balance requirements.

Optimization of air (and CO_2) consumption.

Provision of residues for the optimization of the liquid/solid separation, cyanidation and effluent neutralization stages.

Engineering design information on construction materials, oxygen transfer efficiency and equipment for liquid/solid separation.

Detailed engineering and final economics.

Environmental considerations on residual solids stability

An important characteristic of the refractory gold-bearing sulfide ores is the common presence of arsenopyrite and other sulfide arsenic compounds that are bioleached in the process. One of the arguments for the bio-oxidation process is that after treatment the arsenic is disposed of as an inert precipitate of ferric arsenate. However, the products of the treatment are in fact more complex than this and stoichiometric precipitated $FeAsO_4$ is not stable. As mentioned previously, the decomposition of FeAsS produces arsenate (As(V)) and ferric (Fe(III)), and also arsenite (As(III)) and ferrous (Fe(II)) depending on the mineralogy of the substrate. Ferric arsenate precipitates even during bioleaching, so arsenic in solution may be mainly as arsenite (Morin & Ollivier, 1990). The typical treatment of effluent before recycling is neutralization by addition of calcite (limestone) to about pH 3 and with hydrated lime to pH 7.

Robins (1985, 1987) has constructed thermodynamic stability diagrams for a number of simple metal arsenates, which indicate that an important change in pH, coupled with the effect of atmospheric CO_2, results in decomposition of the various arsenates so that disposal of calcium and ferric arsenate may not be appropriate. Moreover, the systems show a generally higher solubility of the arsenites compared to the arsenates so that none of the metal arsenites is sufficiently stable for disposal purposes.

A study of the system Fe-As-H_2O conducted by Krause & Ettel (1985) showed that the higher the Fe : As molar ratio the lower was the solubility of the arsenic. They also reported that precipitates formed with an Fe : As ratio >1 are not physical mixtures of $FeAsO_4$ and $Fe(OH)_3$ but specific compounds that may be represented by the formulae $FeAsO_4.xFe(OH)_3$. Further evidence for the stability of high iron ferric arsenates has been generated by Papassiopi et al. (1987) and Harris & Monette (1987). The latter have concluded that:

Arsenic can be stabilized in residues over the pH range 4–7, provided that the Fe : As molar ratio is >3 : 1.

The pH range of stability can be increased to 4–10 with the presence of small amounts of coprecipitated base metals, notably Cd + Zn + Cu.

Natural scorodite ($FeAsO_4.2H_2O$) is much less soluble than previously published thermodynamic data would indicate.

In a subsequent paper Harris & Monette (1989) confirmed these results of stability for periods up to 3 years.

It can be concluded from this brief review of the literature that two required conditions for obtaining environmentally safe wastes are that iron and arsenic must be in their most oxidized forms and that the Fe : As molar ratio in the precipitate must be at least 3 : 1.

When pyrite is the only constituent of the sulfide substrate and arsenic is marginal, effluent neutralization poses no problem as it leads to a ferric hydroxide residue that is environmentally acceptable for disposal. However, the question must be taken into consideration when arsenic and iron have similar concentrations in solution.

Published data on testwork on residues freshly produced by bioleaching are extremely rare. Morin & Ollivier (1989) have presented results of stability tests on neutralization precipitates from the effluent from the bioleaching of an arsenopyrite concentrate. It was confirmed that stability was acquired only after the arsenite produced by bioleaching was oxidized (using hydrogen peroxide) and addition of ferric iron. After this treatment the solubility of the arsenic in the residue decreased from about 200 mg/l without posttreatment to 0.2 mg/l.

Hackl (1990) has obtained good results for the tailings solids from cyanidation of a bioresidue having an Fe : As average molar ratio of only 2.2 : 1. Cyanide destruction and lowering of the pH to 7 led to an arsenic solubility of 0.2 mg/l over a period of 300 days.

An important consequence of the necessity to dispose of a high quantity of iron dissolved along with arsenic is that, from the environmental point of view, the selectivity of attack of arsenopyrite versus pyrite can be seen as a drawback rather than an advantage.

Pilot studies and industrial plants

A number of semicommercial and pilot plant operations for the treatment of refractory ores or concentrates by biooxidation have been undertaken in the last decade. Marchant (1986) has reported a pilot plant campaign operated for 9 months to treat a refractory arsenical sulfide concentrate scavenged from flotation tailings at Equity Silver Mines (British Columbia, Canada). The concentrate assayed 5.5–6.0 p.p.m. Au and 75–100 p.p.m. Ag and direct cyanidation indicated 10–20% Au and Ag recovery. The general operating conditions were 10% solids, and 40 h total residence time. Gold recovery after bacterial oxidation was increased to 75%. A partial sulfur oxidation was sufficient to release gold owing to preferential oxidation of arsenopyrite. After this pilot study a feasibility study was made for an 80 tons/day plant including tailings reclaim and flotation, bacterial oxidation and cyanidation.

In the former USSR Karavaiko *et al.* (1986) have carried a pilot campaign with a small continuous unit. The unit consists of two series of cascade Pachuca tanks with a daily capacity of 50–60 kg. The two arsenical sulfide concentrates tested assayed at about 8% arsenic. The pulp density was 16–20% and the culture of *T. ferrooxidans* employed was adapted to develop at a pH as low as 1.2–1.3 and with up to 20 g As/l and 40 g Fe/l in solution. For one concentrate, the gold recovery was 7–10% for the input but, after 87–91% of arsenopyrite oxidation and 120 h residence time, it reached 90%.

The longest continuous bioleaching of refractory sulfide material has been operating since 1986 by GENCOR at Fairview Mines in South Africa. The plant capacity is reported to be 300 tons/month of a pyritic concentrate containing 100 to 150 g Au/ton (Anonymous, 1988). Bacterial pretreatment leads to a 95% gold recovery. This plant is the first commercial-concentrate bacterial-oxidation unit in the world (Sutill, 1990). After this success, GENCOR tested with success a full-scale 580 m³ tank for bioleaching of a sulfide concentrate on the Sao Bento site (Brazil). The objective of the treatment is to preoxidize flotation concentrates ahead of the existing autoclaves to obtain an increase in oxidation capacity. After elimination of mechanical problems and thiocyanate poisoning of the bacteria, the BIOX® plant was operated in series with the autoclaves (van Aswegen, 1993). Another commissioning of a BIOX® plant was successfully carried out in 1992 at Harbour Lights (Western Australia), confirming the flexibility and commercial viability of the bacterial process.

Another semicommercial biooxidation plant with a 5 tons/day nominal capacity is reported to have been in operation at Riverlea Mines, Zimbabwe, since 1987 (Adam *et al.*, 1989). The reactors used in the plant were built and patented by EIMCO. It seems that no information concerning the process performance is available.

The biooxidation plant with the largest capacity built to date is US Gold's Tonkin Springs in Nevada. Its nominal capacity is 1500 tons/day and it consists of four tanks in three stages giving 60 h of residence time. The feed material is an ore containing 1.76% Fe and 1.47% S, and approximately

3.5 p.p.m. gold. Foo *et al.* (1990) have explained that this plant was commissioned in the spring of 1990 and operated for a short time successfully as a bioleach plant, but has temporarily been put on a standby basis for financial reasons.

The Canadian company Giant Bay Biotech Inc., in a joint venture with Giant Yellowknife Mines Ltd, in 1987 operated at 10 tons per day demonstration plant at Salmita mill in the Northwest Territories (Hackl *et al.*, 1990). The gold grade in the ore was 21.04 g/ton, the refractory gold being primarily disseminated within arsenopyrite. Iron, arsenic and total sulfur contents were 2.92, 0.75 and 0.94%, respectively. The nominal conditions achieved during steady-state operation at the design capacity were a 2.5 days' retention time, at a 22.5% pulp density, for a 9.45 tons/day ore feed rate. In these conditions the sulfide oxidation was 75% and gold recovery 95.6%, whereas it was 65% before bioleaching.

Later, Giant Bay operated a full-scale commercial prototype tank at Congress, British Columbia. The tank was 6.55 m in diameter and 7.31 m high and had a capacity of 225 m³. The treatment was performed on a rougher flotation concentrate, bioleaching of raw ore being ruled out because of excessive acid consumption. The tests were carried out by the batch method as the object of the programme was agitation studies (Hackl, 1989).

Bactech (Australia) has built a pilot plant to be transportable to any isolated mine site. This company has successfully tested, and now offers on a commercial basis, the use of a mixed culture of moderate thermophiles for treatment of pyrite–arsenopyrite concentrates (Barrett, 1990). Shamrock Resources and its affiliate, Coastech Research, also possess a mobile bioleach plant for demonstrations in North America (Chapman *et al.*, 1990) A number of other pilot and laboratory-scale continuous plants are reported to indicate that a great variety of refractory ores and concentrates are amenable to bacterial oxidation (Pooley *et al.*, 1987; Morin & Ollivier, 1990).

Description of the other processes and economics

Many processes have been proposed for the treatment of refractory sulfide gold ores or concentrates using pyrometallurgical or hydrometallurgical methods. However, only two processes, roasting and pressure leaching, have been successful on an industrial scale.

As mentioned in the Introduction, roasting has been the only procedure applied in the past to deal with these materials. The most common technique is a two-stage process. During the first stage, the roasting is carried out under oxygen-deficient conditions in order to produce a low calcine that consists mainly of magnetite, Fe_3O_4; in the second stage, magnetite is transformed into porous hematite, Fe_2O_3 (Kontopoulos & Stefanakis, 1988). The arsenic from arsenopyrite is successively transformed to As_3O_4 and then As_2O_3. Afterwards, arsenic trioxide is recovered by condensation downstream. In the same way the gaseous sulfur dioxide released has to be collected and transformed to sulfuric acid. The gold recovery is carried out by cyanidation of the calcine.

The roasting temperature is a crucial factor (Arriagada & Osseo-Asare, 1984) and in a general way the roasting process requires careful fine tuning and specific conditions for the material being treated in order totally to liberate gold. Secondary refractoriness can appear because of retrapping of gold in new mineral phases.

Generally, flotation is required before roasting as an 8% S content in the feed material is necessary for the process to be autothermal (Kontopoulos & Stefanakis, 1990).

The production of H_2SO_4 and As_2O_3 is the troublesome aspect of this process as the economic marketing of sulfuric acid depends strongly on site location and the world market for arsenic trioxide is known to be limited and volatile. Furthermore, even if gas emission regulations are respected, harmful sulfur dioxide may be released.

The advantages of the process are its simplicity, its attractive costs compared with other processes and also the fact that know-how is available worldwide. The second industrial process for the pretreatment of refractory gold ores is pressure leaching. This process involves the use of pure oxygen in an aqueous acidic medium. The reactions of oxidation are similar to those taking place during bacterial leaching and the conceptual process flowsheets are roughly similar.

Two types of pressure treatment exist, corresponding to two areas of working temperature: high temperature (>160 °C), and low temperature (<120 °C). In the first process, the whole sulfide content has to be transformed to sulfates through the action of a high oxygen pressure (up to 2200 kPa). The reaction is carried out in autoclaves in which oxygen is mechanically dispersed and a part of the oxidized products can be recycled to ensure a complete conversion of elemental sulfur in particular. The residence time is maintained within 1–3 h (Weir & Berezowsky, 1986).

The autoclave temperature is sustained without addition of heat, provided that the sulfur content of the fed material is at least 3% (Kontopoulos & Stefanakis, 1990). Treatment of a flotation concentrate is advised in order to minimize fluctuations in sulfur and arsenic contents, which markedly affect operability (da Silva *et al.*, 1989).

Pressure leaching results generally in a high degree of gold liberation, which, together with the fact that wastes can be ultimately confined as stable solids, has brought a rapid commercial success for this technique as a replacement for the roasting process. Moreover, the technical feasibility of the pressure-leaching technique is strongly supported by the fact that it has already been tested and in industrial use for other metallurgical applications (treatment of zinc, nickel and uranium ores).

Since 1985, this type of pressure oxidation has been incorporated into four plants processing refractory gold ores, McLaughlin mine in California, Sao Bento Mineracao in Brazil, Barrick Mercur Gold Mines in Utah, and Getchell Gold mine in Nevada. A fifth plant was scheduled for start-up in early 1990 for the treatment of refractory arsenical pyrite concentrate from the Olympias mine in northern Greece. Three additional plants were scheduled for production before late 1992 (White, 1990).

This technology demands high levels of skill in both operation and maintenance. However, the operating plants have confirmed the technical and economical viability and improved knowledge in the pressure-leaching technique.

The low temperature pressure-leaching process, known as 'ARSENO', is a nitrate-catalysed pressure leach (Kontopoulos & Stefanakis, 1990). The reaction is very fast as the residence time in a batch operation could be 15 min or less using a continuous procedure (Beattie *et al.*, 1985). The process has other favourable features such as simple autoclave construction, while its residue has the same environmental characteristics as that from the high pressure leaching. However, the validity of the process at the industrial scale must be proved and in particular the efficiency of the recycling of the nitrates. The ARSENO process is planned to be used on the 3000 tons/day Cinola project of City Resources in British Columbia (Kontopoulos & Stefanakis, 1990).

Other chemical oxidation processes exist which, according to their inventors, have attractive technical and economic advantages but which have not yet received industrial ratification. Among them must be cited the Nitrox Process (Van Weert, 1988), which utilizes nitric acid to oxidize sulfide minerals as follows:

$$3FeAsS + 14HNO_3 + 2H_2O \rightarrow 3FeAsO_4.2H_2O + 3H_2SO_4 + 14NO$$
$$(2.12)$$

$$3FeS_2 + 18HNO_3 \rightarrow Fe_2(SO_4)_3 + Fe(NO_3)_3 + 3H_2SO_4 + 15NO + 6H_2O$$
$$(2.13)$$

Other processes use Caro's acid oxidation or alkaline oxidation leaching (Bhakta *et al.*, 1989). Pietsch *et al.* (1983) have described testwork on pressure cyanidation in a pipe reactor. This techique has been in use since 1983 to treat antimony flotation concentrates at Consolidated Murchison, South Africa (Hendricks, 1988).

Lastly, ultrafine milling must be mentioned. By using an attrition reactor, the particle size of the refractory material can be lowered so that the d90 (the size at which 90% of particles pass) is less than 10 µm. The proportion of gold accessible to cyanide is thus increased in proportion to the surface of refractory material created by the extra grinding. As Liddell (1989) has pointed out, when gold is in solid solution within a sulfide mineral ultrafine milling may not be sufficient. However, it can be combined with an oxidizing process to improve oxidation rate and also gold recovery when it is trapped in mineral phases inert to the oxidation. Marchant (1989) has concluded that ultrafine milling can be economically justified where overall gold extraction is improved.

This brief review shows that the technical and economical feasibility of bioleaching is usually based on a comparison with the two major existing industrial processes, roasting and pressure leaching.

In such evaluations the main criteria taken into consideration are:

> Capital costs.
> Operating costs.
> Revenues.
> Environmental impact.
> Degree of operator skill required.
> Technological background and scale-up confidence.

Generally, bacterial leaching has the lowest capital cost. It is also true that the devices and construction materials for a bioleach unit are quite common compared with the equipment necessary to operate pressure leaching or roasting. The power for agitation, the air supply and the reagents for neutralization are the major items of the operating costs for bacterial leaching (Barrett, 1990). Oxygen supply causes higher operating costs for pressure leaching. The roasting process is recognized as having the lowest operating costs. According to Litz & Carter (1990) biological oxidation shows significant economic advantages if a limited oxidation of the sulfide sulfur is required. Otherwise the difference of overall costs for the three techniques is fairly small. In the case of the treatment of the Olympias ore, Kontopoulos & Stefanakis (1989) show data giving a clear advantage to bacterial leaching.

It is generally accepted that hydrometallurgical methods usually lead to higher gold recoveries than roasting, and the environmental impact of roasting is negative, whereas the solid residues produced by the hydrometallurgical processes can be satisfactory.

Pressure leaching requires the most qualified personnel.

At this stage of the discussion it is clear that bacterial leaching is very attractive. This is confirmed by the full-scale plants using bioleaching operated recently in South Africa, Brazil and Australia, even if it is surprising that so far only Genmin (South Africa) is putting this new technology into commercial operation (Bruynestyn, 1993). Only industrial units will remove the uncertainties concerning the cost and the efficiency of agitation and aeration in large tanks.

Furthermore, as in all the fields of biotechnology the quest for the best strain, the most efficient microorganism, is a very important aspect and rigorous work on characterizing the properties of the microorganisms in the context of their utilization is still necessary.

The author thanks John Kemp for his careful review of the manuscript. The author also acknowledges BRGM Research Direction for permission to publish the paper.

References

Acevedo, F., Cacciuttolo, M. A. & Gentina, J. C. (1988). Comparative performance of stirred and pachuca tanks in the bioleaching of a copper concentrate. In *Biohydrometallurgy: Proceedings of the International Symposium, Warwick 1987*, ed. P. R. Norris & D. P. Kelly, pp. 385–94. Science and Technical Letters, Kew, Surrey.

Adam, K., Prevosteau, J. M., Kontopoulos, A., Stefanakis, M. & Errington, M. (1990). Applications of process mineralogy on the treatment of Olympias pyrite concentrate, Paper presented at the SME-Gold '90 Congress, 26 February to 1 March 1990, Salt Lake City, UT.

Adam, K., Stefanakis, M. & Kontopoulos, A. (1989). Bacterial oxidation of the

Olympias arsenical pyrite concentrate. In *Biotechnology in Minerals and Metal Processing*, ed. B. J. Scheiner, F. M. Doyle & S. K. Kawatra, pp. 131–8. Society of Mining Engineers, Inc., Littleton, CO.

Adamson, R. J. (1973). *Gold Metallurgy in South Africa*. Chamber of Mines of South Africa, Cape Town, South Africa.

Anonymous (1988). Microbes extract gold. *South African Mining, Coal, Gold and Base Minerals*. February, p. 51.

Arriagada, F. J. & Osseo-Asare, K. (1984). Gold extraction from refractory ores: roasting behavior of pyrite and arsenopyrite. In *Precious Metals: Mining, Extraction, and Processing*, ed. V. Kudryk, D. A. Corrigan & W. W. Liang, pp. 367–85. The Metallurgical Society of AIME, Warrendale, PA.

Barrett, J. (1990). New gold bugs. *International Gold Mining Newsletter*, 17, 44–5.

Barrett, J., Ewart, D. K., Hughes, M. N., Nobar, A. M. & Poole, R. K. (1990). The oxidation of arsenic in arsenopyrite: the toxicity of AS(III) to a moderately thermophilic mixed culture. In *Biohydrometallurgy 89*, ed. J. Salley, R. G. L. McCready & P. L. Wichlacz, pp. 49–57. Canmet, Ottawa.

Beattie, M. J. V., Raudsepp, R., Sarkar, K. M. & Childs, A. M. (1985). The Arseno process for refractory gold ores. In *Impurity Control and Disposal*, Paper no. 9. Canadian Institute of Mining and Metallurgy.

Berry, V. K. & Murr, L. E. (1978). Direct observations of bacteria and quantitative studies of their catalytic role in the leaching of low-grade, copper-bearing waste. In *Metallurgical Applications of Bacterial Leaching and Related Microbiological Phenomena*, ed. L. E. Murr, A. E. Torma & J. A. Brierley, pp. 103–6. Academic Press, New York.

Bhakta, P., Langhans, J. W. Jr & Lei, K. P. V. (1989). *Alkaline Oxidative Leaching of Gold-bearing Arsenopyrite Ores*. Report of Investigations no. 9258. Bureau of Mines, United States Department of the Interior, Washington, DC.

Blancarte-Zurita, M. A. & Branion, R. M. R. (1988). Computer simulation of bioleaching in continuous reactors in series. In *Biohydrometallurgy: Proceedings of the International Symposium Warwick 1987*, ed. P. R. Norris & D. P. Kelly, pp. 517–20. Science and Technical Letters, Kew, Surrey.

Bos, P., Huber, T. F., Kos, C. H., Ras, C. B. & Kuonen, J. G. (1986). A Dutch feasibility study on microbial coal desulphurization. In *Fundamental and Applied Biohydrometallurgy*, ed. R. W. Lawrence, R. M. R. Branion & H. G. Ebner, pp. 129–50. Elsevier, Amsterdam.

Brierley, J. A. & Luinstra, L. (1993). Biooxidation-heap concept for pretreatment of refractory gold ore. In *Biohydrometallurgical Technologies*, ed. A. E. Torma, J. E. Wey & V. L. Lakshmanan, pp. 437–48. The Minerals, Metals & Materials Society, Warrendale, PA.

Bruynesteyn, A. (1993). Biological treatment of refractory ores. In *International Conference and Workshop on Applications of Biotechnology in the Mineral Industry – Conference Proceedings*, pp. 3.1–3.17. Australian Mineral Foundation, Glennside, South Australia.

Budden, J. R. & Spencer, P. A. (1990). Considerations in the monitoring of a moderately thermophilic culture in the oxidation of refractory gold ores and

concentrates. In *EPD Congress 90*, ed. D. R. Gaskell, pp. 315–22. The
   Metallurgical Society of AIME, Warrendale, PA.
Burbank, A., Choi, N. & Prisbey, K. (1990). Biooxidation of refractory gold ores in
   heaps. In *Advances in Gold and Silver Processing*, ed. M. C. Fuersteneau & J. L.
   Hendrix, pp. 151–9. AIME, Littleton, CO.
Chapman, J. T., Marchant, P. B. & Lawrence, R. W. (1990). Bacterial leaching pilot
   study oxidation of a refractory gold bearing high arsenic sulphide concentrate.
   In *Randol Gold Forum Squaw Valley 1990*, pp. 81–7. Randol International
   Ltd, Golden, CO.
Chryssoulis, S. L. & Cabri, L. J. (1990). Significance of gold mineralogical balances.
   Transactions of the Institution of Mining and Metallurgy, Section C, 99, 1–10.
Classen, R., Logan, C. T. & Snyman, C. P. (1993). Bio-oxidation of refractory
   gold-bearing arsenopyritic ores. In *Biohydrometallurgical Technologies*, ed. A. E.
   Torma, J. E. Wey & V. L. Lakshmanan, pp. 479–88. The Minerals, Metals
   & Materials Society.
Collinet, M.-N. & Morin, D. (1990). Characterization of arsenopyrite oxidizing
   Thiobacillus. Tolerance to arsenite, arsenate, ferrous and ferric iron. *Antonie
   van Leeuwenhoek*, 57, 237–44.
da Silva, J. E., Haines, A. K., Carvalho, T. M., de Melo, P. M. & Doyle, B. N.
   (1989). Refractory gold: the role of pressure oxidation. In *Proceedings of World
   Gold '89*, ed. R. Bhappu & R. Harden, pp. 322–32. SME, Littleton, CO.
Dew, D. W. & Godfrey, M. W. (1991). Sao Bento biox reactor. Paper presented at
   Bacterial Oxidation Colloquium of SAIMM, 18 June 1991.
Foo, K. A., Reid, W. W. & Young, J. L. (1990). Designing very large biooxidation
   plants. In *Randol Gold Forum Squaw Valley 1990*, pp. 107–13. Randol
   International Ltd, Golden, CO.
Gormely, L. S. & Branion, R. M. R. (1990). Engineering design of microbiological
   leaching reactors. In *Biohydrometallurgy 89*, ed. J. Salley, R. G. L. McCready
   & P. L. Wichlacz, pp. 499–518. Canmet, Ottawa.
Greenhalgh, P., Riley, R. P. & Baguley, W. (1990). Development of the VelMix
   bioreactor. In *Randol Gold Forum Squaw Valley 1990*, pp. 115–36. Randol
   International Ltd, Golden, CO.
Griffin, E. A. & Luinstra, L. (1990). Bioreactor scaleup: practical considerations for
   biologically assisted gold recovery. In *Biohydrometallurgy 89*, ed. J. Salley,
   R. G. L. McCready & P. L. Wichlacz, pp. 221–30. Canmet, Ottawa.
Grishin, S. I., Skakun, T. O., Adamov, E. V., Pol'kin, S. I., Kovrov, B. G., Denisov,
   G. V. & Kovalenko, T. F. (1985). Intensification of bacterial oxidation of iron
   and sulfide minerals by a *Thiobacillus ferrooxidans* culture at a high cell
   concentration. In *Biogeotechnology of Metals*, ed. G. I. Karavaiko & S. N.
   Groudev, pp. 259–65. Centre of International Projects GKNT, Moscow.
Hackl, R. P. (1989). What to be aware in cyanidation of biooxidized products. In
   Randol Gold Forum Sacramento 1989, pp. 143–4. Randol International Ltd,
   Golden, CO.
Hackl, R. P. (1990). Stability of arsenical tailings from the Salmita Bioleach Pilot
   Project. In *Randol Gold Forum Squaw Valley 1990*, pp. 101–6. Randol
   International Ltd, Golden, CO.

Hackl, R. P. & Wright, F. R. (1989). Scaleup experiences in biooxidation of refractory gold ores and concentrates. In *Randol Gold Forum Sacramento 89*, pp. 123–7. Randol International Ltd, Golden, CO.

Hackl, R. P., Wright, F. R. & Gormely, L. S. (1990). Bioleaching of refractory gold ores – out of the lab and into the plant. In *Biohydrometallurgy 89*, ed. J. Salley, R. G. L. McCready & P. L. Wichlacz, pp. 533–49. Canmet, Ottawa.

Hansford, G. S. & Drossou, M. (1988). A propagating-pore model for the batch bioleach kinetics of refractory gold-bearing pyrite. In *Biohydrometallurgy: Proceedings of the International Symposium Warwick 1987*, ed. P. R. Norris & D. P. Kelly, pp. 345–58. Science and Technical Letters, Kew, Surrey.

Hardwick, W. E., Errington, M. T., Miller, P. C. & McKee, D. (1988). A brief technico-economic assessment of the provision of oxygen to reaction systems for refractory sulfide ores. In *Randol Gold Forum 1988*, pp. 205–8. Randol International Ltd, Golden, CO.

Harris, G. B. & Monette, S. (1987). The stability of arsenic-bearing residues. In *Arsenic Metallurgy Fundamentals and Applications*, ed. R. G. Reddy, J. L. Hendrix & P. B. Queaneau, pp. 469–88. AIME, Warrendale, PA.

Harris, G. B. & Monette, S. (1989). The disposal of arsenical solid residues. Paper presented at the Productivity and Technology in the Metallurgical Industries TMS-AIME/GDMB Joint Symposium, Cologne, West Germany, 17–22 September 1989.

Hausen, D. M. (1989). Processing gold quarry refractory ores. *Journal of Metals*, **41**, 43–5.

Helle, U. & Onken, U. (1988). Continuous bacterial leaching of a pyritic flotation concentrate by mixed cultures. In *Biohydrometallurgy: Proceedings of the International Symposium Warwick 1987*, ed. P. R. Norris & D. P. Kelly, pp. 61–75. Science and Technical Letters, Kew, Surrey.

Hendricks, L. P. (1988). The recovery of gold from refractory materials at Consolidated Murchison using low alkalinity pressure cyanidation. In *Randol Gold Forum 1988*, pp. 227–32. Randol International Ltd, Golden, CO.

Homes, D. S. (1988). Biotechnology in the mining and metal processing industries: challenges and opportunities. *Minerals and Metallurgical Processing*, May, pp. 49–56.

Hutchins, S. R., Brierley, J. A. & Brierley, C. L. (1988). Microbial pretreatment of refractory sulfide and carbonaceous ores improves the economics of gold recovery. *Mining Engineering*, April, pp. 249–54.

Jha, M. C. (1987). Refractoriness of certain gold ores to cyanidation: probable causes and possible solutions. *Mineral Processing and Extractive Metallurgy Review*, **2**, 331–52.

Karavaiko, G., Chuchalin, L. K., Pivovarova, T. A., Yemel'Yanov, B. A. & Dosofeyev, A. G. (1986). Microbiological leaching of metals from arsenopyrite containing concentrates. In *Fundamental and Applied Biohydrometallurgy*, ed. R. W. Lawrence, R. M. R. Branion & H. G. Ebner, pp. 115–26. Elsevier, Amsterdam.

Komnitsas, C. & Pooley, F. D. (1989). Mineralogical characteristics and treatment of refractory gold ores. *Minerals Engineering*, **2**, 449–57.

Komnitsas, C. & Pooley, F. D. (1990). Bacterial oxidation of an arsenical gold sulphide concentrate from Olympias, Greece. *Minerals Engineering*, 3, 295–306.

Kontopoulos, A. & Stefanakis, M. (1988). Process selection for the Olympias refractory gold concentrate. In *Precious Metals '89*, ed. M. C. Jha & S. D. Hill, pp. 179–209. The Minerals, Metals & Materials Society.

Kontopoulos, A. & Stefanakis, M. (1990). Process options for refractory sulfide gold ores: technical, environmental and economic aspects. In *EPD Congress '90*, ed. D. R. Gaskell, pp. 393–412. The Metallurgical Society of AIME, Warrendale, PA.

Krause, E. & Ettel, V. A. (1985). Ferric arsenate compounds: are they environmentally safe? Solubilities of basic ferric arsenates. In *Impurity Control and Disposal*, Paper no. 5. Canadian Institute of Mining and Metallurgy.

Lawrence, R. W. & Gunn, J. D. (1985). Biological preoxidation of a pyrite gold concentrate. In *Frontier Technology in Mineral Processing*, pp. 13–17. AIME, New York.

Lawrence, R. W. & Marchant, P. B. (1987). Biochemical pretreatment in arsenical gold ore processing. In *Arsenic Metallurgy Fundamentals and Applications*, ed. R. G. Reddy, J. L. Hendrix & P. B. Queneau, pp. 199–211. AIME, Warrendale, PA.

Lawrence, R. W. & Marchant, P. B. (1988). Comparison of mesophilic and thermophilic oxidation systems for the treatment of refractory gold ores and concentrates. In *Biohydrometallurgy: Proceedings of the International Symposium Warwick 1987*, ed. P. R. Norris & D. P. Kelly, pp. 359–74. Science and Technical Letters, Kew, Surrey.

Lawson, E. N., Taylor, J. L. & Hulse, G. A. (1990). Biological pretreatment for the recovery of gold from slimes dams. *Journal of the South African Institute of Mining and Metallurgy*, 90, 45–9.

Liddell, K. (1989). Applications of ultra-fine milling and the attrition reactor in the treatment of refractory gold ore. In *Randol Gold Forum Sacramento 1989*, pp. 109–113. Randol International Ltd, Golden, CO.

Litz, J. E. & Carter, R. W. (1990). Economics of refractory gold ore processes. Paper presented at the 119th TMS Annual Meeting in Anaheim, California, 18–22 February.

Liu, M. S., Branion, R. M. R. & Duncan, D. W. (1988). Oxygen transfer to *Thiobacillus* cultures. In *Biohydrometallurgy: Proceedings of the International Symposium Warwick 1987*, ed. P. R. Norris & D. P. Kelly, pp. 375–84. Science and Technical Letters, Kew, Surrey.

Livesey-Goldblatt, E. (1986). Bacterial leaching of gold, uranium, pyrite bearing compacted mine tailing slimes. In *Fundamental and Applied Biohydrometallurgy*, ed. R. W. Lawrence, R. M. R. Branion & H. G. Ebner, pp. 89–96. Elsevier, Amsterdam.

Livesey-Goldblatt, E., Norman, P. F. & Livesey-Goldblatt, D. R. (1983). Gold recovery from arsenopyrite/pyrite ore by bacterial leaching and cyanidation. In *Recent Progress in Biohydrometallurgy*, ed. G. Rossi & A. E. Torma, pp. 627–41. Azzociazione Mineraria Sarda, Iglesias.

Marchant P. B. (1986). Commercial piloting and the economic feasibility of plant scale continuous biological tank leaching at Equity Silver Mines Ltd. In *Fundamental and Applied Biohydrometallurgy*, ed. R. W. Lawrence, R. M. R. Branion & H. G. Ebner, pp. 53–76. Elsevier, Amsterdam.

Marchant, P. B. (1989). Cost benefit considerations for innovative applications of biohydrometallurgy. In *Randol Gold Forum Sacramento 1989*, pp. 115–21. Randol International Ltd, Golden, CO.

Marion, P., Monroy, M., Mustin, C. & Berthelin, J. (1991). Effect of auriferous sulphide minerals structure and composition of their bacterial weathering. In *Source, Transport and Deposition of Metals*, ed. M. Pagel & J. Leroy, pp. 561–4. Balkema, Rotterdam.

McCready, R. G. L. (1988). Progress in bacterial leaching of metals in Canada. In *Biohydrometallurgy: Proceedings of the International Symposium Warwick 1987*, ed. P. R. Norris & D. P. Kelly, pp. 177–95. Science and Technical Letters, Kew, Surrey.

McDonald, W. R., Johnson, J. L. & Sandberg, R. G. (1990). Treatment of Alaskan refractory gold ores. *Engineering and Mining Journal*, **191**, 48–53.

Mihaylov, B. V. & Hendrix, J. L. (1993). Gold recovery from a low-grade ore employing biological pretreatment in columns. In *Biohydrometallurgical Technologies*, ed. A. E. Torma, J. E. Wey & V. L. Lakshmanan, pp. 499–511. The Minerals, Metals & Materials Society.

Miller, P. C. & Errington, M. T. (1989). Influence of ore type and leaching mechanism on the design of bio-leaching plants. In *Extraction Metallurgy 89*, ed. J. D. Gilchrist, pp. 521–32. Pergamon Press, New York.

Miller, P. C., Huberts, R. & Livesey-Goldblatt, E. (1986). The semi-continuous bacterial agitated leaching of nickel sulphide material. In *Fundamental and Applied Biohydrometallurgy*, ed. R. W. Lawrence, R. M. R. Branion & H. G. Ebner, pp. 23–42. Elsevier, Amsterdam.

Monroy, M., Marion, P., Berthelin, J. & Videau, G. (1993). Heap-bioleaching of simulated refractory sulfide gold ores by *Thiobacillus ferrooxidans*: a laboratory approach on the influence of mineralogy. In *Biohydrometallurgical Technologies*, ed. A. E. Torma, J. E. Wey & V. L. Lakshmanan, pp. 489–98. The Minerals, Metals & Materials Society.

Moore, D. C. (1989). Development of a biooxidation leach process at Asamera Minerals (U.S.) Cannon Mine. In *Biotechnology in Minerals and Metal Processing*, B. J. Scheiner, F. M. Doyle & S. K. Kawatra, pp. 123–30. Society of Mining Engineers, Inc., Littleton, CO.

Morin, D., Collinet, M.-N., Ollivier, P., El Kaliobi, F. & Livesey-Goldblatt, E. (1989). Etude de la lixiviation bactérienne de concentré sulfuré arsénié d'or réfractaire en pilote de laboratoire. *Industrie Minérale – Mines et Carrières – Les Techniques*, March–April, pp. 61–9.

Morin, D. & Ollivier, P. (1989). Biolixiviation de concentré arsénié d'or réfractaire pour extraction de l'or et élimination de l'arsenic. Paper presented at the Gold '89 in Europe Congress, Toulouse, France.

Morin, D. & Ollivier, P. (1990) Pilot practice of continuous bioleaching of a refractory gold sulfide concentrate with a high As content. In *Biohydrometallurgy 89*, ed.

J. Salley, R. G. L. McCready & P. L. Wichlacz, pp. 563–76. Canmet, Ottawa.

Murthy, D. S. R. (1990). Microbially enhanced thiourea leaching of gold and silver from lead–zinc sulphide flotation tailings. *Hydrometallurgy*, **25**, 51–60.

Norman, P. F. & Snyman, P. C. (1988). The biological and chemical leaching of an auriferous pyrite/arsenopyrite flotation concentrate: a microscopic examination. *Geomicrobiology Journal*, **6**, 1–10.

Norris, P. R. (1990). Factors affecting bacterial mineral oxidation: the example of carbon dioxide in the context of bacterial diversity. In *Biohydrometallurgy 89*, ed. J. Salley, R. G. L. McCready & P. L. Wichlacz, pp. 3–14. Canmet, Ottawa.

Oolman, T. (1993). Bioreactor design and scale-up in minerals bioleaching. In *Biohydrometallurgical Technologies*, ed. A. E. Torma, J. E. Wey & V. L. Lakshmanan, pp. 401–15. The Minerals, Metals & Materials Society.

Oolman, T., Nagpal, S. & Dahlstrom, D. (1990). O_2 and CO_2 consumption with steady-state continuous flow bioleaching. In *Advances in Gold and Silver Processing*, ed. M. C. Fuersteneau & J. L. Hendrix, pp. 237–45. AIME, Littleton, CO.

Panin, V. V., Karavaiko, G. I. & Pol'kin, S. I. (1985). Mechanism and kinetics of bacterial oxidation of sulphide minerals. In *Biogeotechnology of Metals*, ed. G. I. Karavaiko & S. N. Groudev, pp. 197–215. Centre of International Projects GKNT, Moscow.

Papassiopi, N., Stefanakis, M. & Kontopoulos, A. (1987). Removal of arsenic from solutions by precipitation as ferric arsenate. In *Arsenic Metallurgy Fundamentals and Applications*, ed. R. G. Reddy, J. L. Hendrix & P. B. Queaneau, pp. 321–34. AIME, Warrendale, PA.

Petruck, W. (1989). Recent progress in mineralogical investigations related to gold recovery. *CIM Bulletin*, **82**, 37–9.

Pietsch, H. B., Türke, W. M. & Rathje, G. H. (1983). Research on pressure leaching of ores containing precious metals. *Ertzmetall*, **36**, 261–5.

Pinches, A., Chapman, J. T., Riolo, W. A. M. & Van Staden, M. (1988). The performance of bacterial leach reactors for the preoxidation of refractory gold-bearing sulphide concentrates. In *Biohydrometallurgy: Proceedings of the International Symposium Warwick 1987*, ed. P. R. Norris & D. P. Kelly, pp. 329–44. Science and Technical Letters, Kew, Surrey.

Pooley, F. D., Shrestha, G. N., Errington, M. T. & Gibbs, H. E. (1987). The separate generator concept applied to the bacterial leaching of auriferrous minerals. In *Separation Processes in Hydrometallurgy*, pp. 58–67.

Robins, R. G. (1985). The aqueous chemistry of arsenic in relation to hydrometallurgical processes. In *Impurity Control and Disposal*, Paper no. 1. Canadian Institute of Mining and Metallurgy.

Robins, R. G. (1987). Arsenic hydrometallurgy. In *Arsenic Metallurgy Fundamentals and Applications*, ed. R. G. Reddy, J. L. Hendrix & P. B. Queneau, pp. 215–47. AIME, Warrendale, PA.

Sakagushi, H. & Silver, M. (1976). Microbiological leaching of a chalcopyrite concentrate by *Thiobacillus ferrooxidans*. *Biotechnology and Bioengineering*, **18**, 1091–101.

Shrestha, G. N. (1988). Microbiological pretreatment of refractory gold ores. In *Asian Mining '88 Conference*, pp. 179–87. IMM, London.

Silverman, M. P. & Lundgren, D. G. (1959). Studies on the chemoautotrophic iron bacterium *Ferrobacillus ferrooxidans*. I. An improved medium and a harvesting procedure for securing high cell yields. *Journal of Bacteriology*, **77**, 642–7.

Southwood, M. J. & Southwood. A. J. (1986). Mineralogical observations on the bacterial leaching of an auriferous pyrite: a new mathematical model and implications for the release of gold. In *Fundamental and Applied Biohydrometallurgy*, ed. R. W. Lawrence, R. M. R. Branion & H. G. Ebner, pp. 98–113. Elsevier, Amsterdam.

Spencer, P. A., Budden, J. R. & Sneyd, R. (1990). Use of moderately thermophilic bacterial culture for the treatment of a refractory arsenopyrite concentrate. In *Biohydrometallurgy 89*, ed. J. Salley, R. G. L. McCready & P. L. Wichlacz, pp. 231–42. Canmet, Ottawa.

Sutill, K. R. (1989). Bio-oxidation for refractory gold. *Engineering and Mining Journal*, **190**, 31–2.

Sutill, K. R. (1990). Sao Bento plans biox. *Engineering and Mining Journal*, **191**, 30–4.

Swash, P. M. (1988). A mineralogical investigation of refractory gold ores and their beneficiation, with special reference to arsenical ores. *Journal of South African Institute of Mining and Metallurgy*, **88**, 173–80.

Torma, A. E. (1988). A review of gold biohydrometallurgy. In *Proceedings of the 8th International Biotechnology Symposium, Paris*, ed. G. Durand, L. Bobichon & J. Florent, vol. II, pp. 1158–68. Société Française de Microbiologie, Paris.

van Aswegen, P. C. (1993). Bio-oxidation of refractory gold ores – the Genmin experience. In *International Conference and Workshop on Applications of Biotechnology to the Minerals Industry – Conference Proceedings*, pp. 15.1–15.14. Australian Mineral Foundation, Glennside, South Australia.

Van Veert, G. (1988). An update on the NITROX process. In *Randol Gold Forum 1988*, pp. 209–10. Randol International Ltd, Golden, CO.

Wagner, F. E., Ph, M. and Regnard, J.-R. (1988). [197]Au Mössbauer study of gold ores, mattes, roaster products, and gold minerals. *Hyperfine Interactions*, **41**, 851–4.

Wagner, F. E., Swash, P. M. & Ph, M. (1989). A [197]Au and [57]Fe. Mössbauer study of the roasting of refractory gold ores. *Hyperfine Interactions*, **46**, 681–8.

Weir, D. R. & Berezowsky, R. M. G. S. (1986). Refractory gold: the role of pressure oxidation. In *Gold 100, Proceedings of the International Conference on Gold*, vol. 2, *Extractive Metallurgy of Gold*, pp. 275–85. South African Institute of Mining and Metallurgy, Johannesburg.

White, L. (1990). Treating refractory gold ores. *Mining Engineering*, **42**, 168–74.

3

Development of improved biomining bacteria

DOUGLAS E. RAWLINGS
and DAVID R. WOODS

Introduction

The mining industry is faced with several problems for which bioleaching may provide the solution. The most important problem is the depletion of high grade surface ore deposits. This has forced mining companies to work lower grade surface deposits or to mine at greater depths. Mining companies have been looking for economic methods to recover metals from ores with low metal content, and to ways of recovering the small quantities of metal remaining after the processing of richer ones. The metal content of an ore is a large factor in the cost of metal recovery by conventional mining techniques but is of less importance to the cost of metal recovery when bioleaching technology is used (Debus, 1989). Bioleaching can also reduce the expense of mining at great depths. There are several examples where the bioleaching of deep or low grade deposits has been carried out *in situ*, with large savings in the cost of bringing vast tonnages of ore and waste rock to the surface.

A second benefit of bioleaching processes is that they are carried out under conditions that are close to ambient and therefore require relatively little energy. For example, traditional methods for the processing of difficult-to-treat (recalcitrant) gold-bearing ores involve processes that consume large quantities of energy in the form of heat and pressure, compared with the bioleaching process.

Bioleaching technology can also make a contribution to the control of water, soil and air pollution that results from mining and associated metal recovery processes. The uncontrolled leaching of metals and acid from mine dumps and tailing dams as a result of the activity of naturally occurring bioleaching bacteria is a long-standing problem. The controlled leaching and recovery of metals from waste dumps can result in both the recovery of valuable metals and the protection of the environment from this source of pollution. Many of the high temperature roasting and smelting processes result in sulfur- and arsenic-laden air effluents. Biological oxidation processes produce little or no air effluents. In addition, there are large coal reserves that have a high sulfur content and cannot be burned without unacceptable levels of sulfur dioxide release. The biological removal of most of the inorganic sulfur from these fuels is the subject of much research activity (Monticello & Finnerty, 1985).

Naturally occurring leaching bacteria

A large number of acidophilic bacteria capable of attacking mineral sulfides have been isolated from industrial leaching operations or from sites of natural leaching. These bacteria have been divided according to their preferred temperatures for growth into three groups: mesophiles, moderate thermophiles, and extreme thermophiles, with optimum growth temperatures of 30, 50 and 70 °C, respectively (Norris, 1990).

Mesophilic organisms

The dominant organism in the oxidation of mineral sulfides at temperatures below 40 °C is *Thiobacillus ferrooxidans*. The majority of *T. ferrooxidans* strains have a growth optimum of 25–35 °C, although some Canadian isolates had a greater cold tolerance than most strains and a temperature optimum of 20 °C (McCready, 1988). The bacterium is found ubiquitously in nature and has a physiology that is ideally suited to growth in an inorganic mineral environment. *Thiobacillus ferrooxidans* is autotrophic and obtains the carbon it requires for the synthesis of new cell material by the fixation of carbon dioxide from the atmosphere. It derives its energy from oxidation–

reduction reactions. In these reactions ferrous iron or reduced sulphur compounds serve as the electron donor and oxygen as the preferred electron acceptor. Ferrous iron is oxidized to ferric iron and sulfur to sulfuric acid. Iron pyrite is a typical example of an energy source used by *T. ferrooxidans*.

$$4FeS_2 + 15O_2 + 2H_2O \rightarrow 2Fe_2(SO_4)_3 + 2H_2SO_4 \tag{3.1}$$

The large quantities of sulphuric acid that are produced make the environment in which *T. ferrooxidans* grows inhospitable to most other organisms. The bacterium is itself well adapted to high concentrations of sulfuric acid and grows optimally in the pH range 1.5–2.5. In addition to their ability to fix carbon dioxide, all *T. ferrooxidans* strains examined so far also fix nitrogen (i.e. are diazotrophic). In the absence of oxygen the bacterium is still able to grow on reduced inorganic sulfur compounds using ferric iron as an alternative electron acceptor (Sugio *et al.*, 1985). It has recently been shown that three strains of *T. ferrooxidans* tested were facultative hydrogen oxidizers (Drobner *et al.*, 1990). The ability to oxidize hydrogen was repressed by ferrous iron or sulfur and occurred only in the presence of oxygen. *Thiobacillus ferrooxidans* is also resistant to a wide variety of metal ions such as copper, zinc, nickel and uranium (Tuovinen *et al.*, 1971). The bacterium therefore has a remarkable physiology that allows it to thrive in an inorganic mining environment. Its minimum growth requirements can be satisfied by water, air, an oxidizable iron or sulfur source and trace minerals. The trace elements required are usually present as impurities in the water or ore.

Other important mesophiles are the chemolithotrophic bacteria *Thiobacillus thiooxidans* and *Leptospirillum ferroxidans*. These species are also highly acidophilic (optimum pH 1.5–2.0), obligately autotrophic and grow optimally at temperatures of 25–35 °C. In contrast to *T. ferrooxidans*, *T. thiooxidans* is able to use only reduced sulfur compounds, whereas all *L. ferrooxidans* strains described to date are able to use only ferrous iron. Because of this, neither organism is able to efficiently attack mineral sulfides on its own, although together they can rapidly degrade a variety of ores. In addition, a number of acidophilic heterotrophic bacteria (assigned to the genus *Acidiphilium*) have been isolated; they grow in a close commensal relationship with the chemolithotrophic bacteria. These bacteria are unable to oxidize iron or sulfur and probably grow on organic carbon excreted by the chemolithoautotrophs (Harrison, 1984). Their presence is thought to enhance the growth of the chemoautolithotrophs through the removal of inhibitory organic waste products (Wichlacz & Thompson, 1988).

Moderate thermophiles

Moderately thermophilic bacteria that have been shown to oxidize pyrite, chalcopyrite ($CuFeS_2$) and similar ores at temperatures of 45–60 °C have been isolated (Norris, 1990). In contrast to the Gram-negative, obligately autotrophic *T. ferrooxidans* and *L. ferrooxidans* strains, these bacteria are all Gram-positive and have a wider nutritional versatility. The moderate thermophiles are a genetically diverse group of bacteria, as indicated by the G + C content of their DNA, which ranges between 45 and 69 mol% (Kelly, 1988). In this category are the Th1 strains (G + C = 50%), which have been isolated from many countries and appear to be widespread, as well as strains ALV (G + C = 57%), TH3 (G + C = 69%). Members of the genus *Sulfobacillus* (Karavaiko *et al.*, 1988) that have a DNA G + C content of 45.5 to 49.3 mol% also have a large amount of morphological variation, including branched forms. Many of these moderate thermophiles grow better when supplied with yeast extract or sugars such as glucose, fructose or sucrose. The growth of these thermophiles on iron in the presence of yeast extract is chemolithoheterotrophic without significant utilization of carbon dioxide. For vigorous autotrophic growth, most moderate thermophiles require carbon dioxide-enriched air as well as cysteine or some form of reduced organic sulfur. They are therefore unlikely to play a part in most industrial leaching processes unless a deliberate attempt is made to encourage their growth.

Extreme thermophiles

Extreme thermophiles belonging to the genus *Sulfolobus* were originally isolated from hot acid springs and are able to oxidize either iron or reduced sulfur compounds. These bacteria have been shown to decompose pyrite, chalcopyrite and pyrrhotite (FeS) ores at temperatures of 60–70 °C even more rapidly than does *T. ferrooxidans* (Norris & Parrott, 1986). As is the case with the moderate thermophiles, members of the genus *Sulfolobus* grow more rapidly if provided with organic supplements. They are, however, also able to grow autotrophically and have a pH and metal tolerance similar to that of *T. ferrooxidans*. The most significant aspect of this group is their potential use in rapid high temperature leaching of low value and recalcitrant sulfide ores. *Sulfolobus* is a genus of the Archaebacteria, a group of microorganisms that differs in several respects from all other organisms

(Woese, 1981). An unusual characteristic of the Archaebacteria is that they have cell walls lacking peptidoglycan. These bacteria are therefore more fragile and sensitive than eubacteria to the abrasive forces found in many leaching processes. This may be the reason why, in spite of their rapid mineral-leaching ability, no industrial-scale bioleaching processes using *Sulfolobus* are currently in operation.

A large variety of metal-containing ores may be leached through the bacterially assisted oxidation of insoluble metal sulfides to soluble metal sulfates. Copper, uranium and more recently gold-bearing arsenopyrite are the ores that are leached in the greatest tonnages, although this technology can also be applied to ores containing sulfides of zinc, lead, cobalt, nickel, bismuth and antimony. The chemistry of oxidation and methods of leaching several of the ores has been frequently reviewed (Brierley, 1978; Kelly *et al.*, 1979; Lundgren, 1980).

Genetic improvement of leaching bacteria

Naturally occurring isolates are the starting point for the development of improved leaching bacteria. As leaching bacteria are ubiquitous they may be isolated with little difficulty wherever oxidizable ore bodies are exposed to the surface. Newly isolated natural bacterial populations cannot, however, be expected to oxidize ores at maximum rates. It is likely that these bacteria would have been selected for their ability to grow and survive under a wide range of often adverse conditions rather than for their ability to rapidly oxidize ores under the carefully controlled optimum conditions of an industrial bioleaching process. The challenge to the biotechnologist is to improve the rate of cell growth and ore oxidation by these microbes. Two general approaches to the genetic improvement of bioleaching bacteria are mutation followed by selection, and genetic engineering. Each approach has distinct advantages, and ideally it should be possible to use both techniques.

Mutation with selection

This technique is dependent upon rare spontaneous mutations in the DNA sequence that occur during the replication of the bacterial chromosome. The mutation frequency may be increased through the use of mutagens that interfere with the accuracy of the DNA replication mechanism. Most mutational changes are either neutral or harmful to growth, but occasionally some will occur that are advantageous to the cell. If a selective pressure is placed on a microbial population, those bacteria that have acquired a mutation enabling them to outcompete the rest will eventually dominate the population. The rate of growth and mineral oxidation by a population of leaching bacteria can be improved simply by cultivating a population of bacteria in a continuous flow apparatus. If the flow rate through the apparatus is slowly increased, those bacteria that are capable of the most rapid growth will replace the others.

The advantage of mutation with selection is that it is a simple, low technology procedure that can be applied in an unsophisticated laboratory. Unlike genetic engineering, mutation with selection is not dependent on an in-depth understanding of the biochemistry of the bacterium. The technique can also be applied to both mixed and pure cultures of bacteria. A disadvantage is that it may take a long time to improve the bacterial strain or population to an economically significant extent. Since mutation and selection is essentially an empirical technique, very little information is gained about the bacterium being manipulated. This approach has nevertheless been used to improve the leach rates of *T. ferrooxidans*-dominated cultures several fold over that of the original isolates. The improvement of biomining bacteria by mutation and selection has had a dramatic effect on the economics of the biooxidation of gold-bearing arsenopyrite ores in particular. In order to explain this improvement a brief description of the process is given below.

Biooxidation of gold-bearing arsenopyrite ores

It was not until the 1980s that the potential of bioleaching to assist in the extraction of gold from recalcitrant ores was appreciated. Recalcitrant ores are those in which the gold is encased in a matrix of pyrite/arsenopyrite and cannot be efficiently recovered by cyanidation. Treatment of these ores to decompose the arsenopyrite is required before the gold is accessible to cyanide extraction. Since the volumes of ore to be treated are large and the gold is located in a relatively small pyrite/arsenopyrite fraction, the ore is crushed and a gold-bearing concentrate prepared by flotation. Conventional methods for the treatment of recalcitrant concentrates are the energy-intensive physicochemical procedures of roasting and pressure leaching. During roasting, the ore is heated in a furnace at 700 °C in the presence of oxygen, while pressure leaching involves digestion with acid under pressure in an oxygen-enriched atmosphere. Biooxidation in which chemolithotrophic bacteria such as *T. ferrooxidans* are used to decompose the ore is a low energy alternative to these processes:

$$2FeAsS \text{ (arsenopyrite)} + 7O_2 + 2H_2O \rightarrow 2FeAsO_4 + 2H_2SO_4 \qquad (3.2)$$

Without pretreatment to expose the gold, only 30–50% of the gold is recovered, whereas after biooxidation more than 99% of the gold is recoverable, depending on the mineral composition of the concentrate and the extent of treatment. Gold-bearing concentrates are valuable substrates compared with copper and uranium ores and so leaching is carried out in a vat leaching process. Vat leaching takes place in highly aerated open fermenters that are considerably more efficient than dump, heap or *in situ* leaching processes (Fig. 3.1). As this type of oxidation plant is more expensive to construct and operate, the rate of ore decomposition has a greater effect on the economics of vat leaching processes than on the relatively inefficient gravity leach operations. It is therefore important that the leaching bacteria oxidize the gold-bearing pyrite/arsenopyrite concentrates at the maximum rate possible.

A major difficulty with the first attempts at using the biological processes was that rates of oxidation of the concentrate were too slow for bioleaching to be economically competitive when compared with the physiochemical alternatives of roasting or pressure leaching (Livesey-Goldblatt *et al.*, 1983).

Adaptation of bacterial cultures to arsenopyrite ores

The ability of the bioleaching organisms to adapt when exposed to a selective pressure can be illustrated by the experience of the Genmin Mining Corporation of South Africa. In 1983 this company began a programme to improve the rate of biooxidation of a gold-bearing arsenopyrite concentrate produced by the Fairview Mine in the province of Transvaal. When first isolated, the natural populations of leaching bacteria required a retention time of over 12 days in a continuous flow system in order to oxidize the concentrate sufficiently for complete gold recovery. One of the reasons for the long retention time was that toxic arsenic compounds were leached from the concentrate and inhibited microbial activity. Initially the bacteria were sensitive to less than 1 g total arsenic/l and the concentration of arsenic had to be reduced at frequent intervals by raising the pH to 3.5, followed by removal of the precipitated arsenic. Through a process of mutation with selection in a laboratory chemostat, the rate of oxidation of the concentrate was improved so that, by 1986, the bacteria had become resistant to 13 g total arsenic/l, and the required retention time had been

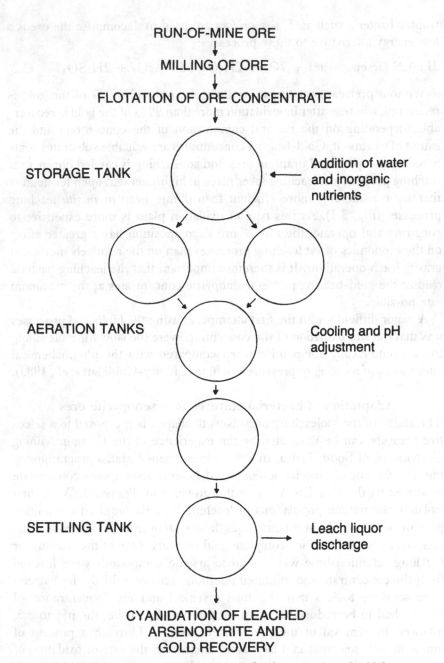

RUN-OF-MINE ORE

↓

MILLING OF ORE

↓

FLOTATION OF ORE CONCENTRATE

↓

STORAGE TANK   Addition of water
                      and inorganic
                      nutrients

AERATION TANKS   Cooling and pH
                      adjustment

SETTLING TANK   Leach liquor
                      discharge

CYANIDATION OF LEACHED
ARSENOPYRITE AND
GOLD RECOVERY

Fig. 3.1 Flow diagram of a vat leaching process for the extraction of gold from arsenopyrite ores.

reduced by 5 days. During 1986 a full-scale continuous biooxidation plant was built, which operated with a retention time of 7 days and treated 10 tons of gold-bearing concentrate per day (van Aswegen & Haines, 1988). By 1989, the growth rate of the leaching bacteria had improved still further so that the plant was operated at a retention time of a little over 3 days, and the same equipment processed 18 tons of concentrate per day. Biooxidation had become considerably more economic than the previously used roasting process and during 1990 the company built a second biooxidation plant at a mine in Sao Bento, Brazil. During 1992 and 1993, two further biooxidation plants were constructed at different sites in Western Australia and development work on the biooxidation of other gold-bearing ore bodies is continuing (A. K. Haines, personal communication).

Genetic engineering

An important difference between mutation with selection and genetic engineering is that during mutation with selection no new genetic material is gained by the bacteria. If a bacterium lacks a certain ability because it does not have the necessary genetic material, mutation with selection will not enable the organism to acquire that property. In contrast, genetic engineering results in the placement of new genetic material in the organism being manipulated.

A substantial amount of information about the biochemistry of the bacterium to be modified is required before genetic engineering is possible. However, once a genetic system is in place, genetic engineering is a more effective procedure for manipulating an organism than is mutation with selection. Because of its importance in the bioleaching process, *T. ferrooxidans* is the obvious choice for the first round of genetic engineering.

There are several reasons why an understanding of molecular genetics and gene structure of a bacterium such as *T. ferrooxidans* is essential for the development of a genetic system. It is important that all the components essential for the genetic engineering of the bacterium are available. These include plasmid vectors that can replicate in *T. ferrooxidans*, selectable genetic markers that are expressed in *T. ferroxidans*, and a method for placing the new genetic material into the organism. Molecular genetic studies are also necessary to investigate the expression and regulation of *T. ferrooxidans* metabolism, particularly those aspects affecting its industrial usefulness.

For example, an understanding of the mechanisms involved in the oxidation of iron and sulfur will be important in the future manipulation of *T. ferrooxidans* because energy production is likely to be a limiting factor in the rates of growth and mineral oxidation.

In addition to studying unique aspects of *T. ferrooxidans* physiology, a certain amount of comparative genetic work is necessary. This will help to identify those organisms to which *T. ferrooxidans* is genetically most closely related. These organisms are likely to serve as the best sources of foreign genetic material for the manipulation of the bacterium. The unique physiology and growth characteristics of *T. ferrooxidans* make it difficult to study genetically. Its sensitivity to organic matter, low pH requirements, relatively slow growth rate and requirement for iron or sulfur media combine to make the organism more difficult to work with than most heterotrophic bacteria.

Components of a *T. ferrooxidans* genetic system

T. ferrooxidans plasmids
A starting point for the development of a genetic system for *T. ferrooxidans* is the construction of shuttle vectors that can replicate in genetically well-characterized *Escherichia coli* strains and in *T. ferrooxidans*. The vectors must also contain selectable genetic markers that are expressed in both organisms. The strategy adopted was to utilize the numerous well-characterized *E. coli* vectors and clone into these vectors the required *T. ferrooxidans* origin of replication and potential markers.

Plasmids are found in a large number of *T. ferrooxidans* strains and these are an obvious source of *T. ferrooxidans* origins of replication. Several workers have isolated and cloned plasmids from the bacterium (Holmes *et al.*, 1984; Rawlings *et al.*, 1984). Four *T. ferrooxidans* plasmids, (pTF35, pTF-FC2, pTF3320-1, pTF3302-2) from three different *T. ferrooxidans* strains (35, FC, 33020) have been successfully cloned into pBR325 and two into pBR322. Two of the plasmids were isolated from the uranium-resistant *T. ferrooxidans* ATCC33020 strain (Holmes *et al.*, 1983) but neither conferred increased uranium resistance to an *E. coli* host strain (D. E. Rawlings, unpublished data). The 12.4 kb pTF-FC2 plasmid was the most prevalent of three plasmids in the *T. ferrooxidans* FC strain, which was isolated from the acid leach liquor of a South African mine and was very resistant to arsenic. However, the recombinant plasmid between pTF-FC2 and the *E. coli* plasmid pBR325 did not express arsenic resistance in *E. coli*.

Although all cloned *T. ferrooxidans* plasmids were cryptic in *E. coli*, plas-

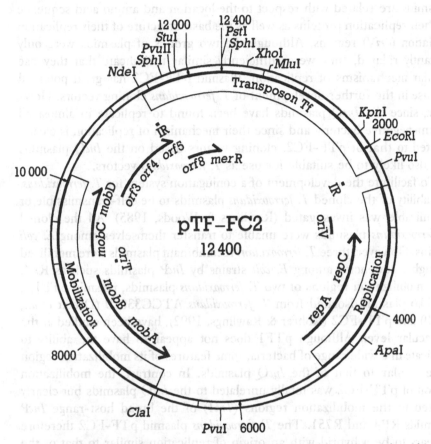

Fig. 3.2 A genetic and restriction enzyme map of the broad host-range plasmid pTF-FC2, which was isolated from *T. ferrooxidans*. IR, inverted repeat. (From Rawlings *et al.*, 1993.)

mid pTF-FC2 was found to have a broad host-range origin of replication (Fig. 3.2; Rawlings *et al.*, 1993), and has been the subject of intensive studies (Dorrington & Rawlings, 1989, 1990). The plasmid has been shown to replicate in *Pseudomonas aeruginosa*, *Thiobacillus novellus*, *Klebsiella pneumoniae*, *Rhizobium meliloti* and *Agrobacterium tumefaciens*. Only a few broad host-range plasmids of Gram-negative bacteria have been discovered. Among the most extensively studied are the almost identical plasmids RSF1010, R1162 and R300B, which belong to the *Inc*Q incompatibility group (Scholz *et al.*, 1989). A comparative analysis of the origins of replication between pTF-FC2 and the *Inc*Q plasmids has shown that the two plasmids are related with respect to the location and amino acid sequence of their replication proteins as well as the basic structure of their replication initiation (*ori*V) regions. Although the two groups of plasmids were only distantly related, they were sufficiently similar to indicate that they use similar mechanisms of replication. Plasmid pTF-FC2 has great potential for use in the further development of *T. ferrooxidans* cloning vectors. However, since the *Inc*Q plasmids have been found to replicate in almost all Gram-negative bacteria and since their mechanism of replication is clearly related to that of pTF-FC2, cloning vectors based on the *Inc*Q plasmids are also likely to be suitable for use as *T. ferrooxidans* vectors.

To facilitate the development of a conjugation system for *T. ferrooxidans*, the ability of the cloned *T. ferrooxidans* plasmids to be self-transmissible or mobilizable was investigated (Rawlings & Woods, 1985). All the cloned *T. ferrooxidans* plasmids were unable to transfer themselves among *E. coli* strains. However, three *T. ferrooxidans* recombinant plasmids were mobilized at high frequencies among *E. coli* strains by *Inc*P plasmids such as RP4. The mobilization regions of two *T. ferrooxidans* plasmids, plasmid pTF1, a 6.65 kb plasmid isolated from *T. ferrooxidans* ATCC33020 (Drolet *et al.*, 1990) and pTF-FC2 (Rohrer & Rawlings, 1992), have been studied at the molecular level. Although pTF1 does not appear to have the ability to replicate in a wide range of bacteria, some features of its mobilization region were similar to that of the *Inc*Q plasmids. In contrast, the mobilization region of pTF-FC2 was totally unrelated to the *Inc*Q plasmids but clearly related to the mobilization regions (*Tra*1) of the broad host-range *Inc*P plasmids RP4 and R751. The *T. ferrooxidans* plasmid pTF-FC2 therefore appears to be a hybrid with an origin of replication similar to that of the *Inc*Q plasmids and a mobilization region related to that of the *Inc*P plasmids. The mobilization studies show that the *ori*T, *nic* and *mob* functions from plasmids isolated from *T. ferrooxidans* are expressed in *E. coli*.

The discovery of mobilizable, broad host-range *T. ferrooxidans* plasmids is encouraging for the development of a genetic system for *T. ferrooxidans* because it suggests that a conjugation system may exist in *T. ferrooxidans*. Although *T. ferrooxidans* plasmids have been mobilized by *Inc*P plasmids among *E. coli*, *P. aeruginosa* and *T. novellus* cells, transfer of these plasmids to *T. ferrooxidans* has not been demonstrated (Rawlings *et al.*, 1986). Various ingenious direct and indirect conjugation strategies have been tried but without success. This may be due to as yet undiscovered specific conditions required for conjugation in *T. ferrooxidans* or the lack of expression of the selectable markers utilized for the isolation of exconjugants.

Vector transfer
The development of a genetic system for *T. ferrooxidans* depends on a
method for transferring plasmid vectors to *T. ferrooxidans* cells. Plasmid
transfer using either conjugation or the transfer of naked DNA into
T. ferrooxidans (with cell treatment using calcium or other substances) has
been attempted by several workers and to date only one of these attempts
has been successful (Kusano *et al.*, 1992). Electroporation of naked DNA
into bacterial cells by the application of a high voltage electrical discharge
is a transformation procedure that is finding increasing application to a
wide range of bacteria. Kusano and co-workers attempted to transform
different *T. ferrooxidans* isolates using electroporation and were able to
demonstrate the successful transformation of one of the 30 isolates tested.
This isolate could be transformed with three of four plasmid vectors constructed using natural *T. ferrooxidans* plasmids or a vector based on an
*Inc*Q-type replicon. Transformation occurred at a low efficiency (less than
200 transformants per microgram of DNA) and was independent of the
vector used. The recombinant plasmids were stable for as many as 110
generations. The reason why only one strain out of 30 tested was amenable
to transformation by electroporation is still uncertain. One of the major
difficulties in the development of a widely applicable transformation system
is the lack of a strong selectable marker.

Selectable markers for *T. ferrooxidans*
The problem of identifying potential markers for genetic studies that could
be selected and utilized in inorganic ferrous sulfate medium at pH 1.8 has
been investigated. Metal ion tolerance is a particularly attractive marker for
genetic studies in *T. ferrooxidans* because it is a useful laboratory marker
for which plasmid-mediated resistance is known to occur, and also has
the potential of conferring an industrially significant characteristic on the
organism. Six *T. ferrooxidans* strains have been shown to be sensitive to
mercury and arsenic (Rawlings *et al.*, 1983). Since genes coding for resistance to these metals have been identified in other bacteria, these resistance
genes could serve as genetic markers in the development of *T. ferrooxidans*
genetic systems.
Antibiotic resistance markers have been widely used as selectable genes
in heterotrophic bacteria. Therefore the sensitivity of *T. ferrooxidans* strains
to a range of antibiotics has been determined (Rawlings *et al.*, 1983).
All the strains tested were sensitive to rifampicin, chloramphenicol, cepha-
loridine and ampicillin, but were resistant to gentamycin, kanamycin,

streptomycin, tetracycline, vancomycin, tobramycin and erythromycin. The apparent resistance of *T. ferrooxidans* to the antibiotics tested was in all cases shown to be due to the instability of the antibiotics in the low pH and high metal ion medium. Shiratori *et al.* (1989) cloned the mercury ion reductase gene (*merA*) from *T. ferrooxidans*. The *merA* gene confers resistance to mercury by reducing mercuric ions to volatile elemental mercury and is the first selectable genetic marker to be isolated from *T. ferrooxidans*. It was this gene that was used by Kusano *et al.* (1992) to isolate transformants following electroporation. However, mercury resistance was not a stringent selectable marker and only 13 out of 22 colonies that grew on mercury-containing media contained the recombinant plasmid.

The cloning and expression of genes from *T. ferrooxidans*

As discussed earlier, studies on the molecular biology of genes from *T. ferrooxidans* can serve two main purposes. An investigation of those genes that are also found in many other bacteria is useful for comparative purposes. Those genes that are involved with unique aspects of *T. ferrooxidans* physiology will not have counterparts in most other bacteria but are more likely to lead to breakthroughs in our understanding of metabolic bottlenecks.

Comparative genetic studies

The first chromosomal gene from *T. ferrooxidans* to be cloned was the gene for glutamine synthetase (*glnA*) (Barros *et al.*, 1985), and the first gene sequenced was the *nifH* gene, which encodes the iron-containing protein of the enzyme nitrogenase (Pretorius *et al.*, 1987). During the past 5 years a number of other *T. ferrooxidans* genes have been sequenced. These include the *glnA* gene (Rawlings *et al.*, 1987), the nitrogenase α and β subunits (*nifDK*) (Rawlings, 1988), the *recA* gene product (Ramesar *et al.*, 1989), mercury ion reductase (*merA*) (Inoue *et al.*, 1989), *merC* (Inoue *et al.*, 1990) and the *ntrA* gene (Berger *et al.*, 1990). In addition a family of repeated sequences (Yates *et al.*, 1988) and the RNA component of RNase P (Takeshima *et al.*, 1989) have been sequenced. A comparison of most of these genes with similar genes of other bacteria has been made and will not be repeated here (Rawlings *et al.*, 1991). As a result of these studies it can be said that in spite of its unusual physiology, most of the *T. ferrooxidans* genes tested appeared to be expressed in *E. coli*. Whether the cloned genes are expressed from identical promoters in *E. coli* and *T. ferrooxidans* has, however, not been proved in all cases. Nevertheless at least some of the signals for *T. ferrooxidans* gene expression are recognized by other bacteria.

All indications are that obtaining expression of many foreign bacterial genes in *T. ferrooxidans* should not present serious difficulties. From these expression studies as well as a comparison of the predicted amino acid sequences of several of the cloned genes, *T. ferrooxidans* appears from a genetic viewpoint to be a typical Gram-negative bacterium.

Molecular investigations of unique aspects of *T. ferrooxidans* physiology

An understanding of the molecular genetics and regulation of energy production in general and iron and sulfur oxidation in particular is one of the areas of research that is most likely to lead to an improvement in the biooxidation performance of *T. ferrooxidans*. Mjoli & Kulpa (1988) showed that when *T. ferrooxidans* was cultivated on iron-containing media the SDS-polyacrylamide gel electrophoresis (PAGE) protein profile was different from when cells were grown on sulfur media. Certain proteins were induced only when the organism was grown in the presence of iron and others only when sulfur was present. A 32 kDa iron-induced protein has been purified, the amino acid sequence of some CNBr-derived peptides determined, and a DNA oligonucleotide probe constructed and used to isolate the gene encoding the protein from a *T. ferrooxidans* gene bank (N. Mjoli, unpublished data; Rawlings *et al.*, 1991). The same approach could be used to isolate other genes involved in iron and sulfur oxidation in order to study the mechanisms by which they are regulated.

It has been shown that *T. ferrooxidans* synthesizes ATP by means of a membrane-associated H^+-translocating ATP synthase (Apel *et al.*, 1980). This enzyme complex consists of two parts, a membrane integral F_0 portion, which forms the H^+-conducting channel, and an F_1 portion, which is located on the cytoplasmic side of the membrane and is the catalytic component responsible for ATP synthesis. It is the passage of protons from the outside of the cell, across the cytoplasmic membrane and through the ATP synthase complex that results in the synthesis of ATP (Fig. 3.3). Since *T. ferrooxidans* grows in a low pH environment (pH 1.5–2.0), but has an internal cytoplasmic pH close to neutrality, the pH gradient across the *T. ferrooxidans* cytoplasmic membrane is one of the greatest in all living organisms (Cox *et al.*, 1979). The *atp* operon from *T. ferrooxidans*, which encodes the ATP synthase enzyme complex, has been cloned and is currently being studied to determine the features that allow *T. ferrooxidans* cells to maintain their unusually large transmembrane pH gradient (L. Brown, author's laboratory).

Thiobacillus ferrooxidans has the ability to fix both carbon dioxide and nitrogen from the atmosphere. These processes require a large input of energy and place a severe metabolic drain on the energy resources of the cell. Several genes involved in nitrogen fixation have been cloned and their

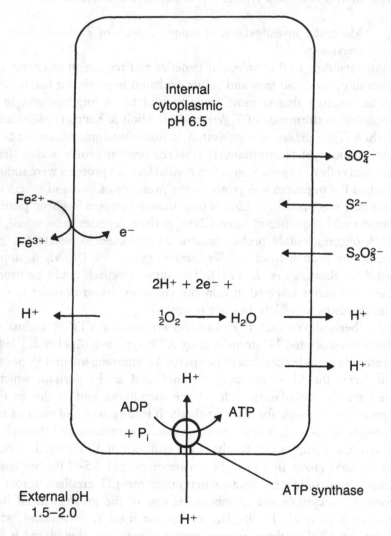

Fig. 3.3 A model for the generation of ATP by *T. ferrooxidans*. Ferrous iron or reduced sulfur compounds serve as the electron donor and oxygen as an electron acceptor. During respiration, protons are pumped out of the cell and enter via the ATP synthase complex.

regulation investigated (for a review, see Rawlings *et al.*, 1991). More recently the structural genes for the *T. ferrooxidans* genes involved in the synthesis of an enzyme involved in carbon dioxide fixation, ribulose biphosphate carboxylase, have been cloned (Kusano *et al.*, 1990). Much of the energy used for the fixation of carbon dioxide and nitrogen is associated with the reduction of these compounds and is of a fundamental chemical nature. Although it will not be possible to lower this component, a deeper understanding of the regulation of the genes of the pathways involved may make a positive contribution to the optimization of the growth conditions for the bacterium.

An interesting discovery made by Yates & Holmes (1987) is that many *T. ferrooxidans* strains have families of mobile repeated sequences that are located on the chromosome. Holmes *et al.* (1988) have speculated that these repeated sequences could be transposon-like elements that could be responsible for switching genes on or off and may be the explanation for the remarkable adaptability that has long been recognized to be a feature of many *T. ferrooxidans* strains. Schrader & Holmes (1988) demonstrated that all six *T. ferrooxidans* strains they tested were able to undergo spontaneous changes in colony morphology from a small colony form to a large spreading colony (LSC). LSC variants lost the ability to oxidize iron but retained the ability to oxidize reduced sulfur compounds. This phenomenon was termed phenotypic switching. Preliminary results indicated that phenotypic switching may be a result of specific changes in position of the mobile genetic elements. A better understanding of phenotypic switching could also lead to unexpected breakthroughs in the ability to alter the performance of *T. ferrooxidans*-based oxidation processes.

Conclusions

Thiobacillus ferrooxidans-dominated cultures have been utilized for the leaching of copper and uranium for centuries (Kelly *et al.*, 1979). Unlike the leaching of copper and uranium, which is usually carried out in relatively inefficient low rate dump, heap and *in situ* leaching processes, the bioleaching of arsenopyrite ores is carried out in high rate vigorously agitated oxidation tanks (van Aswegen *et al.*, 1988). It is in these high rate processes that the need for microbial cultures that are capable of rapidly oxidizing ores becomes most important. There are two main approaches towards improving the performance of bacteria involved in the biooxidation of ores, namely mutation with selection and recombinant DNA technology (genetic engineering).

Natural selection in the laboratory and in pilot and full-scale plants over several years has produced *T. ferrooxidans* strains that are highly resistant to arsenic and capable of rapid oxidation of gold-bearing arsenopyrite ores in a continuous industrial bioleaching process. Highly adapted strains decompose arsenopyrite ores to an extent that allows more than 95% gold recovery in 3½ days compared to the more than 12 days required by the original isolates. Improvement in the performance of natural *T. ferrooxidans* isolates by mutation with selection has, however, reached a plateau and further improvement is likely to require the application of recombinant DNA technology to amplify genes or to enable the introduction of new genetic material.

Molecular genetic studies on a bacterium that does not have an efficient conjugation or transformation system and for which no bacteriophages have been discovered is not an easy undertaking. These studies are further complicated in a bacterium such as *T. ferrooxidans* with a physiology that differs radically from heterotrophic bacteria. The successful application of recombinant DNA technology to *T. ferrooxidans* will depend on an understanding of gene structure, regulation and the development of genetic systems for industrial strains of the bacterium. An encouraging start has been made by relatively few researchers who have developed the basic ingredients for a genetic system and analysed the detailed genetic structure of at least 10 *T. ferrooxidans* genes. In addition, two insertion elements that appear to be part of a natural *T. ferrooxidans* transposon or phenotypic switching mechanism have been investigated. Knowledge of gene structure and codon usage has resulted in a viable reverse genetics system for the isolation of genes involved in sulfur and iron oxidation for which there is no selection technique in heterotrophs. As *T. ferrooxidans* is an autotrophic, chemolithotropic, nitrogen-fixing organism, its ability to generate energy is likely to be a major restraint on its rate of growth. Molecular genetic studies in this area are likely to provide important information on probable bottlenecks in this process.

Industrial processes that are based on microbial activity typically have three main ingredients: a substrate, an organism/group of organisms, and a set of conditions required to ensure optimum growth or metabolic activity of the organisms. There are some major differences between the biooxidation of ores and most other microbial-based industrial fermentations such as the production of ethanol, antibiotics or amino acids. In a typical fermentation, the substrates from different localities can be made relatively similar, whereas in the case of bioleaching almost every ore deposit (substrate) is unique with respect to its mineralogy and chemical composition. This means that a bacterial population that rapidly decomposes one ore deposit may not be as active on a different deposit. Furthermore, it has been observed that natural isolates of *T. ferrooxidans* may be more efficient at oxidizing the ore from which they were isolated than are populations isolated from a different ore body. A second important difference is that, in most industrial processes, fermentation substrates are sterilized prior to inoculation. This means that the inoculated organism does not have to compete with other organisms for limited nutrient and energy resources. As it would be uneconomic to sterilize large tonnages of ore, the genetically manipulated strains would have to outcompete the indigenous strains introduced from non-sterile ores. Irrespective of whether mutation and selection or genetic engineering is to be used to improve bioleaching rates, it may be necessary to use the local isolate as a starting point rather than foreign strains. Molecular genetic studies on this important industrial bacterium with its unique physiology are poised for an interesting and exciting future. These studies should make an important contribution to bioleaching technology as well as advancing our understanding of fundamental biological processes.

References

Apel, W. A., Dugan, P. R. & Tuttle, J. H. (1980). Adenosine 5'-triphosphate formation in *Thiobacillus ferrooxidans* vesicles by H$^+$ ion gradients comparable to those of environmental conditions. *Journal of Bacteriology*, 142, 295–301.

Barros, M. E., Rawlings, D. E. & Woods, D. R. (1985). Cloning and expression of the *Thiobacillus ferrooxidans* glutamine synthetase gene in *Escherichia coli*. *Journal of Bacteriology*, 164, 1386–9.

Berger, D. K., Woods, D. R. & Rawlings, D. E. (1990). Complementation of *Escherichia coli* σ^{54} (*NtrA*) dependent formate-hydrogen-lyase activity by a cloned *Thiobacillus ferrooxidans* ntrA gene. *Journal of Bacteriology*, 172, 4399–406.

Brierley, C. L. (1978). Bacterial leaching. *CRC Critical Reviews in Microbiology*, 6, 207–62.

Cox, J. C., Nicholls, D. G. & Ingledew, W. J. (1979). Transmembrane electrical potential and transmembrane pH gradient in the acidophile *Thiobacillus ferrooxidans*. *Biochemical Journal*, 178, 195–200.

Debus, K. H. (1989). Identifying the biohydrometallurgical processes with the greatest probability of commercial adoption. In *Biohydrometallurgy 89*, ed. J. Salley, R. G. L. McCready & P. Wichlacz, pp. 487–98. Canmet, Ottawa.

Dorrington, R. A. & Rawlings, D. E. (1989). Identification and sequence of the basic replication region of a broad-host-range plasmic isolated from *Thiobacillus ferrooxidans*. *Journal of Bacteriology*, **171**, 2735–9.

Dorrington, R. A. & Rawlings, D. E. (1990). Characterization of the minimum replicon of the broad-host-range plasmid pTF-FC2 and similarity between pTF-FC2 and the *IncQ* plasmids. *Journal of Bacteriology*, **172**, 5697–705.

Drobner, E., Huber, H. & Stetter, K. O. (1990). *Thiobacillus ferrooxidans*, a facultative hydrogen oxidizer. *Applied and Environmental Microbiology*, **56**, 2922–3.

Drolet, M., Zanga, P. & Lau, P. C. K. (1990). The mobilization and origin and transfer regions of a *Thiobacillus ferrooxidans* plasmid: relatedness to plasmids RSF1010 and pSC101. *Molecular Microbiology*, **4**, 1381–91.

Harrison, A. P. (1984). The acidophilic thiobacilli and other acidophilic bacteria that share their habitat. *Annual Review of Microbiology*, **38**, 265–92.

Holmes, D. S., Lobos, J. H., Bopp, L. H. & Welch, G. C. (1983). Setting up a genetic system *de novo* for studying the acidophilic *Thiobacillus*, *T. ferrooxidans*. In *Recent Progress in Biohydrometallurgy*, ed. G. Rossi & A. E. Torma, pp. 541–54. Azzociazione Mineraria Sarda, Iglesias.

Holmes, D. S., Lobos, J. H., Bopp, L. H. & Welch, G. C. (1984). Cloning on a *Thiobacillus ferrooxidans* plasmid in *Escherichia coli*. *Journal of Bacteriology*, **157**, 324–6.

Holmes, D. S., Yates, J. R. & Schrader, J. (1988). Mobile repeated DNA sequences in *Thiobacillus ferrooxidans* and their significance for biomining. In *Biohydrometallurgy*, ed. P. R. Norris & D. P. Kelly, pp. 153–60. Science and Technology Letters, Kew, Surrey.

Inoue, C., Sugawara, K. & Kusano, T. (1990). *Thiobacillus ferrooxidans mer* operon: sequence analysis of the promoter and adjacent genes. *Gene*, **96**, 115–20.

Inoue, C., Sugawara, K., Shiratori, T., Kusano, T. & Kitagawa, Y. (1989). Nucleotide sequence of the *Thiobacillus ferrooxidans* chromosomal gene encoding mercuric reductase. *Gene*, **84**, 47–54.

Karavaiko, G. I., Golovacheva, R. S., Pivovarova, T. A., Tzaplina, I. A. & Vartanjan, N. S. (1988). Thermophilic bacteria of the genus *Sulfobacillus*. In *Biohydrometallurgy*, ed. P. R. Norris & D. P. Kelly, pp. 29–41. Science and Technology Letters, Kew, Surrey.

Kelly, D. P. (1988). Evolution of the understanding of the microbiology and biochemistry of the mineral leaching habitat. In *Biohydrometallurgy*, ed. P. R. Norris & D. P. Kelly, pp. 3–14. Science and Technology Letters, Kew, Surrey.

Kelly, D. P., Norris, P. R. & Brierley, C. L. (1979). Microbiological methods for the extraction and recovery of metals. In *Microbial Technology: Current State, Future Prospects*, ed. A. T. Bull, D. C. Ellwood & C. Ratledge, pp. 263–308. Cambridge University Press, Cambridge.

Kusano, T., Sugawara, K., Inoue, C. & Suzuki, N. (1990). Molecular cloning and expression of *Thiobacillus ferrooxidans* chromosomal ribulose biphosphate carboxylase genes in *Escherichia coli*. *Current Microbiology*, **22**, 35–41.

Kusano, T., Sugawara, K., Inoue, C., Takeshima, T., Numata, M. & Shiratori, T. (1992). Electrotransformation of *Thiobacillus ferrooxidans* with plasmids containing a *mer* determinant as the selective marker by electroporation. *Journal of Bacteriology*, 74, 6617–23.

Livesey-Goldblatt, E., Norman, P. & Livesey-Goldblatt, D. R. (1983). Gold recovery from arsenopyrite/pyrite ore by bacterial leaching and cyanidation. In *Recent Progress in Biohydrometallurgy*, ed. G. Rossi & A. E. Torma, pp. 627–41. Azzociazione Mineraria Sarda, Iglesias.

Lundgren, D. G. & Silver, M. (1980). Ore leaching by bacteria. *Annual Review of Microbiology*, 34, 263–83.

McCready, R. G. L. (1988). Progress in the bacterial leaching of metals in Canada. In *Biohydrometallurgy*, ed. P. R. Norris & D. P. Kelly, pp. 177–95. Science and Technology Letters, Kew, Surrey.

Mjoli, N. & Kulpa, C. R. (1988). The identification of a unique outer membrane protein required for iron oxidation in *Thiobacillus ferrooxidans*. In *Biohydrometallurgy*, ed. P. R. Norris & D. P. Kelly, pp. 89–102. Science and Technology Letters, Kew, Surrey.

Monticello, D. J. & Finnerty, W. R. (1985). Microbial desulfurization of fossil fuels. *Annual Review of Microbiology*, 39, 371–89.

Norris, P. R. (1990). Acidophilic bacteria and their activity in mineral sulphide oxidation. In *Microbial Mineral Recovery*, ed. H. L. Erlich & C. L. Brierley, pp. 3–28. McGraw-Hill, New York.

Norris, P. R. & Parrott, L. (1986). High temperature, mineral concentrate dissolution with *Sulfolobus*. In *Fundamental and Applied Biohydrometallurgy*, ed. R. W. Lawrence, R. M. R. Branion & H. G. Ebner, pp. 355–65. Elsevier, Amsterdam.

Pretorius, I.-M., Rawlings, D. E., O'Neill, E. G., Jones, W. A., Kirby, R. & Woods, D. R. (1987). Nucleotide sequence of the gene encoding the nitrogenase iron protein of *Thiobacillus ferrooxidans*. *Journal of Bacteriology*, 169, 59–65.

Ramesar, R. S., Abratt, V., Woods, D. R. & Rawlings, D. E. (1989). Nucleotide sequence and expression of a cloned *Thiobacillus ferrooxidans recA* gene in *Escherichia coli*. *Gene*, 78, 1–8.

Rawlings, D. E. (1988). Sequence and structural analysis of the α- and β-dinitrogenase subunits of *Thiobacillus ferrooxidans*. *Gene*, 69, 337–43.

Rawlings, D. E., Dorrington, R. A., Rohrer, J. & Clennel, A.-M. (1993). A molecular analysis of a broad-host-range plasmid isolated from *Thiobacillus ferrooxidans*. *FEMS Microbiology Reviews*, 11, 3–8.

Rawlings, D. E., Gawith, C., Petersen, A. & Woods, D. R. (1983). Characterization of plasmids and potential genetic markers in *Thiobacillus ferrooxidans*. In *Recent Progress in Biohydrometallurgy*, ed. G. Rossi & A. E. Torma, pp. 541–54. Azzociazione Mineraria Sarda, Iglesias.

Rawlings, D. E., Jones, W. A., O'Niel, E. & Woods, D. R. (1987). Nucleotide sequence of the glutamine synthetase gene and its controlling region from the acidophilic autotroph *Thiobacillus ferrooxidans*. *Gene*, 53, 211–17.

Rawlings, D. E., Pretorius, I.-M., & Woods, D. R. (1984). Expression of a *Thiobacillus ferrooxidans* origin of replication in *Escherichia coli*. *Journal of Bacteriology*, 158, 737–8.

Rawlings, D. E., Sewcharan, R. & Woods, D. R. (1986). Characterization of a broad-host-range mobilizable *Thiobacillus ferrooxidans* plasmid and the construction of *Thiobacillus* cloning vectors. In *Fundamental and Applied Biohydrometallurgy*, ed. R. W. Lawrence, R. M. R. Branion & H. G. Ebner, pp. 419–27. Elsevier, Amsterdam.

Rawlings, D. E. & Woods, D. R. (1985). Mobilization of *Thiobacillus ferrooxidans* plasmids among *Escherichia coli* strains. *Applied and Environmental Microbiology*, **49**, 1323–5.

Rawlings, D. E., Woods, D. R. & Mjoli, N. P. (1991). The cloning and structure of genes from the autotrophic biomining bacterium, *Thiobacillus ferrooxidans*. In *Advances in Gene Technology*, vol. II, ed. P. J. Greenaway, pp. 215–37. JAI Press, London.

Rohrer, J. & Rawlings, D. E. (1992). Sequence analysis and characterization of the mobilization region of the broad-host-range plasmid pTF-FC2, isolated from *Thiobacillus ferrooxidans*. *Journal of Bacteriology*, **174**, 6230–7.

Scholz, P., Haring, V., Wittmann-Leibold, B., Ashman, K., Bagdasarian, M. & Scherzinger, E. (1989). Complete sequence and gene organization of the broad-host-range plasmid RSF1010. *Gene*, **75**, 271–88.

Schrader, J. & Holmes, D. S. (1988). Phenotypic switching of *Thiobacillus ferrooxidans*. *Journal of Bacteriology*, **170**, 3915–23.

Shiratori, T., Inoue, C., Sugawara, K., Kusano, T. & Kitigawa, Y. (1989). Cloning and expression of *Thiobacillus ferrooxidans* mercury resistance genes in *Escherichia coli*. *Journal of Bacteriology*, **171**, 3458–64.

Sugio, T., Domatsu, C., Munakata, O., Tano, T. & Imai, K. (1985). Role of a ferric ion-reducing system in sulfur oxidation of *Thiobacillus ferrooxidans*. *Applied and Environmental Microbiology*, **49**, 1401–6.

Takeshima, T., Inoue, C., Kitagawa, Y. & Kusano, T. (1989). Nucleotide sequence of a *Thiobacillus ferrooxidans* chromosomal gene which encodes putative RNA component of RNase P. *Nucleic Acids Research*, **17**, 9482.

Tuovinen, O. H., Niemalä, S. I. & Gyllenberg, H. G. (1971). Tolerance of *Thiobacillus ferrooxidans* to some metals. *Antonie van Leeuwenhoek*, **37**, 489–96.

van Aswegen, P. C. & Haines, A. K. (1988). Bacteria enhance gold recovery. *International Mining*, May, pp. 19–23.

van Aswegen, P. C., Haines, A. K. & Marais, H. J. (1988). Design and operation of a commercial bacterial oxidation plant at Fairview. *Randol Perth Gold*, **88**, 144–7.

Wichlacz, P. L. & Thompson, D. L. (1988). The effect of acidophilic bacteria on the leaching of cobalt by *Thiobacillus ferrooxidans*. In *Biohydrometallurgy*, ed. P. R. Norris & D. P. Kelly, pp. 77–86. Science and Technology Letters, Kew, Surrey.

Woese, C. R. (1981). Archaebacteria. *Scientific American*, **244**, 98–122.

Yates, J. R., Cunningham, R. P. & Holmes, D. S. (1988). IST2: an insertion sequence from *Thiobacillus ferrooxidans*. *Proceedings of the National Academy of Science, USA*, **85**, 7284–7.

Yates, J. R. & Holmes, D. S. (1987). Two families of repeated sequences in *Thiobacillus ferrooxidans*. *Journal of Bacteriology*, **169**, 1861–70.

4

Electrochemical aspects of biocorrosion

HÉCTOR A. VIDELA

Introduction

General considerations of electrochemical and biological processes at the metal–solution interface

Many aspects of biological processes involve electrical potentials and currents, both of which are electrochemical in nature. An outstanding example is the cellular potential. Its modification by an external excitation, followed by a selective permeation of ions through the cell membrane, corresponds to a typical electrochemical phenomenon of charge transfer (Bockris & Reddy, 1970). The redox processes and the electron transport chain between a metabolite and oxygen, occurring in mitochondria, involve various specific enzymic systems. Each of these systems involves electron transfer reactions and a well-ordered sequence of redox potentials with electrochemical characteristics.

The interface between a metal and a surrounding electrolyte is characterized by a certain distribution of electrical charges that can be depicted by the electrical double-layer model. Present knowledge of the structure of the electrical double layer is based mainly on data obtained with the dropping-mercury electrode. The behaviour of the interface between mercury and various aqueous electrolyte solutions can be considered as approximately equal to that of an ideally polarizable interface. However, this electrochemical behaviour is far from that presented by the complex metal–solution interfaces associated with biologically influenced corrosion (BIC). Arvia (1986) has applied the electrical double-layer concept to interfacial phenomena in biofilms. In this approach, the various adsorption processes occurring at the interface, the formation of biofilms, their colloidal characteristics, and the influence of the electric field on microorganisms were considered. The structure of the electrochemical interface in BIC processes can be likened to that of a membrane adhering directly or indirectly to the metal surface containing different redox systems within the membrane structure.

General dimensions of microorganisms involved in BIC processes, like bacteria, fungi or yeasts, are of the order of a micrometre in size. This characteristic allows microorganisms to colonize very inaccessible areas, such as the interior of pits or crevices, and to resist the shear stress of the fluid circulating over the metal surface. Moreover, small dimensions and light weight facilitate the rapid and easy dispersion of microorganisms by environmental factors. The synergistic effect of several microbial properties such as growth rate, varied metabolic products (many of them of a corrosive nature), and a high surface to volume ratio, allows the microorganisms to interact very actively with the medium (Videla, 1986a). All these facts can explain why the metal–solution interface can be dramatically changed by microbial activity. The microorganisms add to the corrosion process all the diverse effects derived from microbial interactions with the environment surrounding the metal surface. As this interaction is very active, it can be expected that microbial participation in corrosion will markedly enhance metal damage.

A retrospective overview of BIC studies from an electrochemical point of view

Due to the complex nature of BIC, research in this field demands both an understanding of microbiological effects and a proper knowledge of corrosion science. Although the participation of microorganisms in corrosion has been recognized since the late nineteenth century (Garret, 1891), subsequent publications on BIC rarely interpreted the interaction between microorganisms and metal surfaces adequately. A further hindrance has been a general lack of awareness of the significance of the problem (Iverson, 1987).

The first attempt to explain microbial participation in corrosion electrochemically was the Cathodic Depolarization Theory (CDT, see p. 102) in the early thirties. von Wolzogen Kühr & van der Vlugt (1934) suggested that the enzyme hydrogenase of sulfate-reducing bacteria (SRB) removed hydrogen from cathodic areas on iron surfaces actively corroding in water-logged soils. In such environments, at nearly neutral pH and low oxygen content, corrosion of iron should be negligible, because neither of the two common reactants that bring about depolarization (acceleration) of the corrosion cathodic reaction are available (Booth, 1971). However, thin-walled, mild-steel pipes were rapidly perforated in such situations.

Electrochemical techniques, such as polarization experiments and corrosion potential versus time measurements, were used several years later (Hadley, 1943; Horvath & Solti, 1959; Booth & Tiller, 1960) to assess the action of SRB on iron corrosion. Polarization experiments were used to follow the time-dependent polarization behaviour of steel in the test solutions. This unconventional use of polarization experiments was later repeated by several researchers working with varied experimental conditions (Booth & Tiller, 1960; Costello, 1974) and different kinds of micro-organisms (Edyvean & Terry, 1983; Westlake et al., 1986). Since the chemical composition, pH and redox conditions of the medium are continuously varied by microbial metabolism, electrochemical measurements are difficult to interpret. The present state of knowledge of BIC demands a proper recognition of the importance of fouling of metal surfaces and biofilm formation in natural or industrial environments. The necessity of interpreting the complex interactions taking place at the biofilm–metal interface has been the main reason for the increasing use of a wide variety of modern electrochemical techniques in recent publications.

The use and limitations of these techniques for investigating BIC have been critically reviewed (Dexter et al., 1989; Mansfeld & Little, 1990). Among the diverse electrochemical methods found in the latest literature on BIC, potentiodynamic sweep techniques (Gaylarde & Videla, 1987), electrochemical impedance spectroscopy, electrochemical noise (Mansfeld & Xiao, 1994) and current density mapping (Franklin et al., 1990) are mentioned. A more detailed description of the applications of electrochemical methods in the evaluation of BIC are given on pp. 104–10, below.

Type of corrosion attack found in BIC

Corrosion manifests itself in several characteristic forms, the two main ones being uniform and localized attack. The former occurs evenly over the whole metal surface, whereas localized attack may present as different types: pitting and crevice corrosion, selective dissolution, stress corrosion cracking (SCC), fatigue corrosion, impingement and fretting corrosion. Uniform attack as a rule is not a great problem from the technological point of view if its rate can be determined with reasonable accuracy. Prediction of the expected lifetime is usually not difficult and, if necessary, some corrosion-preventing measure can be taken. Much more insidious and unpredictable are the different types of localized corrosion. These forms of attack cause unexpected, local failures some of which are not of a purely electrochemical nature but may be partially caused by mechanical or metallurgical factors. In all cases of localized corrosion, the total metal loss leading to failure is much greater than for uniform corrosion, which usually corresponds to a much longer life of the metal structure.

The small dimensions of microorganisms, as well as their ubiquity, allows them to form small ecosystems in restricted areas of the metal surface. BIC usually occurs as some type of localized attack (mainly pitting and crevice corrosion) and consequently these forms of attack will be discussed in some detail.

Pitting is a form of localized corrosion in which the metal is removed preferentially from vulnerable areas of the surface (Szklarska-Smialowska, 1986). Pitting corrosion is a local dissolution process leading to the formation of cavities in passivated metals when they are exposed to aqueous, nearly neutral solutions containing aggressive anions such as chlorides. There are internal and external factors influencing pitting. Among the former are the effects derived from alloying elements, the thickness and electronic properties of passive oxide films, cold working, heat treatment and weld effects. The main environmental factors affecting pitting are electrolyte composition, pH and temperature. A detailed description of these effects or the different theories to explain pit initiation is beyond the scope of this chapter and the reader is referred to several specialized publications (Staehle *et al.*, 1974; Szklarska-Smialowska, 1986). Corrosion of stainless steels in chloride-containing media such as seawater, or the corrosive attack of carbon steel by mixtures of SRB metabolites and chlorides, are only two of the many practical cases of BIC in which pitting corrosion is involved.

Local differences in the composition of a solution can be the cause of

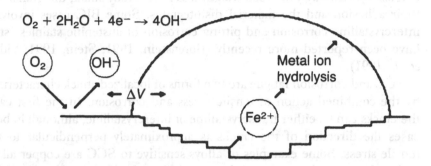

$$O_2 + 2H_2O + 4e^- \rightarrow 4OH^-$$

O_2 OH^- Metal ion hydrolysis

$\leftarrow \Delta V \rightarrow$ Fe^{2+}

Fig. 4.1 Diagram of the differential aeration effects under a microbial colony formed on an iron surface (from Duquette & Ricker, 1986, with permission from NACE International, Houston, TX).

potential differences on an immersed metal and can thus accelerate corrosion. An important example is oxygen concentration differences commonly referred to as differential aeration. In practice, this effect occurs mainly in narrow crevices or under deposits. Bacterial biofilms on metal surfaces generally lead to this type of localized corrosion, which can be considered as one of the more frequent forms of attack found in BIC. In the particular case of passive metals (i.e. stainless steel), crevice corrosion can be severe. In addition, it has been reported that bacterial oxygen depletion in crevice water can be as rapid as a purely electrochemical mechanism (Dexter et al., 1986).

On passivated stainless steel surfaces, oxygen depletion by bacteria is dominant and may accelerate the initiation of crevice corrosion. When the concentration of oxygen is higher at one part of the metal surface and lower at another, the part exposed to the lower concentration will act as the anode of a corrosion cell and will suffer an increased localized attack. A large anode to cathode ratio will favour localized attack within the crevice. Cathodic reduction of oxygen will lead to an alkaline pH outside the crevice, whereas the hydrolysis of metal ions will enhance the pH drop inside the crevice, leading to the formation of a differential aeration cell (Fig. 4.1).

Another common form of localized attack is selective dissolution of the least noble component of an alloy. A BIC case of removal of zinc from brass has been published (Alanis et al., 1986). A similar kind of selective attack is produced when only the narrow boundaries between crystalline regions (crystallites or grains) are preferentially damaged (intercrystalline corrosion). Although the total weight loss is generally small, the grains lose their adhesion and the material disintegrates. Some BIC cases involving intercrystalline corrosion and pitting corrosion of austenitic stainless steel have been reported more recently (Borenstein, 1991; Stein, 1991; Videla *et al.*, 1991).

SCC and corrosion fatigue are two forms of localized attack characterized by the combined action of tensile stress and corrosion. In the first case, the cracks can be either transcrystalline or intercrystalline, although in both cases the direction of the cracks is approximately perpendicular to the tensile stress. Some examples of alloys sensitive to SCC are copper alloys in humid atmospheres containing ammonia or sulfur dioxide, austenitic stainless steel in chloride-contaminated steam and aluminium alloys in seawater.

Corrosion fatigue is a special case of SCC where the simultaneous action of cyclic stress and corrosion leads to failure. It occurs in a wider range of environments than SCC and it is almost always transcrystalline. Microorganisms also participate in these two types of localized corrosion. A typical case is the fatigue corrosion of steel in marine environments containing microbiologically generated hydrogen sulfide (Thomas *et al.*, 1988; Edyvean, 1990).

Electrochemical nature of corrosion

The classical metal–solution interface in corrosion studies

Metallic corrosion can be defined as the attack produced on a metal surface by reaction with an aggressive environment, with the consequent deterioration of the properties of the substratum. Corrosion is an electrochemical process caused by a flow of electricity from one metal either to another metal or to another electron sink. As a result of the interaction with the environment, metals lose their elemental state and tend to a combined form. Corrosion is, then, a natural or spontaneous process because, with the exception of the noble metals, all other metallic substrata display a thermodynamic tendency to revert to the oxides from which they probably came.

An electrochemical reaction involves the transfer of electrons through coupled oxidation and reduction processes. To occur, corrosion needs a

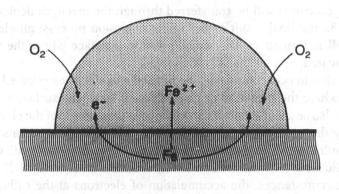

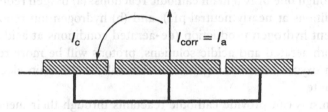

Fig. 4.2 Simple version of the corrosion process on an iron surface under a droplet
of water. The process is modelled underneath, as a short-circuited
electrochemical cell. I_a, anodic current; I_c, cathodic current; I_{corr}, corrosion
current. (Adapted from Atkins, 1986; with permission of Oxford University
Press, Oxford, UK.)

solution able to conduct the electrical flow (the electrolyte). Seawater or
many industrial waters, because of their saline content, are excellent electrolytes, allowing the conduction of electricity from a negative area to a positive
one. Inorganic corrosion is then accomplished in the presence of two
elements: the metal and the electrolyte. By analogy with a reaction taking
place in an electrochemical cell, corrosion is an anodic or oxidation process
and its final result is the dissolution of the metal surface, which enters the
solution as metallic cations. A cathodic area, necessary to return the current
to the metal, can be supplied by the same metal if the electrolyte composition
is varied. The cathodic reaction is, then, an electron-consuming or
reduction reaction. The simplest scheme to illustrate the corrosion process
is that of a droplet of water over a metal surface. Near the boundary of the
water with air, the oxygen concentration is higher and this part will provide
the cathodic reaction of oxygen reduction (Fig. 4.2). In the region under
the droplet, oxygen concentration is lower and the anodic oxidation of iron

takes place. Electrons will be transferred through the metal, as depicted in the figure. As the final result of the whole corrosion process, an electrochemical cell is formed on the metal–solution interface where the water droplet is located.

For corrosion to occur, ions must be formed and electrons released at an anodic site where the oxidation or dissolution of the metal surface occurs. There must also be a simultaneous acceptance at the cathode of the electrons produced by the anodic reaction. Both anodic and cathodic reactions must proceed simultaneously and at equivalent rates. Metal dissolution will occur only at anodic areas (e.g. the area under the droplet shown in Fig. 4.2).

In most circumstances, the accumulation of electrons at the cathode is prevented through one of two main cathodic reactions: (a) oxygen reduction (aerated conditions at nearly neutral pH), and (b) hydrogen ion reduction and consequent hydrogen production (de-aerated conditions at acidic pH values). In both aerated and acidic solutions, protons will be more readily available than oxygen, and hydrogen reduction will be the main electron-consuming route.

Microorganisms can provide cathodic reactants through their metabolic activity, as in the case of SRB. Thus, the production of cathodic reactants such as H_2S or HS^- can lead to alternative cathodic reactions such as the reduction of H_2S to produce HS^- and hydrogen. Costello (1974) suggested an indirect action of SRB in the corrosion of iron through this mechanism.

Metal dissolution and passivation: a kinetic approach to the corrosion process

The current flow induces a change (polarization) at the metal–solution interface that conditions the rate of the overall electrochemical process. Corrosion reactions tend to slow down as corrosion products form at the interface. Conversely, any accelerating effect on the corrosion reaction is called depolarization. Corrosion products formed at the metal–solution interface can alter its structure, leading to a loss of reactivity (passivity). In spite of a copious corrosion literature, the nature of passivity is still under discussion. However, it is generally agreed that this phenomenon is caused by the formation of a surface film (passive film) at the metal surface, acting as a barrier to further corrosion. The extent to which this film is able to adhere firmly to the metal surface, resist removal by turbulence effects, or be restored if broken, finally determines the capability of the alloy to remain in a passive condition. In many cases, the interaction between microbial biofilms and inorganic passive films condition the metal behaviour and its resistance to corrosion attack (Videla, 1991a).

A thermodynamic approach to corrosion reactions is important to determine which reactions are theoretically possible under given practical conditions. It can be said that a metal tends to corrode whenever it is in contact with a solution where a cathodic reaction is possible at an equilibrium potential higher than that of the metal dissolution reaction in that solution. However, it is not sufficient to know whether a certain metal can corrode under given conditions. It is essential to know the rate of a possible reaction. Even if a reaction is thermodynamically possible, it can proceed at so low a rate that, for all practical purposes, it can be said not to occur at all. There are several examples of metal surfaces (e.g. aluminium) that are unstable under equilibrium conditions, but which frequently corrode much more slowly than a relatively more stable metal such as iron.

The rate of the corrosion reaction can be measured by the anodic current, i.e. by the current due to metal ions leaving the metal (see Fig. 4.2). Corrosion effects of current flow on polarization phenomena are related not only to the total amount of current flow, but also to the current density (current flow per unit area). It can be easily understood that the effect of a certain amount of current localized on a small area of metal surface will be greater than when the same amount of current is dispersed over a much larger area.

Since the anodic current must migrate through the solution to return to the metal at the cathode, the cathodic current must be equal to the anodic one. The tendency for a metal to corrode can thus be expressed by an equivalent electrochemical cell (Fig. 4.3). If the external resistor of this cell is short circuited ($R = 0$) and the internal solution resistance is small enough to be neglected, the current that flows through the cell is the current responding to the corrosion process, and its corresponding potential is the corrosion potential, which can be readily measured experimentally. By using separate standard electrodes one can also measure the potentials of each electrode. If it is assumed that the rates of both reactions (anodic and cathodic) are determined by charge transfer processes, the corrosion behaviour of a metal in a given solution can be expressed by a potential–current diagram or polarization diagram. Instead of plotting the cathodic current to the left and the anodic current to the right, it is more convenient to plot both currents to the right as shown in Fig. 4.4. This type of plot is usually called an Evans diagram and the potential–current relationship follows a logarithmic dependence. The intersection point of the potential and current lines corresponds to the current flowing through the cell and to the potential of the metal freely corroding in that medium.

Microbial participation in the corrosion reaction

Microorganisms influence corrosion by changing the electrochemical conditions at the metal–solution interface. These changes may have different effects, ranging from the induction of localized corrosion, through a change in the rate of general corrosion, to corrosion inhibition. Any biological

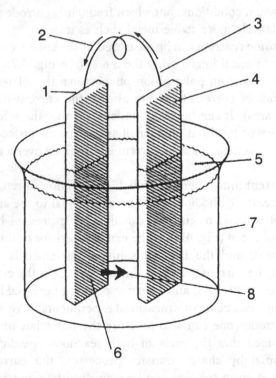

Fig. 4.3 Anodic and cathodic corrosion reactions in an electrochemical cell. 1, Anode (oxidation reaction: metal dissolution); 2, current flux through the conductor; 3, metallic conductor; 4, cathode (reduction reaction); 5, oxygen or other depolarizing agent; 6, metal ions; 7, electrolyte; 8, current flux through the electrolyte.

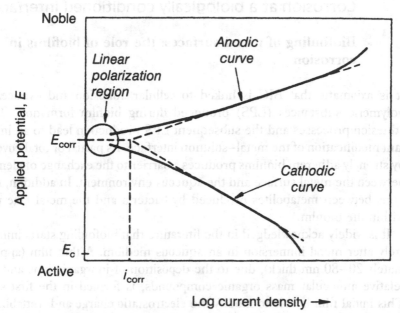

Fig. 4.4 Evans diagram showing corrosion potential and corrosion current values obtained by extrapolation. E_{corr}, corrosion potential; E_c, cathodic potential; i_{corr}, corrosion current density. (From Dexter *et al.*, 1991, with permission from NACE International, Houston, TX.)

influences that either encourage or restrict one of the components (anodic or cathodic) of the corrosion reaction, or permanently separate (localized) anodic and cathodic sites, will increase corrosion. Thus, stimulation of the anodic reaction (e.g. by acidic metabolites) or the cathodic reaction (e.g. by microbial production of a cathodic reactant such as H_2S), disruption of a passivating film, or increasing the conductivity of the electrolyte will increase corrosion.

Even though the electrochemical model of corrosion remains valid for BIC, the participation of microorganisms in the process introduces several unique features, chiefly the modification of the metal–solution interface structure through biofilm accumulation. Because of their important role in BIC, all the changes at the interface, associated with biofouling and microbial metabolic activities within the biofilm, are discussed below in special detail.

Corrosion at a biologically conditioned interface

Biofouling of metal surfaces: the role of biofilms in corrosion

It is axiomatic that BIC is linked to cellular adhesion and extracellular polymeric substances (EPS) produced during biofilm formation. These adhesion processes and the subsequent EPS production lead to an important modification of the metal–solution interface. Its partial or total coverage by strongly adherent biofilms produces a barrier to the exchange of elements between the metal surface and the aqueous environment. In addition, reactions between metabolites produced by bacteria and the metal take place within the biofilm.

It is widely acknowledged in the literature that biofouling starts immediately after metal immersion in an aqueous medium. A thin film (approximately 20–80 nm thick), due to the deposition of inorganic ions and high relative molecular mass organic compounds, is formed in the first stage. This initial film is able to modify the electrostatic charge and wettability of the metal surface (Dexter, 1976), facilitating its further colonization by microorganisms. Hitherto, no visible biofilm will have settled at the metal–solution interface. In a short time, microbial growth and EPS production results in the development of a biofilm consisting of bacterial cells, their EPS and, occasionally, some entrapped particulate material. Thus, a biofilm is the result of a surface accumulation that is not necessarily uniform in time or space (Characklis & Marshall, 1990).

A dynamic system is formed at the biofouled interface, and different transport processes will take place through the biofilm (Characklis, 1981). This is a consequence of the biofilm structure, characterized by a high degree of hydration, with water comprising nearly 90% (Geesey, 1982).

In this way, microbial colonization of metals drastically modifies the classic concept of the electrical interface commonly used in electrochemical studies. Important changes in the type and concentration of ions, pH and redox conditions are induced by the biofilm, altering the passive behaviour of the metal substratum and its corrosion products, as well as the electrochemical parameters used to assess corrosion rates (Videla, 1989a).

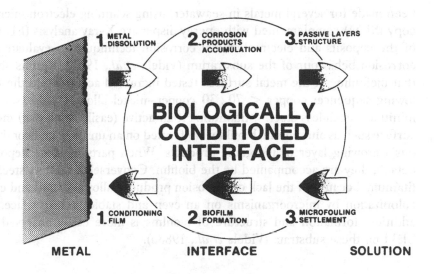

Fig. 4.5 Simplified scheme of biological and inorganic processes at a biologically
conditioned metal–solution interface (from Videla, 1991*b*, with permission
from Elsevier Applied Science, Oxford).

The concept of a new biologically conditioned interface

Simultaneously with the biological changes that lead to biofouling, a
sequence of inorganic changes takes place at the metal surface after its
immersion in an aggressive aqueous medium (e.g. seawater). This sequence
involves the process of metal dissolution (corrosion) and corrosion product
formation (passivation). Thus, corrosion and biofouling of metal surfaces
occur within the same time scale, beginning immediately after the immersion of the metal specimen in the aqueous environment. However, each of
these processes follow opposite directions at the metal–solution interface.
Whereas corrosion and corrosion product accumulation is directed from
the metal surface towards the solution, biofouling is the settlement of planktonic cells that become sessile organisms remaining adsorbed to the metal
surface (Fig. 4.5). A very active interaction between the passive layer and
biofilm at the interface can be expected. The consequent corrosion
behaviour of the metal substratum will vary according to the degree of this
reciprocal interaction.

An assessment of the relationship between corrosion and biofouling has

been made for several metals in seawater, using scanning electron microscopy (SEM) complemented with energy dispersive X-ray analysis (EDXA)
of the deposits and electrochemical corrosion techniques to evaluate the
corrosion behaviour of the substratum (Videla *et al.*, 1987). Results show
that biofouling at the metal surfaces tested increased according to the following sequence: copper < 70 : 30 copper–nickel alloy < brass < aluminium < stainless steel < titanium. At an active (easily corroding) metal
surface such as aluminium, biofilms are formed on an unstable and continuously growing layer of inorganic products. When parts of these deposits
detach, they are accompanied by the biofilm. Conversely, stainless steel or
titanium, because of the lack of corrosion products, allows a rapid and easy
colonization by microorganisms on an even and stable metal surface. In
addition, formation and structure of biofilms is more easily observed by
SEM on these substrata (Videla *et al.*, 1988*a*).

Biofilm–passive layer interactions

Three different metal surfaces are chosen to illustrate the various types of
biofilm–passive layer interactions. A corrosion-resistant metal or alloy (e.g.
titanium or stainless steel) can be severely affected by biofouling. Because of
its technological and economic importance, there have been several publications on biofouling and corrosion of stainless steel in marine environments
(Scotto *et al.*, 1985; Johnsen & Bardal, 1986; Dexter & Gao, 1987). It is
assumed that biofilms can stimulate localized corrosion in two main ways:
(a) by initiating corrosion through the formation of differential aeration cells
and (b) by increasing the rate of the cathodic reaction. Electrochemical reactions are markedly influenced by biofilm formation and by the chemical
microenvironment created at the metal–biofilm interface (Little *et al.*, 1990).
An alteration of the electrode capacitance can be produced by different
adsorption processes occurring on the metal surface (Mansfield *et al.*, 1990).
    Briefly, biofilm–metal interactions on a corrosion-resistant alloy can lead
to corrosion that would not occur in the absence of biofouling. These
conditions will favour the onset of localized attack, mainly by (a) differential
aeration as a result of a patchy distribution of the biofilm, and (b) an
alteration of oxygen gradients within the biofilm. Furthermore, the growth
of microorganisms of different species within adherent biofilms facilitates
the development of structured consortia that enhance the effects of single
microbial species on metal corrosion (Costerton *et al.*, 1988).

However, an easily corrodible surface such as mild steel in saline media is rapidly covered by abundant deposits of corrosion products of varied chemical composition.

In marine environments, a complex fouling layer consisting of bacteria and microalgae embedded in EPS generally consolidates the corrosion product passive layers. Such a cohesive effect of microbial EPS depends on several environmental and biological factors, and will finally determine the extent of passive layer–biofouling interaction (Videla, 1989b). It has been reported (Gaylarde & Videla, 1987) that microbial dissolution of ferric oxides and hydroxides by the reduction of Fe^{3+} species by certain types of marine bacterium can eventually expose the metal surface to the direct action of aggressive species (e.g. sulfides, chlorides) existing in the medium. Microbial consortia can also markedly enhance the localized attack.

Cupronickels (90 : 10 and 70 : 30 copper–nickel alloys) exhibit a behaviour intermediate between those of corrosion-resistant and easily corrodible metal surfaces. In spite of their well-documented antifouling properties, copper–nickel alloys are colonized by marine bacteria after exposure periods of several months (Blunn, 1986). Microorganisms are generally entrapped between corrosion product layers and EPS, leading to a sandwiched structure. In this way, biofilm detachment, due to water flow or marine currents, will influence the removal of inorganic passive layers, resulting in a patchy distribution of the biofilm itself. This causes an increase of the corrosion rate through a differential aeration effect. The effect of biogenic sulfide, altering the cuprous oxide passive layer structure in copper–nickel alloys exposed to saline media, can also act as an alternative BIC mechanism (Videla et al., 1989). Thus, biofouling–passive layer interactions can affect passivity by:

1. Hindering the transport of chemical species to the metal surface.
2. Facilitating the removal of passive layers as biofilm detachment occurs.
3. Leading to differential aeration as a result of a patchy distribution of the biofilm.
4. Altering redox conditions through the direct use of oxygen in bacterial respiration.
5. Facilitating the dissolution and removal of inorganic passive layers on the metal surface.

Biologically induced corrosion from an electrochemical point of view

Classic mechanisms of BIC

Although differing from one metal to another, classic mechanisms proposed for BIC can be summarized as follows:

1. Metabolic production of aggressive compounds that, once produced in the medium, change this from an inert to an aggressive environment.
2. Creation of differential aeration cells on the metal surface.
3. Metabolic disruption of protective coatings.
4. Metabolic uptake of corrosion inhibitors present in the medium.
5. Acceleration of one of the reactions of the corrosion process by a depolarization effect.

Due to the wide variety of substances produced by the metabolic activity of microorganisms, the first mechanism can be subdivided according to Miller (1981) as follows:

(i) Production of substances with surfactant properties.
(ii) Production of inorganic acids.
(iii) Production of carboxylic acids as metabolic end products or by leakage of tricarboxylic acid cycle intermediates.
(iv) Production of sulfide ions, as in the case of SRB.

Mechanism (1) can be illustrated by BIC of iron and carbon steel by *Thiobacillus*. Several oxidation reactions have been presented for this genus, involving many intermediate inorganic sulfur compounds that are susceptible to microbial oxidation (Cragnolino & Tuovinen, 1984). Sulfur oxyanions as metastable intermediates do not persist in oxidative, bacteria-containing environments. Some intermediates such as tetrathionates may accumulate until the substrate is virtually completely oxidized, but the ensuing oxidation leads to the formation of sulfuric acid (Tuovinen & Kelly, 1974).

Mechanism (2), differential aeration, is particularly relevant for corrosion-resistant alloys (e.g. stainless steel) in the presence of biofilms, as was explained in the previous section. A simplified scheme to illustrate this type of differential aeration effect under a microbial colony was shown in Fig. 4.1, above. In such an aeration cell, active growth of the microorganisms keeps oxygen concentrations at a low level under the colony, which thus acts as an anodic area, whereas the surrounding zone, with higher oxygen concentration, acts as a cathodic area. Once the electrochemical cell is established, even the death of microorganisms does not extinguish the cell, since a substantial barrier to the intake of oxygen has been established. A similar situation frequently occurs in the iron pipework of industrial cooling systems, as well as in water mains and water distribution pipes and deposits, caused by the action of iron-oxidizing bacteria generally associated with SRB in the interior of tubercles (Tuovinen et al., 1980).

The third BIC mechanism (3) can be illustrated by the metabolic consumption of the protective coatings of integral aircraft tanks by fungal contaminants of jet fuels (Davis, 1967). Adhesion and surfacial effects of microorganisms in corrosion processes through a preferential dissolution of protective inorganic deposits on the metal surface have been reported (Ghiorse, 1988; Westlake et al., 1986; Gaylarde & Videla, 1987). In this way, a depassivation of the metal surface, later exposed to the corrosive action of microbial metabolites, is achieved.

The practical case of fungal contamination of jet fuels and subsequent BIC of aluminium alloys in fuel water systems can be used to illustrate mechanism (4). Fungal consumption of nitrates (very effective inhibitors of aluminium corrosion in aqueous media) leads to an increase in the chloride : nitrate ratio, thus facilitating the initiation of pitting attack.

The accelerating effect of the corrosion reaction by the depolarization action of microorganisms has been ascribed to the cathodic reaction to explain corrosion of iron and carbon steel by SRB through the CDT of von Wolzogen Kühr and van der Vlugt (1934). A more detailed discussion of CDT as well as an updated overview on the anaerobic corrosion of iron and steel will be made at the end of this section.

An electrochemical classification of BIC processes

From an electrochemical point of view, two types of mechanism can be distinguished: (a) those involving a modification of the anodic corrosion rate, and (b) those that modify the cathodic rate. BIC mechanisms related to anodic effects include:

1. Production of corrosive metabolites (e.g. sulfuric acid by sulfur-oxidizing bacteria).

2. Production of metabolites that enhance the corrosive action of other chemical species already present in the medium (e.g. biogenic sulfides in chloride-containing media such as seawater).
3. Uptake or degradation of corrosion inhibitors (e.g. nitrate consumption by *Hormoconis resinae* in BIC of aluminium alloys).

The mechanisms related to cathodic effects include:

1. Production of cathodic reactants (e.g. protons derived from acidic metabolites).
2. Uptake or degradation of cathodic reactants (e.g. oxygen consumption by microbial respiration leading to differential aeration).
3. Indirect acceleration of the cathodic reaction (e.g. cathodic effects owing to Fe₂S in the anaerobic corrosion of iron).

Several of these mechanisms can operate simultaneously or consecutively, but no single cause can account for all of the corrosive effects of micro-organisms. A multiple mechanism involving synergistic effects between microorganisms, metal surfaces and each environment must be invoked to explain the BIC process (Videla, 1986a). It should be emphasized that one of the main biological effects inducing corrosion is the modification of the metal–solution interface through biofouling (Videla & Characklis, 1992).

The Cathodic Depolarization Theory

The basic idea of the CDT was that hydrogen reduction (and removal), coupled to the bacterial reduction of sulfate to sulfide, could account for the severe pitting attack observed on cast iron pipes. The microbial influence on corrosion would be indirect, causing cathodic depolarization and the consequent enhancement of iron dissolution. The term depolarization was not used in a strict electrochemical sense, but merely to indicate that there was an undefined change in the electrochemical behaviour of the system (Duquette, 1986). The CDT sequence of reactions is depicted in Fig. 4.6.

Overall reaction	$4\,Fe + SO_4^{2-} + 4\,H_2O \rightarrow 3\,Fe(OH)_2 + FeS + 2\,OH^-$		
Metal	$4\,Fe \rightarrow 4\,Fe^{2+} + 8e^-$	Anode	Electro-chemical cell
	$8\,H^+ + 8\,e^- \rightarrow 8\,H_{ad.}$	Cathode	
Solution	$8\,H_2O \rightarrow 8\,H^+ + 8\,OH^-$	Electrolyte	
Microorganism	$SO_4^{2-} + 8\,H \rightarrow S^{2-} + 4\,H_2O$		Microbial depolarization
Corrosion products	$Fe^{2+} + S^{2-} \rightarrow FeS \quad 3Fe^{2+} + 6\,OH^- \rightarrow 3\,Fe(OH)_2$		

Fig. 4.6 Cathodic Depolarization Theory: sequence of reactions.

This indirect role of SRB in anaerobic corrosion of iron is very hard to sustain in the light of present electrochemical knowledge. Several additional factors must be taken into account:

1. The anodic effects of biogenic sulfides, bisulfides, and hydrogen sulfide derived from sulfate reduction.
2. The presence of alternative cathodic reactants such as hydrogen sulfide or bisulfides.
3. The possible role of metabolic intermediates (tetrathionate, thiosulfate) on corrosion.
4. The effect of elemental sulfur derived from the inorganic or biological oxidation of sulfide, as an alternative cathodic path (Schaschl, 1980).

In spite of its omissions and misstatements, the CDT represented a pioneering attempt in the BIC literature to understand electrochemically the anaerobic corrosion of iron. Much of the literature published later was devoted to support or to discuss the assumptions of this theory.

The complexity of biological environments involved with SRB activity makes it very difficult to assess microbial effects by means of electrochemical methods, since chemical composition and pH of the solution are continuously varied by microbial metabolism. Additionally, one important fact generally not taken into account in the formulation of a mechanism for explaining the anaerobic corrosion of iron is that, in practical situations, metal surfaces are generally covered with various deposits (oxides, sulfides, hydroxides and biofilms). Thus, the mechanism proposed to explain the BIC process must include the breakdown of passivity by microbial activity.

An updated overview of the anaerobic corrosion of iron and steel

A bioelectrochemical interpretation of the passivity breakdown process by SRB has been published (Videla, 1988). An updated overview can be summarized in this way:

1. The metabolic activity of SRB adds to the environment several sulfur-containing anions of corrosive characteristics (sulfides, bisulfides, hydrogen sulfide, thiosulfates, tetrathionates).
2. Intermediate metabolic compounds are corrosive for mild steel mainly through their transformation into sulfide anions (Vasquez Moll et al., 1984).
3. The characteristics and intensity of sulfide corrosion on mild steel are closely related to the nature of the passive film already present on the metal surface (Videla, 1986b). The corrosive action of sulfides would be enhanced by other aggressive ions such as chlorides already present in the medium.
4. Physicochemical characteristics of the liquid environment (pH, ionic composition, redox potential) condition the effects of SRB, which may eventually change from corrosive to passivating (Moreno et al., 1992).
5. Biofilms and microbial consortia within biofilms can markedly enhance the corrosive effects of sulfur compounds produced by SRB.

Electrochemical methods to evaluate BIC: use and limitations

In every case the BIC process is electrochemical and electrochemical techniques can be useful, when carefully applied, for investigating microbial effects on metal behaviour. BIC is rarely linked to a single mechanism or to single species of microorganisms. Hence, it is necessary to be cautious in the interpretation of data supplied by electrochemical methods. Electrochemical techniques have often been used in complex media where the characteristics and properties of passive films are not well understood. The presence of complex deposits of corrosion products and EPS may dramatically reduce the usefulness of some electrochemical techniques. Notwithstanding this, the use

of appropriate electrochemical methods, coupled with a careful characterization of the microbial species present and of the metal–solution interface,
can lead to a better understanding of BIC mechanisms.

A detailed description of electrochemical methods for evaluating BIC is
out of the scope of this chapter. A wide variety of electrochemical techniques
such as corrosion and critical pitting potential measurements, Tafel and
potentiodynamic polarization, linear polarization resistance, split-cell current measurements, and several modern electrochemical techniques have
been reviewed by several authors (Dexter *et al.*, 1989; Mansfeld & Little,
1990; Pope, 1991) and the reader is referred to any of these excellent
articles. Three different examples are used below to illustrate the application of electrochemical techniques to BIC.

BIC of aluminium alloys

Aluminium and its alloys show a particularly high resistance to environmental factors, and therefore form a group of widely used materials for vehicles,
aircrafts, buildings, etc. Their corrosion resistance is due to a strong, adherent and very stable passive layer, which in oxidizing surroundings leads to
extremely low corrosion rates. However, like stainless steel, aluminium
alloys show a tendency for pitting corrosion, especially in different chloride-
containing media. The pit morphology observed on Al–Mg alloys (e.g. 2024
type) is similar to that observed for pure aluminium in chloride solutions.
This morphology corresponds to etched shapes presenting crystallographic
facets, their orientation varying from one grain to another (Szklarska-
Smialowska, 1986).

Due to its economic and technological importance, microbial deterioration of jet fuel and subsequent corrosion of aluminium alloys has been
extensively studied during the last two decades. Microorganisms isolated
from contaminated jet fuels include different species of fungi, bacteria and
yeasts, but the fungus *H. resinae* is believed to be the main organism responsible for the corrosion of aluminium and its alloys in fuel/water systems
(Videla *et al.*, 1993*a*).

Microbial contamination is the cause of serious problems in product
quality and corrosion of metals and alloys used in the process of extraction,
production, distribution and storage of hydrocarbon fuels. The attack is
generally located at the bottom of the tanks, where there is an active
microbial population associated with free water. Any free water, such as

droplets or thin films, is sufficient for microbial growth and the subsequent BIC. Low pH values are reached during fungal growth as a consequence of organic acid production by hydrocarbon degradation. Gas chromatographic analysis reveals the presence of monocarboxylic, dicarboxylic and several tricarboxylic acids (McKenzie *et al.*, 1977). Surface active agents are also produced during growth, and this degradation pattern seems to be the same for different fungi (Videla *et al.*, 1988*b*). pH is important as acidity can prevent the repassivation of the aluminium.

Among the different electrochemical techniques used to study this case of BIC, corrosion potential measurements have been utilized to study the behaviour of aluminium alloy 2024 in the presence of aggressive metabolites produced by *H. resinae* during the degradation of hydrocarbon chain molecules (Salvarezza *et al.*, 1983).

The magnitude and sign of the corrosion potential (the voltage difference between a metal immersed in a corrosive medium and an appropriate reference electrode) are functions of the metal itself, as well as the composition, temperature and hydrodynamics of the electrolyte (Dexter *et al.*, 1989). Measurements of the open circuit corrosion potential with time allowed the detection of the transition between the typical behaviour of a passive metal (stable potential) and the onset of localized pitting (strong oscillations). Subsequent observation of the samples indicated the presence of pits and general corrosion areas, confirming the results suggested by the electrochemical measurements.

The redox potential (the relative potential of an electrochemical reaction under equilibrium conditions where there is no net flow of current) can be a useful parameter to study the role played by different microbial species in the modification of the environment. In the case of active/passive metals such as aluminium and its alloys, where a localized form of attack is predominant, the use of redox potentials together with an electrochemical parameter (e.g. the corrosion potential or the pitting potential (E_p)), can be of great importance in assessing whether or not the oxidizing conditions of the medium can reach the values needed to initiate localized corrosion (Salvarezza *et al.*, 1981).

The general term 'pitting potential' or E_p is used to denote several electrochemical parameters related to the initiation of pitting corrosion. Microorganisms generally induce localized corrosion (i.e. pitting). Therefore, different methods for determining characteristic pitting potential values can be very useful to assess the tendency of microorganisms to accelerate pitting on a metal surface.

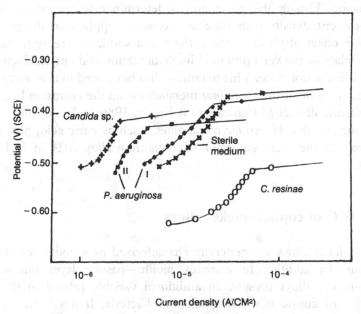

Fig. 4.7 Anodic polarization curves for aluminium alloy 2024 in cultures of different isolates from fuel/water systems. Potentials in volts are referred to a saturated calomel electrode (SCE). The point at which each curve changes suddenly in form corresponds to the E_p. (From Salvarezza *et al.*, 1979.)

The E_p depends strongly on the experimental technique used to measure it and it is usually defined as the most noble potential at which the passive current density remains stable and pits do not nucleate on a surface. This parameter is measured potentiostatically (varying the current at different constant potential values) in the laboratory under controlled experimental conditions.

By comparing E_p values obtained by means of anodic polarization curves performed in cultures of several microbial isolates from fuel storage tanks (Salvarezza *et al.*, 1979), it was possible to differentiate the role played by each microorganism in the corrosion process (Fig. 4.7). These values were in good agreement with weight loss and ionic aluminium measurements, showing conclusively that, among the different isolates (*H. resinae, Pseudomonas aeruginosa, Candida* sp.), the fungus *H. resinae* was the main organism responsible for attack on the metal.

The time it takes to form the first pit on a passive metal exposed to a solution containing aggressive anions is defined as the induction time for pit initiation. Usually this parameter is determined by recording changes in the current density with time at a constant applied anodic potential. When the onset of pitting occurs, there is a sudden increase in current; the time elapsed between potential implementation and current increase is called the induction time. This parameter has been used to assess the effect of citric acid (one of the *H. resinae* metabolites) on the corrosion behaviour of aluminium alloy 2024 (Salvarezza & Videla, 1986; Videla, 1986*c*). These results suggest that *H. resinae* metabolites, such as citric acid, play a very active role in the localized attack of aluminium alloy 2024 in fuel/water systems.

BIC of copper–nickel alloys

Copper–nickel alloys are generally characterized by a complex corrosion behaviour. In addition to complex biofilm–passive layer interactions, copper–nickel alloys present an additional variable related to the toxic properties of cupric (Cu(II)) species on bacteria. It has been reported (Blunn, 1986) that after exposure of the metal to seawater for periods of several months, bacteria can be found entrapped between corrosion product layers and EPS. Thus, a characteristic sandwiched passive layer structure can usually be found. Biofilm detachment could influence the removal of inorganic layers, resulting in a patchy distribution of the biofilm that causes an increase of the corrosion rate through differential aeration (Videla, 1989*b*). A laboratory assessment of the early stages of microfouling and corrosion of 70 : 30 copper–nickel alloy in the presence of two species of marine bacteria has been published (Gomez de Saravia *et al.*, 1989). The corrosion behaviour of the alloy was studied by corrosion potential versus time measurements made in both sterile and contaminated seawater. The corrosion potential of copper–nickel differed when the metal surfaces were immersed in bacterial cultures in artificial seawater or in sterile artificial seawater. Corrosion potential measurements on copper–nickel samples incubated separately over 7 days in bacterial cultures showed a wide range of scatter when compared with the same alloy samples in identical but sterile medium. The scattering in the corrosion potential values could have been induced by the formation of microbial deposits (colonies) on the metal surface (verified by scanning electron microscopy (SEM)). Microbial metabolic activity leads to passive film dissolution beneath these colonies. Corrosion potential values obtained in the culture media, as well as *in situ* measurements, showed tendencies similar to those reported in the literature for stainless steel in seawater (Dexter & Gao, 1987). The decrease in the corrosion potential is due to polarizing currents supplied by the pits. These effects are not observed in sterile media.

The relationship between biofilms and inorganic passive layers in the corrosion of copper–nickel alloys in chloride environments has been studied using different electrochemical techniques such as corrosion potential versus time measurements and potentiodynamic sweep techniques (Videla et al., 1989). The potentiodynamic sweep techniques are most useful in characterizing, and sometimes predicting, the corrosion behaviour for metal/electrolyte systems in which the metal passivates by the formation of a protective film (Dexter et al., 1989). The basic techniques can be found in the ASTM Standards G3 (ASTM, 1981; ASTM, 1982). One of the main experimental variables that can be manipulated is the sweep rate. The scan rate, which can affect the concentration of oxygen and hydrogen as well as the formation of films at the metal surface, is very important in the application of potentiodynamic techniques to BIC.

A synergistic effect of chloride and sulfide anions on copper–nickel alloy dissolution was found by using potentiodynamic techniques and corrosion potential versus time measurements. Modification of the structural characteristics of the corrosion product layers by metabolic products of bacteria and biofilms can dramatically increase localized attack on 70 : 30 and 90 : 10 copper–nickel alloys in seawater or other chloride-containing media (Videla, 1994). These effects can be seen clearly through the modification of the anodic current peaks, corresponding to different corrosion products of copper–nickel, in potentiodynamic measurements (Gomez de Saravia et al., 1990).

BIC of stainless steel

Some recent attempts to interpret the effect of biofilms on corrosion have been made on stainless steels exposed to seawater using corrosion potential versus time measurements (Mollica et al., 1984; Johnsen & Bardal, 1986). The corrosion potential of an AISI type 316 stainless steel and the rate of oxygen reduction, as measured by the cathodic polarization curve, have been determined with and without the presence of a natural marine bacterial film on the metal surface (Dexter & Gao, 1987). It is assumed that microbial biofilms on stainless steel can stimulate localized corrosion in natural seawater in two main ways: (a) by initiating corrosion through the formation of oxygen concentration cells, and (b) by increasing the rate of the cathodic reduction reaction. These two effects combine to make the corrosion potential of the stainless steel highly irreproducible within a week of exposure to natural seawater. When localized corrosion is in progress the potential becomes active, but, on electrodes that remain passive, biofilm causes the potential to be shifted in the noble direction. This effect can be ascribed to a probable change in the kinetics of the oxygen reaction. If the E_p of the metal is more active than the reversible oxygen potential under exposure conditions, the corrosion potential may shift enough to initiate pitting corrosion (see Chapter 5, Fig. 5.16). Even if E_p values were not noble enough to avoid pitting of stainless steel in the presence of a biofilm, the increasingly nobler corrosion potential would make the initiation of crevice corrosion under the film more likely. Thus, microbial participation in corrosion, in this case through the effects derived from biofilm formation and detachment at the metal surface, could change the environmental conditions in the vicinity of the metal surface, allowing or enhancing localized attack. This attack proceeds by typical electrochemical corrosion due to differential aeration.

BIC in industry

What to measure and how to do it

An industrial plant comprises many environments where BIC and biofouling processes are potentially troublesome. Some examples are cooling-water or injection-water systems used in process industry or oil production, respectively, storage tanks, water and wastewater treatment facilities and piping, hydroelectric, thermal or nuclear power plants, etc.

A recirculating cooling-water system provides a good example of an industrial environment where biofouling and BIC can develop. Corrosion and scaling control and monitoring have been the two major objectives of cooling water treatment specialists in the past. However, good corrosion inhibition alone does not guarantee that adverse effects on heat-exchanger effectiveness will be overcome. The major concern now is to improve methods for maintaining heat transfer performance by controlling biological deposits, while still preserving corrosion inhibition and avoiding scale formation. An adequate understanding of the biological effects of biofilms on the corrosion process is still needed to guarantee effective water treatment for cooling water systems. The interrelationship between inorganic corrosion and biofouling of heat transfer equipment must be controlled if long-term reliability is to be achieved.

A monitoring programme based on laboratory and field measurements for assessing biodeterioration (biofouling and BIC) on mild steel and stainless steel in recirculating cooling water systems has been reported (Videla *et al.*, 1990). This programme was based on: (a) water quality control; (b) corrosion monitoring in the field (weight loss and linear polarization probe); (c) laboratory corrosion tests (polarization techniques and corrosion potential versus time measurements); and (d) use of a new multipurpose sampling device that allows monitoring of sessile populations, biofilms, corrosive attack morphology and intensity, and biological and inorganic deposits analysis.

The new side-stream sampling device (Renaprobe) allows reliable biofilm and corrosion sampling without introducing important modifications in the system. Renaprobe is located in a corrosion rack (Fig. 4.8), without altering conventional standards, and allows eight different samples to be taken simultaneously or at different exposure periods.

Two open circulating systems of a chemical processing plant were treated using an organic phosphonate (PBTC) and zinc salt blend for corrosion control (Videla *et al.*, 1990). Selective dispersant agents were also added. To assess biodeterioration effects, chlorine was used only in one of the cooling systems whereas no biocide was added to the water of the other circuit. Over a testing period of 15 days, sessile bacterial counts were dramatically different in each system. SEM observations of the biofilm were in good agreement with these results. Comparison of the corrosive attack on carbon steel coupons withdrawn from both systems revealed that there was little metal attack in the biocide-treated cooling system. Conversely, carbon steel coupons exposed to water without biocide treatment (with hazardous levels of aerobic and anaerobic bacteria) presented copious corrosion products and significant pitting attack. Since the cooling-water and operating conditions (corrosion and scale inhibition treatment) in both systems were identical, the biological source of the metal attack was obvious.

The preceding results demonstrate the importance of adequate monitoring and interpretation of the interrelationship between biofilms and inorganic passive layers (Videla, 1989*b*). Experimental evidence shows that the adverse effects derived from biofouling deposits can defeat the protective action of an otherwise efficient water control treatment. Microbial

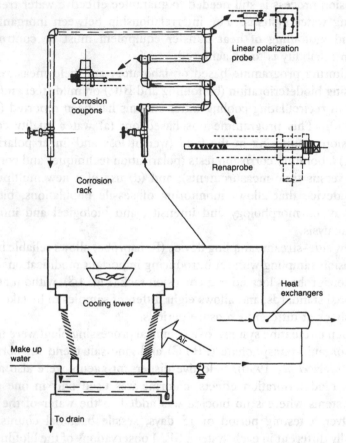

Fig. 4.8 Renaprobe multipurpose sampling device and other corrosion monitoring devices implanted in a side-stream in the corrosion rack of a cooling-water system (from Videla *et al.*, 1990, with permission from NACE International, Houston, TX).

colonization of metal surfaces can change the corrosion behaviour and resistance to breakdown in localized areas, facilitating the onset of pitting attack.

Monitoring devices

In spite of the diversity of biofouling and BIC problems, sampling and monitoring devices can be classified into two main groups: (a) those for monitoring microbial effects in biofilms, and (b) those for monitoring corrosion.

An increasing awareness of the detrimental effects of biofouling has led to the requirement for devices for *in situ* sampling that can facilitate further examination of the microbial components of the biofilm. This is particularly important not only for normal monitoring purposes, but also to evaluate the effectiveness of possible control measures (e.g. biocides). Formerly, measurement of microbial populations in industrial waters was restricted largely to the planktonic microorganisms. However, more recently special emphasis has been laid on the role of sessile microorganisms (Costerton & Lashen, 1983; Sanders & Hamilton, 1986). It is now widely recognized that the attached, sessile bacterial population is more numerous and important than the planktonic one, and misleading results can be obtained if this fact is overlooked. This assertion is supported by the following character-istics of sessile microorganisms: (a) biofilms represent the bulk of micro-organisms in industrial systems either in terms of numbers or biomass; (b) physiological activity and growth rate of microbial species in the bulk water phase may markedly differ from those in the biofilm; (c) the suscepti-bility of sessile microorganisms to biocides is considerably lower than that of planktonic cells mainly because of the protective effects of EPS within the biofilm matrix (Costerton *et al.*, 1988).

Sampling devices for monitoring microbial effects in biofilms fall into two main types: (a) directly implanted in the system or (b) side-stream devices (Gilbert & Herbert, 1987). The first type of device is designed to be fitted directly into the pipe wall and sometimes (e.g. in water-injection lines for oil production) it is required to make them compatible with existing high pressure fittings to avoid partial shutdown and depressurization. Metal coupons of a predetermined surface area can be manufactured with differ-ent materials, usually identical with the constructional material of the system. Sample removal after different exposure periods is generally by means of special tools to avoid any direct contact with the biofilm on the coupon surface. Side-stream sampling and monitoring devices are installed in parallel to the main system, taking a proportion of its flow in identical operating conditions. Metal coupons, similar to those used in the directly implanted devices, are used, although generally they are present in a greater number and sometimes mounted individually in separate holders. The pioneer of this type of tool was the Robbins device, originally constructed from Admiralty brass (Ruseska *et al.*, 1982; see also Chapter 8).

Generally, side-stream sampling systems provide a greater flexibility than directly implanted assemblies. In addition side-stream devices can be isolated from the main flow and subsequently connected to laboratory flow loops for biocide or corrosion testing. A wide variety of side-stream samplers developed in recent years are described in BIC literature (Sanders & Hamilton, 1986; Surinach, 1986; Videla *et al.*, 1990). Once metal coupons have been withdrawn from the system, examination and quantification of sessile populations can be prosecuted by means of different methods for determining the biomass:

1. Microscopic methods: brightfield or epifluorescence optical microscopy (Marshall, 1986); SEM (Videla, 1989*a*); or transmission electron microscopy (TEM: Costerton *et al.*, 1978).
2. Spectroscopic methods (Fletcher, 1976).
3. Weight (dry at 103 °C or volatile at 550 °C) (Greensberg *et al.*, 1985).
4. Biofilm thickness (Bakke & Olson, 1986).
5. Biofilm mass (Trulear & Characklis, 1982; Bakke *et al.*, 1990).
6. ATP measurements (Prasad, 1988).

Enumeration of viable bacteria by culture techniques and microscopic methods has been widely used as a means of determining population density (viable cells). Among the latter are vital dyes such as fluorescein diacetate (Pope, 1986) or tetrazolium salts (Oren, 1987) and also molecular probes for ribosomal RNA or immunological probes (Ward, 1989).

Metabolic activity within the biofilm can also be used to determine the gross activity. In this respect radiorespirometric techniques provide a sensitive method for determining microbial activity *in situ* within the biofilm, after recovering the sampling coupon. One of these techniques has been successfully used to assess the activity of sessile SRB within biofilms isolated from water-injection systems in off-shore oil production (Rosser & Hamilton, 1983; Sanders & Hamilton, 1986).

ELISA methods have been recently used (Bobowski & Nedwell, 1987; Cook & Gaylarde, 1987) as a rapid technique for detecting and enumerating SRB within biofilms. These methods have the advantages of speed and/or simplicity compared with the commonly used enumeration technique by the most probable number (MPN) method (see Chapter 10).

In addition to the monitoring devices mentioned above, other dynamic systems, based on a large suspension volume with respect to substratum, have been developed for assessing the effectiveness of chemical treatments for prevention, inactivation and removal of unwanted biofilms. Some of these laboratory biofilm reactors are: the RotoTorque or rotating annular reactor (Bakke *et al.*, 1984), illustrated schematically in Fig. 4.9; the constant

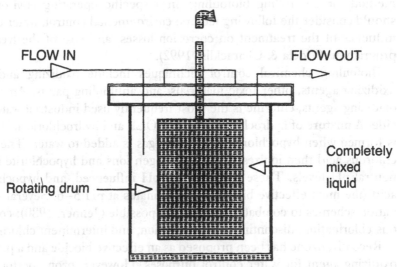

FLOW IN

FLOW OUT

Completely
mixed
liquid

Rotating drum

Fig. 4.9 Schematic diagram of the RotoTorque, consisting of a rotating inner drum
within a stationary outer drum, operating as a continuous flow reactor (from
Characklis, 1990, with permission from Wiley Interscience, New York).

depth film fermentor (Peters & Wimpenny, 1988); the rotating biological
reactor (Kinner *et al.*, 1983); and the multi-tubular flow reactor (Characklis,
1990). Several of these sampling devices can also be used for corrosion monitoring: to assess the intensity and morphology of localized attack, for biofilms
or corrosion products analysis, or as a complement to field and laboratory
corrosion measurements. The practical case described at the beginning of
this section gives a good illustration of the simultaneous assessment of biofouling and corrosion, by using the same side-stream sampling device.

Protective methods and countermeasures

Although there are several physical and chemical methods available for
preventing or controlling undesirable biofouling and BIC effects, there is
no universal remedy against both biodeterioration processes. Moreover, an
effective treatment in one operating environment may be quite ineffective
in another environment or even enhance a particular fouling effect (e.g.
corrosion). Finally, an effective countermeasure for one type of fouling
(e.g. scaling) may be rendered ineffective by the presence of another type
of deposit (e.g. biofouling) (Characklis, 1986). The decision regarding a

method for controlling biofouling, in a specific operating environment, should consider the following factors: environmental control, water quality, influence of the treatment on corrosion losses, and cost of the treatment programme (Videla & Characklis, 1992).

Biofouling chemical control techniques include oxidizing and non-oxidizing agents, other toxic materials, and antifouling paints. Among the oxidizing agents, chlorine is the most frequently used industrial water biocide. A mixture of hydrochlorous acid (HOCl) and hydrochloric acid (HCl) is formed when hypochlorite or chlorine gas is added to water. The hypochlorous acid then ionizes to form hydrogen ions and hypochlorite ions at neutral pH levels. These reactions are pH influenced, and hypochlorous acid (the most effective biocide) predominates at pH 5–6. Several chlorination schemes to combat biofouling are possible (Jenner, 1980): continuous chlorination, discontinuous chlorination, and intermittent chlorination.

Recently, ozone has been proposed as an effective biocide and a powerful oxidizing agent for water control purposes. However, ozone performance in recirculating cooling-water systems, its effects on corrosion of copper and steel and its generation and feed methods are still being explored (Hettiarachi, 1991; Wilkes & Rice, 1991; Videla et al., 1994).

Non-oxidizing agents are often organic-based biocides such as aldehydes, arsenates, ammonia and amines, cyano compounds, organometallics, and chlorophenols. Non-oxidizing biocides can be more effective than oxidizing biocides, owing to their greater persistence, their general control of algae, fungi and bacteria, and because the effectiveness of many of them is independent of pH. The use of a combination of oxidizing and non-oxidizing biocides or a synergistic mixture of two non-oxidizing biocides is frequently adopted in industrial systems to optimize microbiological control programmes.

Among the most frequently used non-oxidizing biocides, methylene bisthiocyanate (MBT) is effective in controlling algae, fungi and bacteria, most notably SRB. However, MBT is not recommended for use at pH values above 8, because of its rapid hydrolysis in the alkaline pH range. Conversely, quaternary ammonium salts are generally most effective against algae and bacteria at alkaline pH values. Because of their surface-active nature, these chemicals become ineffective in heavily fouled systems, but are frequently used in synergistic mixtures with biocides such as glutaraldehyde for specific action against biofilms.

Isothiazoline is a sulfur-containing biocide, very effective in controlling both algae and bacteria over a wide pH range and easily compatible with other chemicals used for water treatment. Glutaraldehyde is one of the most effective weapons for controlling a wide diversity of slime-forming bacteria, SRB, algae and fungi. Nowadays it is widely used in water-injection systems for oil production because of its effectiveness against biofilms over broad pH and temperature ranges. However, glutaraldehyde can be rendered ineffective when high concentrations of compounds containing $-NH_2$ groups are present (e.g. ammonia, amines, etc.).

Finally, it can be emphasized that with environmental and toxicological concerns increasing, careful control and monitoring of biocide use is becoming critically important. Further information on biocides is presented by Gaylarde in Chapter 10.

Toxic alloys presenting antifouling properties have long been used to control the growth of marine fouling organisms. Copper–nickel alloys of the 90 : 10 and 70 : 30 types are examples of antifouling materials. Copper–nickel alloys are used in cooling-water systems of coastal power plants, as well as in the piping and components designed for marine service. When exposed to marine environments, copper–nickel alloys form an adherent cuprous oxide corrosion-resistant film. The copper ions in this film, when released into seawater, are toxic to marine biofouling organisms and inhibit their attachment to the metal surface. However, after long exposures, copper–nickel antifouling properties are counterbalanced by the protective action of microbial EPS in the biofilm.

Antifouling paints consist of various toxic compounds (copper oxides, pesticides, etc.) incorporated into vinyl-chlorinated rubber, coal-tar epoxy, and other types of paint bases. They act by a slow release into the water to inhibit or kill attaching organisms. However, because of the characteristics of their activity, their effectiveness decreases with time, especially in seawater, and regular renewal is mandatory. Antifouling paints or coatings, in association with cathodic protection of metallic structures immersed in seawater, have proved effective in avoiding biodeterioration effects in offshore oil production (Edyvean, 1987).

There are some non-chemical control technologies aimed at the control of biofouling in industrial environments:

> *Thermal backwash*: As an antifouling technique, thermal backwash requires that the cooling-water temperature be raised above the thermal tolerance level of the fouling organisms. The effectiveness of this countermeasure is dependent on the appropriate choice of water temperature, exposure duration and frequency of backwash.

Non-thermal energy antifouling techniques: Some of these techniques such as gamma irradiation and ultraviolet radiation have been proposed as possible antifouling alternatives because of their success in killing microorganisms. The engineering feasibility of effectively irradiating large volumes of water with gamma rays has not been developed sufficiently to consider its use in large-scale industrial systems.

Hydraulic methods: The use of high velocity to prevent the attachment and subsequent growth of fouling organisms has been discussed for many years. The idea has merit and has proved effective under controlled conditions of high velocity and uninterrupted flow over relatively smooth surfaces (Mitchell & Belson, 1980).

Mechanical methods: Mechanical devices able to stop biofouling influx into industrial cooling systems and remove inorganic and organic debris on the inner walls of heat-exchanger tubes have been developed to avoid long plant downtime for manual cleaning. Among the latter, some frequently used online mechanical cleaning systems are continuous sponge ball, batch sponge ball and brush systems. In sponge ball methods, cleaning occurs via the whipping action of slightly oversized sponge rubber balls propelled through tubes using the cooling-water flow. In the brush system, a captive brush is shuttled intermittently back and forth through each tube of the heat exchanger by reversing the direction of water flow. The brushes remove fouling and corrosion products by an abrasive action.

Finally, it must be emphasized that only through an adequate understanding of biofouling dynamics and its interaction with corrosion will the development of successful control strategies be possible.

A present perspective on biocorrosion

Important improvements in analytical, microbiological, electrochemical and microscopical instrumentation have facilitated the development of new methods for laboratory and field assessment of biocorrosion effects in industrial systems. An overview on these advances can be found in recent books on biofouling and biocorrosion in industrial water systems (Videla *et al.*, 1993*b*; Geesey *et al.*, 1994; Kerns & Little, 1994) as well as in several papers presented in recent years at the annual meetings of NACE International.

Chemical analysis inside the biofilms by means of microsensors is one of the most exciting advances in instrumentation. As biofilm systems are diffusion limited, chemical conditions near and inside biofilms can vary dramatically over a distance of only a few micrometres. Thus, the information obtained from analysis of bulk water is limited, and must be closely analysed before any conclusions are drawn about the biofilm. Direct measurements inside biofilms are restricted by: (a) the relatively small thickness of the biofilm; (b) concentration profiles developed across the biofilm where many processes are diffusion limited; (c) the heterogeneous nature of the biofilm. The latter aspect is particularly interesting in microbial colonization of a metal surface and, consequently, in biocorrosion. An example of microsensor technology applied to the evaluation of dissolved oxygen gradients near microbially colonized surfaces has been published recently (Lewandowski, 1994).

Advanced microbiological techniques such as DNA probes have been applied to biocorrosion and biofouling research. Although these techniques are restricted to the laboratory at present, a complementation with microbiological field measurements can be highly useful for monitoring biocorrosion. The use of nucleic acid probes for assessing the community structure of SRB in Western Canadian oil field fluids has been presented recently (Westlake *et al.*, 1993). The development of a chromosomal DNA hybridization technique, reverse sample genome probing (RSGP), permits rapid identification of different bacteria in a sample, with a single probing step. The use of this technique in 31 Canadian oil field samples indicated that there were at least 20 genetically distinct SRB strains in the samples. Among the recent improvements in microscopes, the environmental scanning electron microscope (ESEM), the confocal scanning laser microscope (CSLM) and the atomic force microscope (AFM) are probably the most interesting tools recently developed for biofilm observation and assessment. The use of SEM and transmission electron microscope (TEM) requires the rigorous removal of water from the specimen, and, whenever these techniques are used, the viewer should try to envisage the images rehydrated. The CSLM has allowed the examination of hydrated biofilms by a totally non-intrusive technique that yields clean, three-dimensional images of living biofilms in real time (Costerton, 1994). This innovative technique has shown that approximately 75% to 95% of the volume of bacterial biofilms is occupied by the matrix, and bacterial cells may be concentrated in either the lower or the upper regions of the biofilms, restricted solely to approximately 5% to 25% of the biofilm. ESEM observations for the study of biocorrosion and protective coatings and the use of AFM for the study of copper biocorrosion have been reported recently (Wagner *et al.*, 1992; Bremer *et al.*, 1992).

The development of new electrochemical test methods for the study of localized corrosion phenomena in biocorrosion analysis and monitoring has been presented (Winters *et al.*, 1993; Mansfeld & Xiao, 1994). In addition, innovative field electrochemical devices to monitor the effects of biofilms on biocorrosion of steel in cooling water and seawater have been reported (Licina & Nekoska, 1994; Mollica & Ventura, 1993).

References

Alanis, I., Berardo, L., deCristofaro, N., Moina, C. & Valentini, C. (1986). A case of localized corrosion in underground brass pipes. In *Biologically Induced Corrosion*, ed. S. C. Dexter, pp. 102–8. NACE, Houston, TX.

Arvia, A. J. (1986). Electrochemical approach of metal/solution interface in biodeterioration. In *Proceedings of the Argentine–USA Workshop on Biodeterioration* (CONICET-NSF), ed. H. A. Videla, pp. 5–14. Aquatec Quimica S.A., Sao Paulo, Brazil.

ASTM (1981). *Recent Practice for Conventions Applicable to Electrochemical Measurements in Corrosion Testing*. Standard G3. ASTM, Philadelphia.

ASTM (1982). *Polarization Practice for Standard Reference Method for Making Potentiostatic and Potentiodynamic Polarization Measurements*. Standard G5. ASTM, Philadelphia.

Atkins, D. W. (1986). *Physical Chemistry*, 3rd edn. Oxford University Press, Oxford.

Bakke, R., Characklis, W. G., Turakhia, M. H. & Yeh, A. (1990). Modeling a monopopulation biofilm system: *Pseudomonas aeruginosa*. In *Biofilms*, ed. W. G. Characklis & K. C. Marshall, pp. 487–520. John Wiley & Sons Inc., New York.

Bakke, R. & Olson, P. Q. (1986). Biofilm thickness measurements by light microscopy. *Journal of Microbiological Methods*, **5**, 93–8.

Bakke, R., Trulear, M. G., Robinson, J. A. & Characklis, W. G. (1984). Activity of *Pseudomonas aeruginosa* in biofilms: steady state. *Biotechnology and Bioengineering*, **26**, 1418–24.

Blunn, G. (1986). Biological fouling of copper and copper alloys. In *Biodeterioration 6*, ed. S. Barry, D. R. Houghton, G. C. Llewellyn & C. E. O'Rear, pp. 567–75. CAB International, London.

Bobowski, S. & Nedwell, D. B. (1987). A serological method, using a microELISA technique, for detecting and enumerating sulphate-reducing bacteria. In *Industrial Microbiological Testing*, ed. J. W. Hopton & E. C. Hill, pp. 171–9. Blackwell Scientific Publications, London.

Bockris, J. O'M. & Reddy, A. K. N. (1970). The current across biological membranes. In *Modern Electrochemistry*, pp. 937–47. Macdonald, London.

Booth, G. H. (1971). *Microbiological Corrosion*, pp. 27–40. Mills & Boon Ltd, London.

Booth, G. H. & Tiller, A. K. (1960). Polarisation studies of mild steel in cultures of sulphate-reducing bacteria. *Transactions of the Faraday Society*, 56, 1689–96.

Borenstein, S. W. (1991). Why does microbiologically influenced corrosion occur at or adjacent to austenitic stainless steel weldments? In *Corrosion 91*, Paper no. 286. NACE, Houston, TX.

Bremer, P. J., Geesey, G. G. & Drake, B. (1992). Atomic force microscopy examination of the topography of a hydrated bacterial biofilm on a copper surface. *Current Microbiology*, 24, 1471–80.

Characklis, W. G. (1981). Fouling biofilm development: a process analysis. *Biotechnology and Bioengineering*, 23, 1923–60.

Characklis, W. G. (1986). Influence of microbial films on industrial processes. In *Proceedings of the Argentine–USA Workshop on Biodeterioration* (CONICET-NSF), ed. H. A. Videla, pp. 181–216. Aquatec Quimica S.A., Sao Paulo.

Characklis, W. G. (1990). Laboratory biofilm reactors. In *Biofilms*, ed. W. G. Characklis & K. C. Marshall, pp. 55–89. Wiley Interscience, New York.

Characklis, W. G. & Marshall, K. C. (1990). Biofilms: a basis for an interdisciplinary approach. In *Biofilms*, ed. W. G. Characklis & K. C. Marshall, pp. 3–15. Wiley Interscience, New York.

Cook, P. E. & Gaylarde, C. C. (1987). Rapid techniques for the detection and quantification of sulphate-reducing bacteria. In *Microbial Problems in the Offshore Oil Industry*, ed. E. C. Hill, J. L. Shennan & R. J. Watkinson, p. 245. John Wiley & Sons, Chichester.

Costello, J. A. (1974). Cathodic depolarization by sulphate-reducing bacteria. *South Africa Journal of Science*, 70, 202–4.

Costerton, J. W. (1994). Structure of biofilms. In *Biofouling and Biocorrosion in Industrial Water Systems*, ed. G. G. Geesey, Z. Lewandowski & H. C. Flemming, pp. 1–14. Lewis Publishers, Boca Raton, FL.

Costerton, J. W., Geesey, G. G. & Cheng, K. J. (1978). How bacteria stick. *Scientific American*, 238, 86–95.

Costerton, J. W., Geesey, G. G. & Jones, P. A. (1988). Bacterial biofilms in relation to internal corrosion monitoring and biocide strategies. *Materials Performance*, 27, 49–53.

Costerton, J. W. & Lashen, E. S. (1983). The inherent biocide resistance of corrosion-causing biofilm bacteria. In *Corrosion 83*, Paper no. 246. NACE, Houston, TX.

Cragnolino, G. & Tuovinen, O. H. (1984). The role of sulphate-reducing and sulphur-oxidizing bacteria in the localized corrosion of iron-base alloys. A review. *International Biodeterioration*, 20, 9–26.

Davis, J. B. (1967). Microbial contamination and deterioration of petroleum products. In *Petroleum Microbiology*, pp. 499–540. Elsevier, Amsterdam.

Dexter, S. C. (1976). Influence of substrate wettability on the formation of bacterial slime films on solid surfaces immersed in natural seawater. In *Proceedings of* the 4th International Congress on Marine Corrosion and Fouling, pp. 137–44. Juan les Pins, Antibes, France.

Dexter, S. C., Duquette, D. J., Siebert, O. W. & Videla, H. A. (1989). Use and limitations of electrochemical techniques for investigating microbiological corrosion. In Corrosion 89, Paper no. 616. NACE, Houston, TX.

Dexter, S. C. & Gao, G. Y. (1987). Effect of seawater biofilms on corrosion potential and oxygen reduction of stainless steel. In Corrosion 87, Paper no. 377. NACE, Houston, TX.

Dexter, S. C., Lucas, K. E. & Gao, G. Y. (1986). The role of marine bacteria in crevice corrosion initiation. In Biologically Induced Corrosion, ed. S. C. Dexter, pp. 144–53. NACE, Houston, TX.

Duquette, D. J. (1986). Electrochemical techniques for evaluation of microbiologically influenced corrosion processes. Advantages and disadvantages. In Proceedings of the Argentine–USA Workshop on Biodeterioration (CONICET-NSF), ed. H. A. Videla, pp. 15–32. Aquatec Quimica S.A., Sao Paulo.

Duquette, D. J. & Ricker, R. E. (1986). Electrochemical aspects of microbially induced corrosion. In Biologically Induced Corrosion, ed. S. C. Dexter, pp. 121–30. NACE, Houston, TX.

Edyvean, R. G. J. (1987). Biodeterioration problems of north sea oil and gas production. A review. International Biodeterioration, 23, 199–231.

Edyvean, R. G. J. (1990). The effects of microbiologically generated hydrogen sulfide in marine corrosion. MTS Journal, 24, 5–9.

Eydvean, R. G. J. & Terry, L. A. (1983). Polarisation studies of 50D steel in cultures of marine algae. International Biodeterioration Bulletin, 19, 1–11.

Fletcher, M. (1976). The effect of proteins on bacterial attachment to polystyrene. Journal of General Microbiology, 94, 400–4.

Franklin, M. J., White, D. C. & Isaacs, H. S. (1990). The use of current density mapping in the study of microbial influenced corrosion. In Corrosion 90, Paper no. 104. NACE, Houston, TX.

Garret, J. H. (1891). The Action of Water on Lead. H. K. Lewis, London.

Gaylarde, C. C. & Videla, H. A. (1987). Localised corrosion induced by a marine Vibrio. International Biodeterioration, 23, 91–104.

Geesey, G. G. (1982). Microbial exopolymers: ecological and economic considerations. American Society for Microbiology News, 48, 9–14.

Geesey, G. G., Lewandowski, Z. & Flemming, H. C. (eds.) (1994). Biofouling and Biocorrosion in Industrial Water Systems. Lewis Publishers, Boca Raton, FL.

Ghiorse, W. C. (1988). Microbial reduction of manganese and iron. In Biology of Anaerobic Microorganisms, ed. A. J. B. Zehnder, pp. 305–31. John Wiley and Sons, New York.

Gilbert, P. D. & Herbert, B. N. (1987). Monitoring microbial fouling in flowing systems using coupons. In Industrial Microbiological Testing, ed. J. W. Hopton & E. C. Hill, pp. 79–98. Blackwell Scientific Publications, London.

Gomez de Saravia, S. G., Mele, M. F. L. de & Videla, H. A. (1989). An assessment of the early stages of microfouling and corrosion of 70 : 30 copper nickel alloy in the presence of two marine bacteria. Biofouling, 1, 213–22.

Gomez de Saravia, S. G., Mele, M. F. L. de & Videla, H. A. (1990). Interactions of biofilms and inorganic passive layers in the corrosion of Cu/Ni alloys in chloride environments. *Corrosion*, 46, 302–306.

Greensberg, A. E., Trussel, R. R. & Clesceri, L. S. (1985). *Standard Methods for the Examination of Water and Wastewater*, 16th edn. American Public Health Assocation, Washington, DC.

Hadley, R. F. (1943). The influence of *Sporovibrio desulfuricans* on the current and potential behaviour of corroding iron. In *National Bureau of Standards Corrosion Conference*. National Bureau of Standards, Gaithersburg, MD.

Hettiarachi, S. (1991). The effects of ozone on the corrosion of steel and copper in cooling water systems. In *Corrosion 91*, Paper no. 206. NACE, Houston, TX.

Horvath, J. & Solti, M. (1959). Mechanisms of anaerobic microbiological corrosion of metals in soil. *Werkstoffe und Korrosion*, 10, 624–30.

Iverson, W. P. (1987). Microbial corrosion of metals. *Advances in Applied Microbiology*, 32, 1–36.

Jenner, H. A. (1980). The biology of the mussel *Mytilus edulus* in relation to fouling problems in industrial cooling water systems. *Cebedeau*, 33, 13–19.

Johnsen, R. & Bardal, E. (1986). The effect of a microbiological slime layer on stainless steel in natural seawater. In *Corrosion 86*, Paper no. 227. NACE, Houston, TX.

Kerns, J. R. & Little, B. J. (eds.) (1994). *Microbiologically Influenced Corrosion Testing*, ASTM STP 1232. ASTM, Philadelphia.

Kinner, N. E., Balkwill, D. L. & Bishop, P. (1983). Light and electron microscopic studies of microorganisms growing in rotating biological contactor biofilms. *Applied and Environmental Microbiology*, 45, 1659–69.

Lewandowski, Z. (1994). Dissolved oxygen gradients near microbially colonized surfaces. In *Biofouling and Biocorrosion in Industrial Water Systems*, ed. G. G. Geesey, Z. Lewandowski & H. C. Flemming, pp. 175–88. Lewis Publishers, Boca Raton, FL.

Licina, G. & Nekoska, G. (1994). Experience with on-line monitoring of biofilms in power plant environments. In *Corrosion 94*, Paper no. 257. NACE, Houston, TX.

Little, B. J., Ray, R., Wagner, P., Lewandowski, Z., Lee, W. C., Characklis, W. G. & Mansfeld, F. (1990). Electrochemical behaviour of stainless steel in natural seawater. In *Corrosion 90*, Paper no. 150. NACE, Houston, TX.

Mansfeld, F. & Little, B. J. (1990). The application of electrochemical techniques for the study of MIC. A critical review. In *Corrosion 90*, Paper no. 108. NACE, Houston, TX.

Mansfeld, F., Shih, H. & Tsai, C. (1990). Results of exposure of stainless steel and titanium to natural seawater. In *Corrosion 90*, Paper no. 109. NACE, Houston, TX.

Mansfeld, F. & Xiao, H. (1994). Development of electrochemical test methods for the study of localized corrosion phenomena in biocorrosion. In *Biofouling and Biocorrosion in Industrial Water Systems*, ed. G. G. Geesey, Z. Lewandowski & H. C. Flemming, pp. 265–87. Lewis Publishers, Boca Raton, FL.

Marshall, K. C. (1986). Microscopic methods for the study of bacterial behaviour at inert surfaces. *Journal of Microbiological Methods*, 4, 217–27.

McKenzie, P., Akbar, A. S. & Miller, J. D. (1977). Fungal corrosion of aircraft fuel tank alloys. In *Proceedings of a Symposium on Microbial Corrosion Affecting the Petroleum Industry*, Sunbury, UK, pp. 37–50. Instiute of Petroleum, London.

Miller, J. D. A. (1981). Metals. In *Microbial Biodeterioration*, ed. A. H. Rose, pp. 149–202. Academic Press, London.

Mitchell, R. & Benson, P. H. (1980). *Micro and Macrofouling in the OTEC Program: An Overview*. Argonne National Laboratory Publication ANL/OTEC-BMC-011.

Mollica, A., Trevis, A., Traverso, E., Ventura, G., Scotto, V., Alabisio, G., Marcenaro, G., Montini, U., DeCarolis, G. & Dellepiane, R. (1984). Interaction between biofouling and oxygen reduction rate on stainless steel in seawater. In *Proceedings of the 6th International Congress on Marine Corrosion and Fouling*, pp. 269–81, Athens.

Mollica, A. & Ventura, G. (1993). Use of a biofilm electrochemical monitoring device for an automatic application of antifouling procedures in seawater. In *Proceedings of the 12th International Corrosion Congress*, pp. 3807–12. NACE, Houston, TX.

Moreno, D. A., Ibars, J. R., Ranninger, C. & Videla, H. A. (1992). Use of potentiodynamic polarization to assess pitting of stainless steel by sulphate-reducing bacteria. *Corrosion*, 48, 226–9.

Oren, A. (1987). On the use of tetrazolium salts for measurements of microbial activity in sediments. *FEMS Microbiology and Ecology*, 45, 127–33.

Peters, A. C. & Wimpenny, J. W. T. (1988). A constant depth laboratory model film fermentor. *Biotechnology and Bioengineering*, 32, 263–70.

Pope, D. H. (1986). MIC in U.S. industries. Detection and prevention. In *Proceedings of the Argentine–USA Workshop on Biodeterioration* (CONICET-NSF), ed. H. A. Videla, pp. 105–18. Aquatec Quimica S.A., Sao Paulo.

Pope, D. H. (1991). Biological, chemical, metallurgical, and electrochemical methods for investigating microbiologically influenced corrosion. In *Corrosion 91*, Paper no. 87. NACE, Houston, TX.

Prasad, R. (1988). Pros and cons of ATP measurement in oil field waters. In *Corrosion 88*, Paper no. 87. NACE, Houston, TX.

Rosser, H. R. & Hamilton, W. A. (1983). Simple assay for accurate determination of [^{35}S]sulfate reduction activity. *Applied and Environmental Microbiology*, 45, 1956–9.

Ruseska, I., Robbins, J. & Costerton, J. W. (1982). Biocide testing against corrosion-causing oil-field bacteria helps control plugging. *Oil and Gas Journal*, March, 253–64.

Salvarezza, R. C., Mele, M. F. L. de & Videla, H. A. (1979). The use of pitting potential to study the microbial corrosion of 2024 aluminium alloy. *International Biodeterioration Bulletin*, 15, 125–32.

Salvarezza, R. C., Mele, M. F. L. de & Videla, H. A. (1981). Redox potential and the microbiological corrosion of aluminium and its alloys in fuel/water systems. *British Corrosion Journal*, 16, 162–8.

Salvarezza, R. C., Mele, M. F. L. de & Videla, H. A. (1983). Mechanisms of the microbial corrosion of aluminium alloys. *Corrosion*, 39, 26–32.

Salvarezza, R. C. & Videla, H. A. (1986). Electrochemical behaviour of aluminium in *Cladosporium resinae* cultures. In *Biodeterioration 6*, ed. S. Barry, D. R. Houghton, G. C. Llewellyn & C. E. O'Rear, pp. 212–18. CAB International, London.

Sanders, P. F. & Hamilton, W. A. (1986). Biological and corrosion activities of sulphate-reducing bacteria in industrial process plant. In *Biologically Induced Corrosion*, ed. S. C. Dexter, pp. 47–68. NACE, Houston, TX.

Schaschl, E. (1980). Elemental sulphur as a corrodent in deaerated, neutral aqueous solutions. *Materials Performance*, **19**, 9–12.

Scotto, V., DiCintio, R. & Marcenaro, G. (1985). The influence of marine aerobic microbial film on stainless steel corrosion behaviour. *Corrosion Science*, **25**, 185–94.

Staehle, R. W., Brown, B. F., Kruger, J. & Agrawal, A. (eds.) (1974). *Localized Corrosion*. NACE, Houston, TX.

Stein, A. (1991). Metallurgical factors in stainless steel affecting microbiologically influenced corrosion. In *Corrosion 91*, Paper no. 107. NACE, Houston, TX.

Surinach, P. P. (1986). *A New Concept of Treating Surfaces Exposed to Oilfield Water Systems*. Tech. publication, Hoechst, Frankfurt am Main.

Szklarska-Smialowska, Z. (1986). *Pitting Corrosion of Metals*. NACE, Houston, TX.

Thomas, C. J., Edyvean, R. G. J. & Brook, R. (1988). Biologically enhanced corrosion fatigue. *Biofouling*, **1**, 65–77.

Trulear, M. G. & Characklis, W. G. (1982). Dynamics of biofilm processes. *Journal of the Water Pollution Control Federation*, **54**, 1288–301.

Tuovinen, O. H., Button, K. S., Vuorinen, A., Carlson, L., Mair, D. M. & Yut, L. A. (1980). Bacterial, chemical and mineralogical characteristics of tubercles in distribution pipelines. *Journal of the American Water Works Association*, **72**, 626–35.

Tuovinen, O. H. & Kelly, D. P. (1974). Studies on the growth of *Thiobacillus ferrooxidans*. V. Factors affecting growth in liquid culture and development of colonies on solid media containing inorganic sulphur compounds. *Archives of Microbiology*, **98**, 351–64.

Vasquez Moll, D. V., Salvarezza, R. C., Videla, H. A. & Arvia, A. J. (1984). A comparative pitting corrosion study of mild steel in different alkaline solutions containing salts with sulphur-containing anions. *Corrosion Science*, **24**, 751–67.

Videla, H. A. (1986a). Mechanisms of MIC. In *Proceedings of the Argentine–USA Workshop on Biodeterioration* (CONICET-NSF), ed. H. A. Videla, pp. 43–63. Aquatec Quimica, S.A., Sao Paulo.

Videla, H. A. (1986b). Corrosion of mild steel induced by sulfate reducing bacteria. A study of the passivity breakdown by biogenic sulfides. In *Biologically Induced Corrosion*, ed. S. C. Dexter, pp. 162–71. NACE, Houston, TX.

Videla, H. A. (1986c). The action of *Cladosporium resinae* growth on the electrochemical behaviour of aluminium. In *Biologically Induced Corrosion*, ed. S. C. Dexter, pp. 215–22. NACE, Houston, TX.

Videla, H. A. (1988). Electrochemical interpretation of the role of microorganisms in corrosion. In *Biodeterioration 7*, ed. D. R. Houghton, R. N. Smith & H. O. W. Eggins, pp. 359–71. Elsevier Applied Science, London.

Videla, H. A. (1989a). Metal dissolution/redox in biofilms. In *Structure and Function of Biofilms*, ed. W. G. Characklis & P. A. Wilderer, pp. 301–20. Wiley Interscience, Chichester.

Videla, H. A. (1989b). Biological corrosion and biofilms effects on metal biodeterioration. In *Biodeterioration Research 2*, ed. C. E. O'Rear & G. C. Llewellyn, pp. 39–50. Plenum Press, New York.

Videla, H. A. (1991a). Biofilms and inorganic passive layers interactions in MIC. In *Corrosion 91: Corrosion Research in Progress Symposium, Extended Abstracts*, pp. 7–8. NACE, Houston, TX

Videla, H. A. (1991b). Microbially induced corrosion: an updated overview. In *Biodeterioration and Biodegradation*, vol. 8, ed. H. W. Rossmoore, pp. 63–88. Elsevier Applied Science, London.

Videla, H. A. (1994). Biocorrosion of nonferrous metal surfaces. In *Biofouling and Biocorrosion in Industrial Water Systems*, ed. G. G. Geesey, Z. Lewandowski & H. C. Flemming, pp. 231–41. Lewis Publishers, Boca Raton, FL.

Videla, H. A. & Characklis, W. G. (1992). Biofouling and microbiologically influenced corrosion. *International Biodeterioration and Biodegradation*, 29, 195–212.

Videla, H. A., Gomez de Saravia, S. G. & de Mele, M. F. L. (1989). Relationship between biofilms and inorganic passive layers in the corrosion of copper–nickel alloys in chloride environments. In *Corrosion 89*, Paper no. 185. NACE, Houston, TX.

Videla, H. A., Guiamet, P. S., DoValle, S. & Reinoso, E. H. (1988b). Effects of fungal and bacterial contaminants of kerosene fuels on the corrosion of storage and distribution systems. In *Corrosion 88*, Paper no. 91. NACE, Houston, TX.

Videla, H. A., Guiamet, P. S., DoValle, S. & Reinoso, E. H. (1993a). Effects of fungal and bacterial contaminants of kerosene fuels on the corrosion of storage and distribution systems. In *Microbially Influenced Corrosion*, ed. G. Kobrin, pp. 125–39. NACE, Houston, TX.

Videla, H. A., Lewandowski, Z., Lutey, R. (eds.) (1993b). *Proceedings of the NSF-CONICET Workshop on Biocorrosion & Biofouling: Metal/Microbe Interactions*. Buckman Laboratories International, Memphis, TN.

Videla, H. A., Mele, M. F. L. de & Brankevich, G. (1987). Microfouling of several metal surfaces in polluted seawater and its relation with corrosion. In *Corrosion 87*, Paper no. 365. NACE, Houston, TX.

Videla, H. A., Mele, M. F. L. de & Brankevich, J. (1988a). Assessment of corrosion and microfouling of several metals in polluted seawater. *Corrosion*, 44, 423–6.

Videla, H. A., Mele, M. F. L. de, Moreno, D. A., Ibars, J. & Ranninger, C. (1991). Influence of microstructure on the corrosion behaviour of different stainless steels. In *Corrosion 91*, Paper no. 104. NACE, Houston, TX.

Videla, H. A., Mele, M. F. L. de, Silva, R. A., Bianchi, F. & Gonzales Canales, C. (1990). A practical approach to the study of the interaction between biofouling and passive layers on mild steel and stainless steel in cooling water. In *Corrosion 90*, Paper no. 124. NACE, Houston, TX.

Videla, H. A., Viera, M., Guiamet, P. S. & Staibano, J. C. (1994). Combined action of oxidizing biocides for controlling biofilms and MIC. In *Corrosion 94*, Paper no. 260. NACE, Houston, TX.

von Wolzogen Kühr, G. A. H. & van der Vlugt, L. R. (1934). De Grafiteering van gietijzer als electrobiochemisch proces in anaerobe gronden. *Water (den Haag)*, 18, 147–65. (Translation in *Corrosion*, 17, 293–9, 1961.)

Wagner, P., Little, B. J., Ray, R. I. & Jones-Meehan, J. (1992). Investigations of microbiologically influenced corrosion using environmental scanning electron microscopy. In *Corrosion 92*, Paper no. 185. NACE, Houston, TX.

Ward, D. M. (1989). Molecular probes for analysis of microbial communities. In *Structure and Function of Biofilms*, ed. W. G. Characklis & P. A. Wilderer, pp. 129–44. Wiley Interscience, Chichester.

Westlake, D. W. S., Semple, K. M. & Obuekwe, C. D. (1986). Corrosion by ferric iron reducing bacteria isolated from oil production systems. In *Biologically Induced Corrosion*, ed. S. C. Dexter, pp. 195–200. NACE, Houston, TX.

Westlake, D. W. S., Voordouw, G. & Jack, T. R. (1993). Use of nucleic acid probes in assessing the community structure of sulphate-reducing acteria in Western Canadian oil field fluids. In *Proceedings of the 12th International Corrosion Congress*, pp. 3794–802. NACE, Houston, TX.

Wilkes, J. F. & Rice, R. G. (1991). Fundamental aspects of ozone chemistry in recirculating cooling water systems. In *Corrosion 91*, Paper No. 205. NACE, Houston, TX.

Winters, M. A., Stokes, P. S. N., Zuniga, P. O. & Schlottenmier, D. J. (1993). Developments in on-line corrosion and fouling monitoring in cooling water systems. In *Corrosion 93*, Paper no. 392. NACE, Houston, TX.

5

Effect of biofilms on marine corrosion of passive alloys

STEPHEN C. DEXTER

Introduction

It has been known for many decades that films of microscopic fouling organisms begin to form on structural metals and alloys within a few hours of the immersion of the latter in natural waters. Such film formation starts with the adsorption of a non-living macromolecular conditioning film (Loeb & Neihof, 1975). The conditioned surface is then colonized by a variety of bacteria and other microorganisms (see e.g. Corpe, 1980; Fletcher *et al.*, 1980; Baier, 1984; Characklis & Marshall, 1990, p. 521) followed eventually (in sea and estuarine waters) by the settlement of macroinvertebrate larvae and the development of a diverse macrofouling layer (Crisp, 1984).

Simultaneously with biofilm formation, electrochemical corrosion reactions take place on the same metal surface. Both biological and electrochemical events depend on the pH, temperature and concentrations of various organic and inorganic chemical species at the metal–water interface. Both events can also change the pH and chemical composition of the water at the interface. Thus, it is reasonable that these two processes should influence each other when they take place on the same surface.

Investigators such as the late Frank LaQue have often stated that artificial seawaters and sodium chloride solutions are not as corrosive as the natural waters they are meant to simulate, and that the results of short-term laboratory tests are not easily applied to much longer exposures in the field. Such statements are supported by the bulk of the published literature. Money & Kain (1988) and Dexter (1988) presented summaries of the data and arguments. People have often nodded their assent to these statements without really grasping the significance of their implication to the relation between fouling and corrosion.

Scientists in the UK and the United States have studied the effects of sulfate-reducing bacteria (SRB) on corrosion in marine and buried soil environments since the 1940s (for reviews, see Iverson, 1968; Starkey, 1986; Tiller, 1986), but it is only since about 1980 that many investigators world-wide have begun to study formally the interactions between microbiology and various forms of electrochemical corrosion in marine systems.

In this chapter I discuss many aspects of the interaction between microbial films and electrochemical corrosion. I begin by looking at various ways in which a growing marine microbial film can influence water chemistry at the metal–film interface, and the reverse, how electrochemistry at the interface can affect biofilm formation. I then consider the effects of microbial films on corrosion of passive alloys such as the stainless steels and superalloys, titanium and platinum, examining the effects of both the generally distributed primary film and discrete biodeposits. I touch on the effects of microbial films on many of the familiar types of marine corrosion. In fact, it should be emphasized that microorganisms do not cause some new, mysterious type of corrosion, but rather they influence the types of corrosion already known (Dexter, 1985).

Moreover, just because corrosion in natural marine environments always takes place in the presence of microorganisms does not mean that the organisms always influence corrosion in a significant way. The presence of the organisms is easy to prove. Cause and effect is much more difficult to establish. Sometimes the organisms may be innocent bystanders, attracted to the corrosion site because the electrochemistry has created a favourable environment for their growth. How is it then, that a film of microscopic organisms on the metal can influence an electrochemical process like corrosion? Basically, it is because of their ability to change the chemistry of the environment at the metal surface, where the corrosion takes place.

Table 5.1. *Solubility of oxygen in seawater as a function of temperature and salinity*

$T(°C)$	Solubility of O_2 (ml/1) at three salinities		
	0 p.p.t.	24 p.p.t.	36 p.p.t.
0	10.2	8.7	8.0
15	7.1	6.1	5.7
30	5.3	4.6	4.3

Note: p.p.t., parts per thousand.

Interactions between the biofilm and water chemistry

The presence of a microbial film on the metal surface can create chemical conditions at the metal–film interface that are quite different from those of the ambient environment. Consider, for instance, dissolved oxygen. The surface waters of the world's ocean, where most marine corrosion takes place, are usually saturated (Table 5.1) with oxygen at a value depending on the water temperature and salinity (Kester, 1978, p. 498). These values vary from less than 5 ml/1 in warm saline waters to over 10 ml/1 in cold fresh water. Surface oxygen in the Pacific Ocean varies (Dexter & Culberson, 1980) from about 5 to 8 ml/1. The effect such variations can have on the corrosion rates of many materials is widely recognized (LaQue, 1975, p. 110).

Much larger variations than these, however, can be produced on the metal surface by a marine microbial film. Even in cases where the oxygen concentration in the water is at air saturation, the oxygen tension at the metal surface under a microbial film can be zero (Hamilton & Maxwell, 1986). In bringing this about, the biofilm acts both as a physical oxygen diffusion barrier and as an active oxygen sink in which the living bacteria consume oxygen during respiration.

In contrast to the case for dissolved oxygen, variations in pH of ocean water are quite small (Dexter & Culberson, 1980), ranging from 8.1–8.3 in open ocean surface water to less than 7.6 in deep water. In coastal and estuarine waters, pH values from 7.8 to 8.0 are fairly common. Such pH variations are insignificant to corrosion in seawater, with two exceptions: (a) in the formation and stability of calcareous deposits (Lin & Dexter, 1987, 1988), and (b) in the pitting corrosion of aluminium alloys (Rowland & Dexter, 1980).

The pH changes under marine biofilms, however, can again be much larger and more important than those in the ambient environment. pH values as low as 5 can be expected under aerobic biofilms containing acid-producing bacteria (Pope *et al.*, 1988), and values of 2.8 to 3 have been hypothesized (Chandrasekaran & Dexter, 1993). Even more acid pH values, in the range 1 to 2, can be expected under discrete biodeposits (Pope & Zintel, 1988). Actual measurements of the pH under biofilms and biodeposits are now being made in several laboratories by microelectrode techniques (Lewandowski *et al.*, 1988).

The effect of microorganisms on corrosion depends not only on their metabolic capabilities, but also on the numbers and distribution of organisms on the metal surface. A scatter of individual bacteria as shown in Fig. 5.1 is typical of the film that forms on metals immersed in natural temperate seawaters for less than about 12 h. This type of film, with very small total surface coverage, is unlikely to have much effect on corrosion. As the film grows, however, it takes on one of several appearances: (a) it may become more continuous as shown in Fig. 5.2, where the bacteria have begun to produce the characteristic extracellular polymeric substances (EPS) commonly called 'slime' or 'polymer'; (b) it may provide nearly complete surface coverage (as in Fig. 5.3); or (c) it may take the form of discrete colonies (as in Fig. 5.4), leaving much of the surface uncovered. In the case of either complete film or discrete colonies, the film of organisms and slime is able to produce a localized environment at the metal surface which is utterly different from that of the bulk liquid environment. Moreover, when the surface coverage is incomplete, the film will produce oxygen and other chemical concentration cells, thus increasing the likelihood of localized corrosion.

In natural waters, where many species of microorganisms are present, it is common to find them working in consortia; that is, one organism will create a set of environmental conditions in which another organism can flourish and grow. Perhaps the classic example, presented by Costerton & Geesey (1986; see also Fig. 5.5), is the creation, in a nominally aerated environment, of an anaerobic microenvironment under a mature film or colony. The aerobic organisms in the outer part of the film have created conditions favourable for the growth of the anaerobic sulfate reducers below

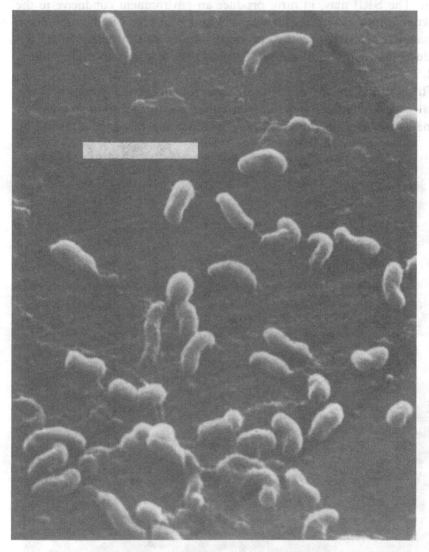

Fig. 5.1 Scatter of individual bacteria attached to a metal surface after about 12 h of immersion in seawater; the scale bar indicates 3 μm (from Dexter, 1987a, reprinted with permission from ASM International).

them. The SRB may, in turn, produce an environment conducive to the growth of other anaerobes such as at A and B in Fig. 5.5, thus forming a consortia. The SRB may also produce sulfides and other metabolic by-products that can be utilized by aerobic sulfur oxidizers to make sulfuric acid.

The electrochemistry of corrosion can also change the chemistry at the metal–water interface, and this can either encourage or inhibit biofilm formation. Corrosion can encourage bacterial attachment and growth by

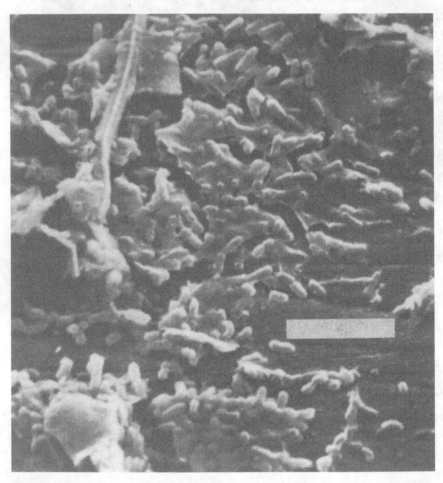

Fig. 5.2 Semicontinuous film of bacteria in slime on metal surface after 2 days of immersion; the scale bar indicates 5 μm (from Dexter, 1987a, reprinted with permission from ASM International).

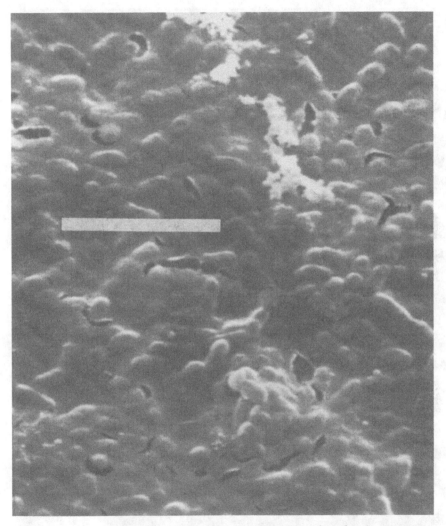

Fig. 5.3 Nearly complete film of bacteria in slime on a metal surface in seawater; the scale bar indicates 5 µm (from Dexter, 1993, reprinted with permission).

producing chemical species that are useful to the organisms as nutrients or energy sources. Conversely, electrochemistry can produce chemical species that will inhibit biofilm formation. Corrosion of copper-based alloys produces toxic copper ions. Cathodic protection can produce enough OH^-

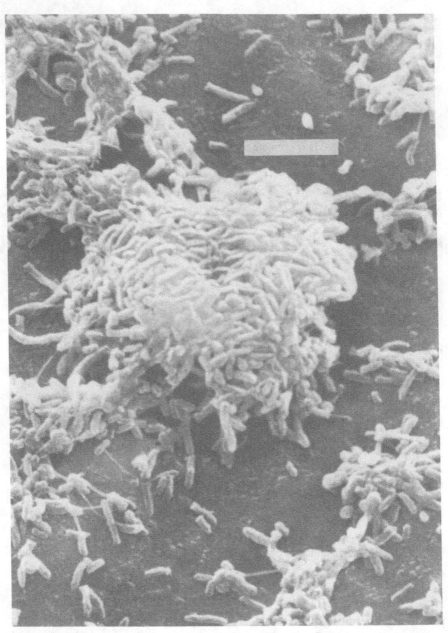

Fig. 5.4 Discrete microcolony of bacteria on metal surface immersed in seawater; the scale bar indicates 5 μm (from Dexter, 1987a, reprinted with permission from ASM International).

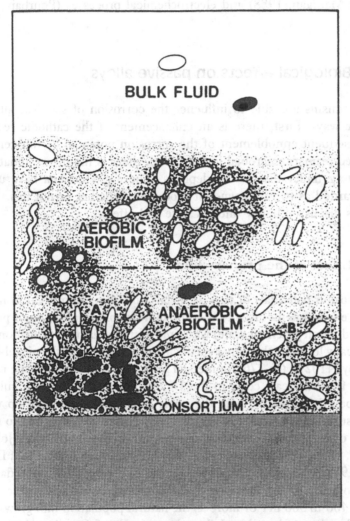

Fig. 5.5 Consortia of aerobic and anaerobic organisms in a mature biofilm (from Costerton & Geesey, 1986, © Copyright by NACE International. All Rights Reserved by NACE, reprinted with permission).

to shift the pH at the metal surface to values above 10 (see e.g. Lin & Dexter, 1988; Dexter & Lin, 1991). pH values more basic than about 9.5 are detrimental to most marine bacteria (Gaudy & Gaudy, 1980, p. 183). Another interesting chemical is hydrogen peroxide, which can be produced on a biofilmed metal surface by both biological (Gottschalk, 1986, p. 34;

Brock & Madigan, 1988) and electrochemical processes (Pourbaix, 1974, p. 106).

Biological effects on passive alloys

Microorganisms are able to influence the corrosion of stainless alloys in two basic ways. First, there is an enhancement of the cathodic reaction, with consequent ennoblement of the corrosion potential by the generally distributed primary microbial film. Second, there is the direct initiation of deep pitting under discrete biodeposits. These phenomena have usually been regarded as two independent processes. Whether or not this view is correct is discussed below under Cause and effect.

Effect of the primary film

The corrosion potentials of passive metals and alloys immersed in natural aqueous environments usually become more noble (that is, more positive on the reduction potential scale) with time of microbial film formation. The data typically look like the upper set of curves in Fig. 5.6 for the nickel-based superalloy N10276 (C-276), immersed for 1 month in summertime natural seawater from the east coast of the United States. The open circuit corrosion potential is plotted with the noble (or positive) direction up versus the exposure time in days. Mollica & Tervis (1976) were the first to report this type of result, and many others have published similar data (Johnsen & Bardal, 1985, 1986; Scotto et al., 1985; Mollica et al., 1987, 1989; Dexter & Gao, 1988; Gallagher et al., 1988; Dexter & Zhang, 1990; Motoda et al., 1990; Mollica, 1992). The open circuit corrosion potential becomes more noble by 400 to 500 mV or more as the natural population film grows. The initial delay time of less than 1 day, shown in Fig. 5.6, varies widely up to about 15 days depending on geographical location, water temperature and flow conditions (Mollica & Trevis, 1976; Johnsen & Bardal, 1985, 1986; Scotto et al., 1985).

It has been shown in several different ways that ennoblement of the corrosion potential is directly attributable to the microbial film. First, the control samples shown in Fig. 5.6, represented by the lower set of curves, were immersed in the same coastal seawater as the test samples, except that the control water had been treated by passing it through a 0.2 μm

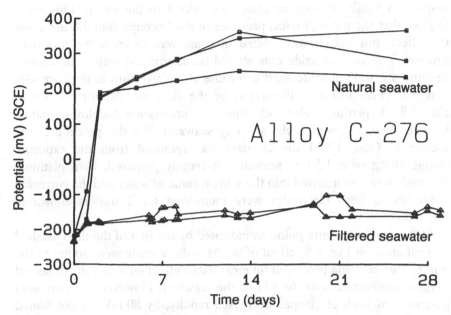

Fig. 5.6 Corrosion potential of superalloy N10276 as a function of time in natural
and filtered seawaters (from Dexter, 1989, © Copyright by NACE
International. All Rights Reserved by NACE, reprinted with permission).

mesh Millipore filter. This treatment did not sterilize the water, but it
removed enough of the film-forming bacteria to delay significant biofilm
formation on the control samples for the duration of the experiment. Note
that the corrosion potentials of the control samples immersed in the filtered
water showed no ennoblement.

Another type of evidence that the effect is biological has been presented
by Mollica & Trevis (1976), who showed that the amount of ennoblement
was decreased and the delay time increased by increasing the flow speed
of water past the surface. Increasing the flow speed retards formation of
the microbial film. The same investigators have also shown that
ennoblement can be prevented by raising the water temperature sufficiently
(to 40 °C) to inactivate the bacteria (Mollica et al., 1989). This does not
mean there will be no microbial effects on corrosion at elevated temperatures. Little et al. (1984) have shown that thermophilic bacteria can stimulate
corrosion at temperatures up to at least 80 °C.

In still another type of experiment, Scotto et al. (1985) published the
important result that the ennoblement disappeared (Fig. 5.7) when a

respiration inhibitor, sodium azide, was added to the water. This result implied that the mere physical presence of the bacterial film did not cause the effect, but that it was related in some way to an active metabolic process. The sodium azide data should be interpreted with some caution because the sodium azide itself can cause a negative shift in the corrosion potential. This effect is illustrated by the data on platinum shown in Fig. 5.8. A platinum electrode that had undergone biofilm formation in summertime Lower Delaware Bay seawater (for the procedure, see Dexter & Gao, 1988) for 26 days was removed from the exposure trough along with 1.5 l of seawater. A freshly prepared, bare platinum electrode was also inserted into the same volume of water and the corrosion potentials of both electrodes were monitored for 1 day as shown in Fig. 5.8.

At the day 1 exposure point, as indicated by the first of the three dashed vertical lines on Fig. 5.8, 20 ml of 0.1 M sodium azide were added to the water. This addition produced no measurable effect on either the dissolved oxygen concentration or the pH of the seawater. However, the corrosion potentials of both electrodes decreased rapidly, by 80 mV for the filmed

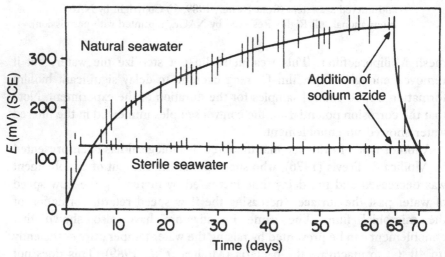

Fig. 5.7 Free corrosion potentials of stainless steel in natural and sterilized seawater showing the effect of sodium azide additions to the water (reprinted from *Corrosion Science*, 25, V. Scotto, R. DiCintio & G. Marcenaro, The influence of marine aerobic microbial film on stainless steel corrosion behaviour, pp. 185–94, Copyright (1985), with kind permission of Elsevier Science Ltd, The Boulevard, Langford Lane, Kidlington OX5 1GB, UK).

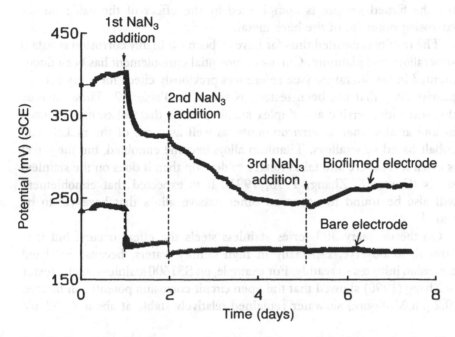

Fig. 5.8 Potentials of biofilm-covered and bare platinum electrodes as a function of
time after sodium azide additions.

electrode and by 40 mV for the bare platinum. At the end of day 2, another
20 ml of the sodium azide solution was added. The corrosion potential of
the bare electrode immediately decreased by another 20 mV but then
remained steady. In contrast, the potential of the biofilmed electrode gradually decreased by 75 to 80 mV over the next 2 days. A final addition of
20 ml of the sodium azide solution at day 5 produced no further effect on
the bare electrode and very little effect on the filmed electrode. In addition,
Fig. 5.9 shows that sodium azide additions to the water affect the platinum
potential in approximately the same way, regardless of whether or not the
solution is aerated. Thus, the effect of the azide on the corrosion potential
cannot be explained by an interaction with dissolved oxygen either in solution or at the metal surface.

The differences in behaviour of the bare and filmed electrodes in Fig.
5.8, particularly after the day 2 injection of sodium azide, confirm Scotto's
earlier conclusion that bacterial metabolism, rather than the mere physical
presence of the film, is necessary for corrosion potential ennoblement.
These results show, however, that interpretation of the sodium azide effect

for the filmed sample is complicated by the effect of the azide on the corrosion potential of the bare metal.

The results presented thus far have all been for highly corrosion resistant superalloys and platinum. Corrosion potential ennoblement has been documented in the literature (see references previously cited) for every active–passive alloy that has been tested, as shown in Table 5.2. These include the austenitic, ferritic and duplex stainless steels that are commonly used in and around marine environments, as well as some of the nickel- and cobalt-based superalloys. Titanium alloys become ennobled, but the effect is often less severe and takes longer to develop than it does on the stainless steels (Dexter & Zhang, 1990, 1991). It is expected that ennoblement will also be found to occur on other passive alloys that have yet to be tested.

On the ordinary 300 series stainless steels the effect occurs, but it is difficult to observe, especially in high salinity waters, because localized corrosion initiates so readily. For example, on S31600 stainless steel, Dexter & Zhang (1990) showed that the open circuit corrosion potential in filtered (0.2 μm Millipore) seawater remained relatively stable at about +150 mV

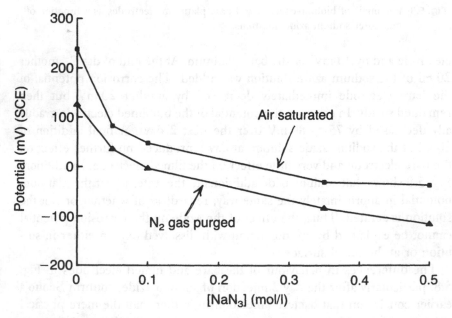

Fig. 5.9 Potentials of bare platinum electrodes in air-saturated and deaerated filtered seawater as a function of sodium azide concentration.

Table 5.2. *Nominal compositions of iron and nickel-based active–passive alloys on which corrosion potential ennoblement has been documented*

UNS no.	Common name	Nominal composition (% by wt)						
		Cr	Ni	Mo	Mn	Fe	C	Other
S30400	304	19	9	—	2	Bal	0.08	1 Si
S31600	316	17	12	2	2	Bal	0.08	1 Si
S31700	317	19	12	3	2	Bal	0.08	1 Si
S43000	430	17	—	—	1	Bal	0.12	1 Si
N08904	904L	22	25	4	2	Bal	0.02	1 Si, 2 Cu
N08367	6XN	21	25	6.5	2	Bal	0.03	1 Si
N08028	Alloy 28	27	31	3.5	2.5	Bal	0.03	1 Si, 1 Cu
S31254	254 SMO	20	18	6	1	Bal	0.02	1 Si, 1 Cu
S31803	2205	22	5.5	3	2	Bal	0.03	1 Si
S32550	Ferralium 255	26	5.5	3	1.5	Bal	0.04	1 Si, 2 Cu
S44635	Monit	25	4	4	1	Bal	0.25	1 Si
S44660	Sea Cure	27	2.5	3	1	Bal	0.03	1 Si
S44735	29–4C	29	1	4	1	Bal	0.03	1 Si
N10276	C–276	15.5	59	16	—	5	0.02	3.7 W
N06625	Alloy 625	21.5	61	9	—	2.5	0.05	3.6 Nb
R30035	MP 35N	20	35	10	—	—	—	35 Co

Note: UNS, Unified numbering system; Bal, balance (i.e. remainder).

(saturated calomel electrode, SCE), as shown by the filled circles in Fig. 5.10. In natural Delaware Bay seawater, however, the corrosion potentials of all three test samples became more noble than that of the control within about the first 200 h of immersion. The amount of ennoblement varied from sample to sample, ranging from nearly insignificant to about 250 mV.

On one sample (represented by the solid triangles in Fig. 5.10) localized corrosion initiated, and the potential dropped to about −125 mV (SCE). For this sample, the data points have been connected so one can see that there were a number of fluctuations in the potential before it came to a steady negative value. These fluctuations were interpreted as corresponding to successive nucleation and repassivation events for localized corrosion on the sample. The incipient localized corrosion finally stabilized after several such cycles, and the corroding region supplied enough current to polarize the entire specimen to the steady negative potential. Similar results were observed for S30400 stainless steel.

Dexter & Gao (1988) showed that the pitted areas on such samples are typically covered (Fig. 5.11) by volcano-like mounds that are just visible to the naked eye and are composed of corrosion products and microorganisms. Examination of these mounds at higher magnification in Fig. 5.12 revealed large numbers of bacteria. The general surface of these samples was covered by a heterogeneous primary microbial film containing much detrital material, as seen in the areas surrounding the mound in Fig. 5.11.

Effects of sunlight and photosynthesis

Recently, Dexter & Zhang (1990) have shown that corrosion potential ennoblement is less likely to occur if photosynthetic algae are present as a significant portion of the biofilm. Figure 5.13 compares two sets of data on samples of the superalloy N10276, taken in Lower Delaware Bay seawater.

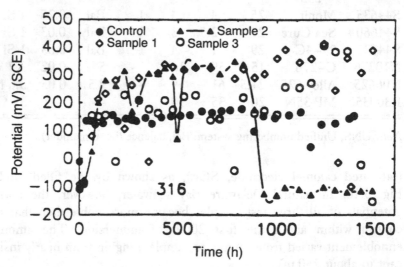

Fig. 5.10 Corrosion potentials of S31600 stainless steel in natural coastal seawater versus time of exposure. The sample represented by the solid triangles suffered crevice corrosion initiation at about 900 h (from Dexter & Zhang, 1991, Copyright © 1991. Electric Power Research Institute. EPRI NP-7275 *Effect of Biofilms, Sunlight and Salinity on Corrosion Potential and Corrosion Initiation of Stainless Alloys*, reprinted with permission).

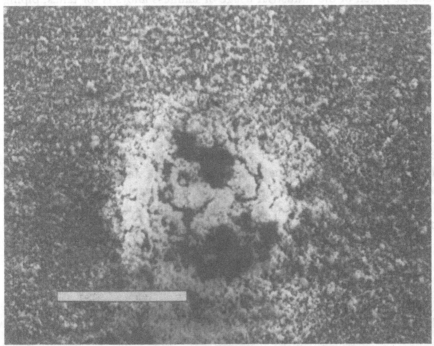

Fig. 5.11 Biofilm and corrosion product on S31600 stainless steel exposed to natural seawater for 7 days; the scale bar indicates 100 µm (from Dexter & Gao, 1988, © Copyright by NACE International. All Rights Reserved by NACE, reprinted with permission).

The upper curve (dashed line) represents the action of a predominantly bacterial film, grown in a darkened laboratory. This is similar to the upper curves in Fig. 5.6. The circles represent data on the same alloy exposed to natural sunlight and the daily light–dark cycle. The biofilm in this latter case was a mixture of bacteria and blue-green algae. Data points shown by open circles were taken in daylight, whereas those shown by solid circles were taken at night. The data for the sample exposed to the light–dark cycle showed large fluctuations throughout the experiment. Only eight points within the 700 h data record showed ennoblement comparable to that observed in the darkened laboratory, and all but one of those eight readings were taken at night.

Thus, an investigator taking measurements on a stainless alloy exposed outdoors in shallow water might well see no significant ennoblement, especially if the data points were all taken in the daylight hours. This is significant because much of the industrial usage of stainless alloys is for tanks, piping and heat-exchanger tubing, for which the continuously immersed portion of the structure is in the dark, where ennoblement is most readily observed. Corrosion measurements, however, in both the laboratory and the field are often taken in daylight, when the effect is greatly reduced.

Effects of salinity and coverage

The same type of ennoblement usually observed in seawater was also found to occur in fresh and brackish waters (Dexter & Zhang, 1990). Exposure tests were performed on a series of austenitic, ferritic and duplex stainless alloys, superalloys and titanium. The amount and reproducibility of ennoblement were found to be largest in fresh water (nearly 500 mV for S30400), and the amount of ennoblement decreased nearly linearly with increasing salinity.

The phenomenon of corrosion potential ennoblement due to the action

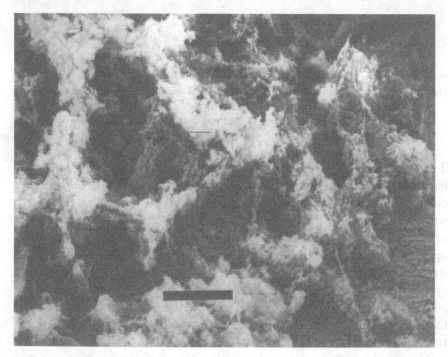

Fig. 5.12 Bacteria within the corrosion product mound of Fig. 5.11; the scale bar indicates 20 μm (from Dexter & Gao, 1988, © Copyright by NACE International. All Rights Reserved by NACE, reprinted with permission).

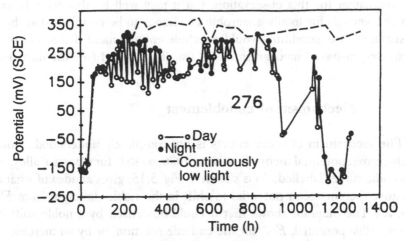

Fig. 5.13 Corrosion potentials for superalloy N10276. The dashed line shows data
taken under continuously low light conditions; circles, under natural light/
dark cycling. Open circles show data taken in daylight. Filled circles show
data taken at night (from Dexter & Zhang, 1991, Copyright © 1991. Electric
Power Research Institute. EPRI NP-7275 *Effect of Biofilms, Sunlight and
Salinity on Corrosion Potential and Corrosion Initiation of Stainless Alloys*,
reprinted with permission).

of a biofilm is inherently variable. It has already been noted there is considerable variability from sample to sample exposed under the same conditions, and that both sunlight and salinity are influential. Variability can
also arise from the degree of coverage of the biofilm on the metal surface.
Mansfeld *et al.* (1992) showed that no ennoblement was observed under
conditions of scant biofilm formation. This agrees with data from my own
laboratory (Fig. 5.14) showing amount of ennoblement with coverage of the
metal surface (Dexter *et al.*, 1993). These data were obtained by galvanically
connecting 1 cm² of a biofilmed and ennobled sample of the nickel-based
superalloy N10276, successively to larger and larger bare samples of the
same metal and measuring the couple potential (Dexter & Zhang, 1990).
From these data, one can see that ennoblement above the usual control
level (about +100 mV (SCE)) in seawater was not achieved at less than
30% coverage.

Complete coverage, however, does not guarantee that ennoblement
will be observed, as was shown by Little *et al.* (1991). The tests they ran
in the waters of the Gulf of Mexico showed little ennoblement, in spite
of the development of very thick biofilms. They did not give a definitive

explanation for this observation, but it may well be that their films were thick enough for totally anaerobic conditions to be established at the metal surface. This condition would preclude ennoblement if it is the result of an oxygen-based mechanism, as is usually assumed (see the next section).

Mechanism of ennoblement

The mechanism of these effects is not completely understood. However, the mixed potential theory (Fontana, 1986, p. 462) for a passive alloy, whose anodic curve (labelled, A) is shown in Fig. 5.15, gives an idea of what could cause the corrosion potential to shift in the noble direction from E^1_{cor} to E^2_{cor}. The diagram shows that it could be caused by a noble shift in the reversible potential, E_{O_2}, for the cathode reaction, or by an increase in the exchange current density, i_o, or a decrease in the Tafel slope, β, or a

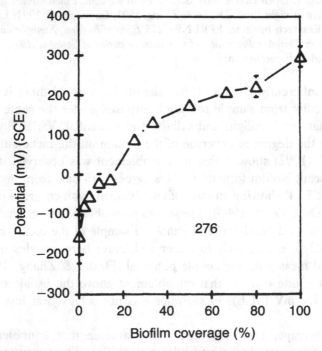

Fig. 5.14 Effect of percentage cover by the biofilm on the corrosion potential of superalloy N10276 in coastal seawater (from Dexter *et al.*, 1993, reprinted with permission).

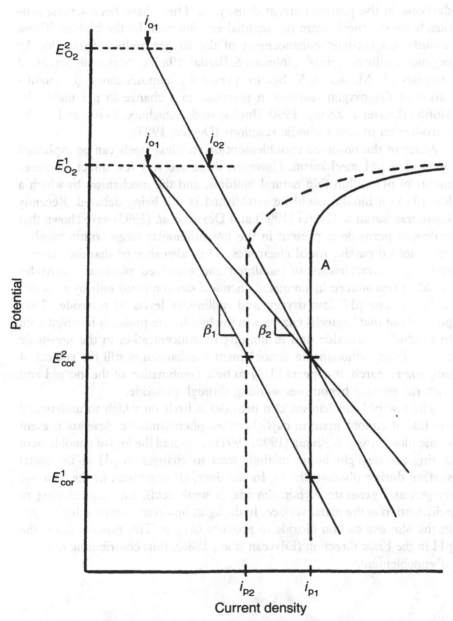

Fig. 5.15 Diagram to show how corrosion potential of stainless alloys may be ennobled. For explanation of symbols, see the text (from Dexter, 1989, © Copyright by NACE International. All Rights Reserved by NACE, reprinted with permission).

decrease in the passive current density, i_p. There have been several proposals for the mechanism of potential ennoblement by the biofilm. These include: (a) catalytic enhancement of the oxygen reduction reaction by organometallic complexes (Johnsen & Bardal, 1985) or bacterially produced enzymes (A. Mollica & V. Scotto, personal communication); (b) modification of the oxygen reaction in response to a change in pH under the biofilm (Dexter & Zhang, 1990; Buchanan & Stansbury, 1990); and (c) the introduction of new cathodic reactions (Dexter, 1993).

Much of the observed ennoblement on stainless steels can be explained by the low pH mechanism. However, there are very few direct measurements of pH within thin natural biofilms, and the mechanism by which a low pH in a biofilm could be established is still being debated. Recently Chandrasekaran & Dexter (1993) and Dexter et al. (1993) have shown that hydrogen peroxide is present in the low millimolar range within biofilms on ennobled passive metal electrodes. They also showed that the electrochemical characteristics of biofilmed and ennobled platinum electrodes could be reproduced in simulated chemical environments only by a combination of low pH, low oxygen and millimolar levels of peroxide. They pointed out that bacterial enzymes in the biofilm are probably involved both in producing peroxide and in limiting its concentration to the non-toxic range. Thus, although the ennoblement mechanism is still the subject of ongoing research, it appears likely to be a combination of the low pH and bacterial enzyme hypotheses working through peroxide.

The low pH mechanism also provides a basis on which to understand the loss of ennoblement in daylight when photosynthetic algae are present in the film. Dexter & Zhang (1990, 1991) attributed the loss of ennoblement during the daylight hours in their tests to changes in pH at the metal surface during photosynthesis. In the dark, all organisms in the film use oxygen and generate carbon dioxide (a weak acid), thus contributing to acidification at the metal surface. In daylight, however, photosynthetic algae in the film use carbon dioxide to produce oxygen. This process drives the pH in the basic direction (Edyvean et al., 1986), thus contributing to a loss of ennoblement.

Consequences of ennoblement

Even though the mechanisms of the biofilm effect are not completely under-stood, the consequences of the effect can be predicted from the mixed potential theory.

Localized corrosion initiation

Dexter & Gao (1988) have used schematic Evans diagrams (Fig. 5.16) to show that the consequence for passive, corrosion-resistant alloys (SS_p) is merely a change in corrosion potential. For less resistant metals (SS_a), the consequence is a decrease in the initiation time for localized corrosion. These two effects were demonstrated by the data presented in Figs. 5.6 and 5.10. Initiation of pitting occurs when the open circuit corrosion poten-tial exceeds the pitting potential. An attempt was made by Dexter & Zhang (1990) to predict the incidence of pitting by comparing the maximum ennobled potentials for stainless steels to their critical pitting potentials in waters of varying salinity. The difficulties of this are two-fold. First, the water chemistry at the metal surface under a biofilm is complex, and it is not yet well enough understood for realistic pitting potential measurements to be made. Second, on practical structures in marine environments, crevice corrosion, which can initiate at any potential, starts preferentially to pitting. An ennoblement of the corrosion potential, while not having the same significance for crevice corrosion as it does for pitting, will increase the probability of both pit and crevice initiation. This may not be important on alloys such as S30400 and S31600 that initiate crevice attack readily in seawater. On the newer, more resistant stainless alloys, however, the degree to which the corrosion potential is ennobled may be critical in determining whether or not crevice corrosion initiates in a given application with a given geometry.

The induction time for crevice corrosion to begin is dependent on the time needed for depletion of dissolved oxygen in the crevice water. Dexter et al. (1986) showed that aerobic bacteria in the crevice solution could deplete the oxygen by respiration within about 15 min. This was judged to be of little practical significance, however, because the electrochemical reaction involved in maintaining the passive film depletes the oxygen by itself in about 10 min. Thus, biological utilization of oxygen in the crevice solution will only be important in cases where electrochemical oxygen reduction is very slow.

The data for initiation of crevice corrosion in the presence of biofilms

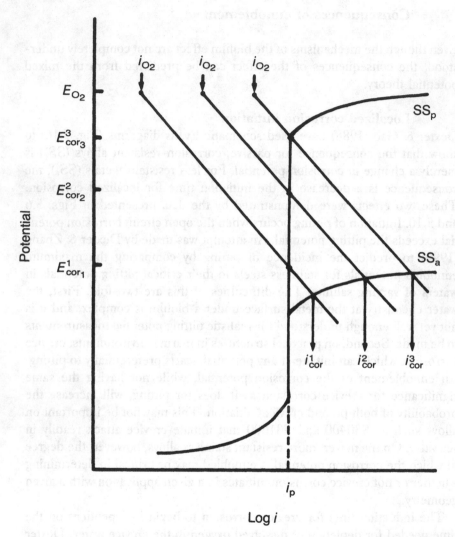

Fig. 5.16 Diagram of the effect of an increase in cathodic kinetics on an active stainless alloy, SS_a, and a resistant alloy, SS_p. For explanation of symbols, see the text (from Dexter & Gao, 1988, © Copyright by NACE International. All Rights Reserved by NACE, reprinted with permission).

are mixed. Kain & Lee (1985) found that initiation times for crevice corrosion on S31600 and N08904 were about the same in natural and artificial seawaters, although they made no analysis of biofilms. Zhang & Dexter (1992) reported that crevice initiation times were often two to five times

shorter for a variety of stainless steels, but the results were not very repro-
ducible. More consistent results have been reported for the effect of biofilms
on propagation of crevice corrosion.

Localized corrosion propagation

Consider next how a primary microbiological film on the boldly exposed
cathode surface might affect the propagation of pitting and crevice corrosion. In the case of stainless steels, not only does the corrosion potential
usually shift in the noble direction in response to the action of a predominantly bacterial biofilm, but Scotto (1989) has shown that the cathodic
kinetics are also affected (Fig. 5.17). The cathodic polarization behaviour
of metal specimens with little or no biofilm is shown as curve no. 1. After
two weeks of film-forming immersion, the cathodic curve (no. 2) is shifted
to higher currents and potentials. At the potential range of this diagram, it
appears that the limiting diffusion current for oxygen is also increased.
After longer immersion times (curve no. 3), however, the limiting current
appears to decrease somewhat, and it is uncertain whether the limiting
current is really affected over the long term, especially at more active potentials than are shown here.

The propagation rate for crevice corrosion has been shown by several
investigators to increase in the presence of a biofilm. Gallagher et al. (1988)
studied crevice corrosion of several stainless alloys in natural and artificial
seawaters. They found that crevice corrosion of several alloys was dramatically less in artificial than in natural seawater. They attributed the difference
to microorganisms in natural seawater but made no analysis of biofilms.
Zhang & Dexter (1992) used the remote crevice assembly technique to
separate the anode and cathode areas during crevice corrosion, so that the
current flow between them can be measured by a zero resistance ammeter.
They found that the measured currents (i.e. the crevice propagation rate)
on a variety of alloys were up two orders of magnitude higher when the
cathode was ennobled by a biofilm. Moreover, Holthe et al. (1989) found that
this relationship still held even when the samples with film had a lower wetted
surface area outside the crevice compared with that inside the crevice. In the
absence of a biofilm, one would expect a decrease in the outside-to-inside
surface area ratio to decrease the crevice propagation rate.

Galvanic corrosion

Data presented by Mollica et al. (1987) and Scotto (1989) predict that there
may be another consequence related to the increase in cathodic kinetics.

Figure 5.18 shows two schematic cathodic polarization curves for stainless steel, first with and then without a biofilm. Both the open circuit potential and the cathodic kinetics of the stainless steel were increased in the presence of the biofilm, as was also shown in Fig. 5.17. Anodic dissolution curves

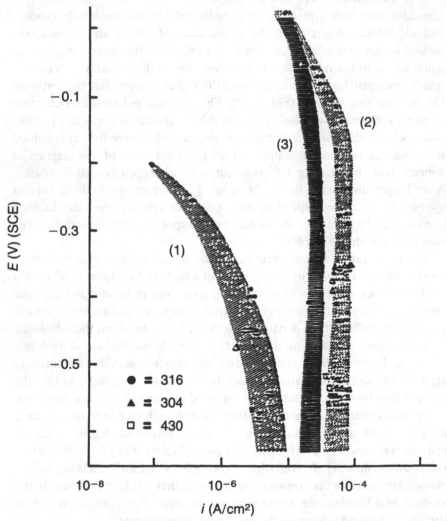

Fig. 5.17 Effect of biofilm on cathodic polarization curves of stainless steels after immersion in seawater for: (1) 1–2 days, (2) 2 weeks and (3) several months (after Scotto, 1989, Copyright © 1989. Electric Power Institute. EPRI ER-6345. *Microbial Corrosion: 1988 Workshop Proceedings*, reprinted with permission).

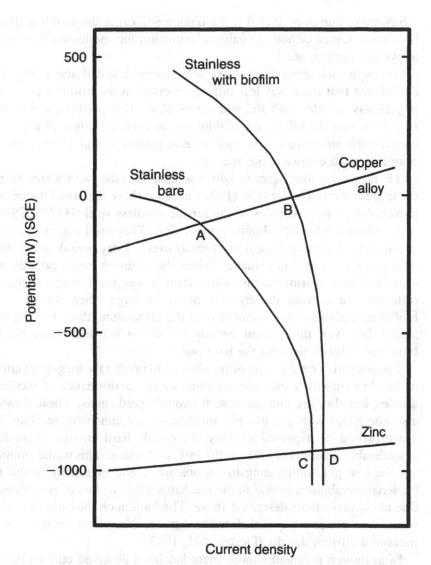

Fig. 5.18 Schematic anodic and cathodic polarization curves showing the predicted
effect of biofilms on galvanic current density with and without a biofilm on
the stainless alloy cathode.

are also shown for a copper alloy and zinc undergoing general corrosion.
If the copper alloy was joined to the stainless steel in a galvanic couple,
these curves predict that the corrosion current density for the couple with
a biofilm (point B) would be higher than that without the film (point A).

Thus, these curves predict that the biofilm will cause the stainless alloy to be a more severe cathode in galvanic corrosion for anodes such as copper alloys and perhaps steel.

At couple potentials more active than points A and B above, Fig. 5.17 had shown that there was less difference between the cathodic properties of stainless samples with and without biofilms. This predicts, as shown in Fig. 5.18, that the effect of a biofilm on the current density of a galvanic couple with an active anode such as zinc (points C and D) may be less than that for the more noble anodes.

There are no long-term weight loss data available with which to test these predictions. Dexter *et al.* (1993), however, have measured the current density for galvanic couples of the ferritic stainless steel S44735 (29-4C) with carbon steel, 3003 aluminium and zinc. They used a zero resistance ammeter to show that the current density over a 1 day period stayed about one order of magnitude higher when the stainless steel cathode was ennobled by a marine biofilm than when it was bare. Surprisingly, the difference in current density was nearly as large when the bare and biofilmed cathodes were connected to the aluminium alloy. For the zinc anode, however, the current density was about two-fold lower for the biofilmed cathode than for the bare one.

These short-term data do not yet allow us to predict the long-term effects of biofilms on either galvanic corrosion or the performance of sacrificial anodes, but they are consistent with Scotto's predictions. These data are also consistent with the low pH mechanism for ennoblement. The zinc anode would be expected to drive the couple hard enough to produce considerable amounts of OH^- at the cathode surface. This would counteract the low pH contributing to ennoblement, and eventually inhibit the bacterial metabolism similar to the mechanism for the loss of ennoblement due to photosynthesis described above. The biofilm on the cathode surface would now act as a physical diffusion barrier, accounting for the drop in measured current density (Dexter *et al.*, 1993).

Even though potential ennoblement has been observed only on passive metals, an increase in cathodic kinetics due to biofilms has been observed on the non-passive copper–nickel alloys as well. Mollica (1992) noted that cathodic polarization curves for 70 : 30 Cu–Ni were shifted progressively to the right with increasing exposure time, even though the corrosion potential was unaffected. This means that an increase in severity of the copper–nickel family of alloys as cathodes in galvanic couples is also predicted by the laboratory data.

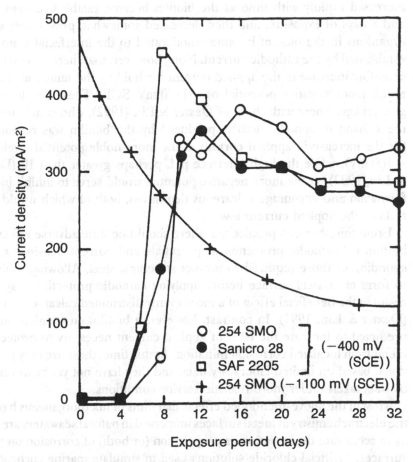

Fig. 5.19 Cathodic current density needed for polarizing stainless steels to various
potentials in quiescent seawater at 20($\pm$2) °C (from Johnsen & Bardal, 1986,
© Copyright by NACE International. All Rights Reserved by NACE,
reprinted with permission).

Cathodic protection

As a final consequence, consider the effect of a biofilm on the current
density for cathodic protection. Johnsen & Bardal (1985, 1986) showed the
effects of a biofilm on the applied current necessary to hold stainless steel
samples at potentials of −400 and −1100 mV (SCE) (see Fig. 5.19). The
necessary applied current was plotted as a function of time for biofilm
formation. For samples held at −400 mV, corresponding to the potential
for cathodically protecting stainless steel from pitting, the applied current

increased rapidly with time as the biofilm became established between 4 and 8 days of exposure, and then decreased somewhat, presumably as the organisms in the biofilm became equilibrated to the interfacial conditions established by the cathodic current. Note, however, that there was no corresponding increase in the applied current for holding the same metal at the much more negative potential of -1100 mV SCE. These results are in general agreement with those of Dexter & Lin (1992), who concluded that the enhanced cathodic activity produced by the biofilm was responsible for the increase in applied current at the more noble potential levels (i.e. -400 mV), while the high interface pH, perhaps greater than 10 (Dexter & Lin, 1992), at the more negative potential would serve to inhibit biofilm formation and encourage calcareous deposition, both of which would tend to keep the applied current low.

From this, one can predict that there should be little adverse effect of a biofilm on cathodic protection at potentials and current densities corresponding to those required to protect structural steel. Allowing a biofilm to form on a steel surface before applying cathodic protection may even result in the beneficial effect of a more evenly distributed calcareous deposit (Dexter & Lin, 1991). In contrast, however, a biofilm on stainless steel is predicted to increase the level of applied current necessary to protect the metal from localized corrosion initiation. At this time, these are only predictions, based on limited laboratory data, and they have not yet been verified by data taken under more realistic service conditions.

Most of the above-mentioned effects that films of microorganisms have on the electrochemistry at metal surfaces immersed in natural seawaters are such as to accelerate the initiation or propagation (or both) of corrosion on those surfaces. Artificial chloride solutions used to simulate marine corrosion in the laboratory cannot reproduce these biological effects. Therefore, it is believed that the living microbial component of natural seawater is responsible for the frequent observation (summarized by Money & Kain, 1988) that such natural seawater is more corrosive than the artificial laboratory solutions.

Effect of discrete biodeposits

The second type of effect that microorganisms can have on stainless alloys is related to the formation of discrete biodeposits. Figure 5.20 shows three examples (Tatnall, 1986) of corrosion problems experienced with stainless steels in natural and industrial freshwater environments. First, there is

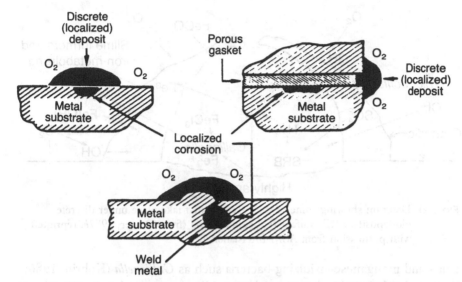

Fig. 5.20 The three most common forms of biocorrosion associated with discrete biodeposits (from Tatnall, 1986, © Copyright by NACE International. All Rights Reserved by NACE, reprinted with permission).

pitting on an open surface under a macroscopic bacterial colony or tubercule. Second, there is a similar situation in which the attack is concentrated in the vicinity of welds and, third, there is crevice attack associated with porous gaskets.

In contrast to the microscopic colonies and biofilms discussed above, the deposits under consideration here are much larger (typically 2 to 4 cm in diameter). They have been found most often when newly fabricated stainless steel tank or piping systems have been filled with fresh water from a local well or river for the purpose of hydrostatic leak testing (Kobrin, 1986). Usually, stainless steels are considered to be resistant to localized corrosion in fresh waters. However, if there is a delay of more than several weeks from the time of hydrotesting until the structure is placed in service, and if the hydrotest water has not been completely drained, then discrete biodeposits may form along the welds. Under the deposit a small pin hole opening leading to a large bottle-shaped subsurface pit has typically been found. Depending upon the metallurgical structure of the weld, selective attack on both the austenitic and ferritic phases of the metal has been reported (Tatnall, 1981; Borenstein, 1988) within these pits.

The active microorganisms under the mound are believed to be the

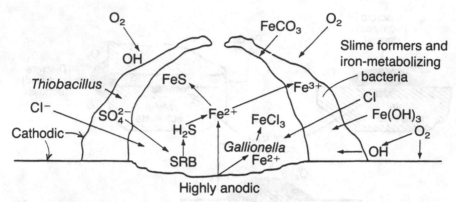

Fig. 5.21 Diagram showing some of the reactions that take place under discrete biodeposits. SRB, sulfate-reducing bacteria (from Dexter, 1987*b*, reprinted with permission from ASM International).

iron- and manganese-oxidizing bacteria such as *Gallionella* (Kobrin, 1986; Tatnall, 1981, 1986). These organisms oxidize ferrous and manganous ions from the metal surface to ferric and manganic. If there are chloride ions in the water, an acid ferric chloride solution then forms under the biodeposit, as shown schematically in Fig. 5.21. SRB have also been isolated from these deposits, although their role in the corrosion is not clear. This type of attack is of major importance in the chemical process and nuclear power industries (Pope *et al.*, 1984; Pope, 1986; Pope & Stoecker, 1986), but to date it has only been reported in fresh waters containing the iron- and manganese-oxidizing bacteria. This is an example of a case where cause and effect have been considered relatively easy to establish by most investigators because the alloy does not suffer the same attack in these low chloride waters without the metal-oxidizing bacteria. In the next section, however, the difficulties of establishing cause and effect are discussed, and reasons will be given why it may not even be as clear as is usually assumed for corrosion under discrete biodeposits.

Cause and effect

The information shown in Figs. 5.10 to 5.12 provide a good example of a case in which the relationship between the bacteria in the corrosion product mound and the initiation of the pit is unknown. It is suspected that pits on biofilm-covered metal surfaces in sea and brackish waters are nucleated by the usual chloride penetration of the passive film in response to corrosion potential ennoblement from the biofilm. It is further suspected that the bacteria in the corrosion product mounds are not directly involved in corrosion initiation, but become associated with the corrosion site after initiation, perhaps because the electrochemistry creates a favourable environment for their growth.

In support of this idea is the well-known sequence of events in the fouling and corrosion of stainless alloys in natural marine systems. The distributed, primary biofilm is well developed within the first week or two of immersion (see Corpe, 1980), while the initiation of localized corrosion usually takes several weeks longer than this, depending on alloy composition and chloride ion activity. Furthermore, the formation of corrosion product/bacterial mounds at the localized corrosion site takes place after, rather than before, corrosion initiation. This sequence would seem to preclude the initiation of corrosion in marine systems by the organisms in discrete biodeposits similar to that often described in industrial fresh water systems (see e.g. Kobrin, 1986). From this point of view then, the bacteria that influence initiation of localized corrosion in natural marine waters are those in the generally distributed primary film remote from the corrosion site.

Now consider the case of corrosion initiation on stainless steels in hydrotest waters. Most of the published work on this type of corrosion associated with discrete biodeposits does not record any information about the distributed biofilm that may have been on the metal surface in addition to the biodeposits. The data of Dexter & Zhang (1990) on stainless steels in fresh water mentioned earlier in this chapter, however, give us good reason to expect that there should be a distributed biofilm, and that the corrosion potential of the alloy should have been ennobled by that film. If there are no chlorides in the hydrotest water, then such ennoblement may be of no consequence, but chlorides in the water, together with the action of the metal-oxidizing bacteria, are usually considered to be responsible for the observed attack under the discrete biodeposits.

The question then must be posed as to what is the causative event for corrosion initiation in hydrotest waters (or at least those containing some minimal level of chlorides). Are the microorganisms first attracted to the vicinity of the weld for some as yet unidentified reason, where they form a discrete deposit, change the water chemistry and initiate corrosion as is generally assumed? Or, rather, does the distributed biofilm form first, ennoble the general corrosion potential, thereby stimulating the initiation of micropits by chloride penetration of the passive film at the most susceptible sites on the metal surface? The sites most vulnerable to pit initiation upon corrosion potential ennoblement would most likely be at or near the welds due to the heterogeneous nature of the metallurgy in those areas, coupled with the introduction of contaminants during the welding process. Under this scenario, is it possible that the electrochemistry taking place at these initial pit sites creates a favourable environment (i.e. plentiful ferrous ions) for growth of discrete biodeposits? The formation of such deposits would then almost certainly stabilize the pit and create a chemistry suitable for rapid pit growth. More information is needed before it will be possible to determine the relative contributions of these two biological mechanisms in the process of pit initiation after hydrotesting.

Summary

It has been shown that the growth of distributed (primary) microbiological films over time on the surface of metals and alloys immersed in natural seawater environments can ennoble the open circuit corrosion potentials of passive metals and alloys, as well as increasing the kinetics of the cathodic reaction. These effects in turn influence the initiation and propagation of pitting and crevice corrosion, the severity of noble metals and alloys as the cathodes in galvanic corrosion and the current density for cathodic protection.

The mechanism by which the effect of biofilms is thought to be established was described as involving a combination of low pH, low oxygen and low millimolar concentrations of hydrogen peroxide at the metal–biofilm interface. Additional experimental data are needed, particularly to establish the pH, before this mechanism can be generally accepted. Bacterially produced enzymes were seen as being the agent through which the peroxide is both produced and regulated. The low pH mechanism also allows one to understand how the ennoblement effect is diminished under natural sunlight when photosynthetic microorganisms form a substantial component of the active biofilm community.

The effects of the primary film in seawater have been contrasted with the severe localized corrosion that has been reported under discrete biodeposits in fresh industrial waters. In marine systems it is clear that the microorganisms responsible for accelerating pit and crevice initiation on stainless alloys are those in the distributed film on the generally exposed metal surface, rather than those at the corrosion site itself. The data presented here have also been used to argue that the organisms responsible for initiation of pitting at the welds under discrete biodeposits may also be those in the distributed biofilm, although additional research will be required to establish whether or not this is true.

The case has been made that the effects of the primary film are at least part of the reason why natural seawater tends to be more corrosive than artificial seawaters, and why the results of short-term laboratory tests are so difficult to apply to the prediction of corrosion under service conditions.

The portion of the research in this paper that was done by the author was supported by NOAA Office of Sea Grant, US Department of Commerce, under grant no. NA86-AA-D-SG040 and the US Office of Naval Research under contract no. N0014-87-K-0108. The US government is authorized to produce and distribute reprints for government purposes, not withstanding any copyright notation that may appear hereon.

References

Baier, R. E. (1984). Initial events in microbial film formation. In *Marine Biodeterioration*, ed. J. D. Costlow & R. C. Tipper, pp. 57–62. Naval Institute Press, Annapolis, MD.

Borenstein, S. W. (1988). Microbiologically influenced corrosion failures of austenitic stainless steel welds. In *Corrosion 88*, Paper no. 78. NACE, Houston, TX.

Brock, T. D. & Madigan, M. T. (1988). *Biology of Microorganisms*, 5th edn, pp. 338–40. Prentice Hall, Englewood Cliffs, NJ.

Buchanan, R. A. & Stansbury, E. E. (1990). Fundamentals of coupled electrochemical reactions as related to microbially influenced corrosion. *In Proceedings of an International Congress on Microbially Influenced Corrosion and Biodeterioration*, ed. N. J. Dowling, M. W. Mittleman & J. C. Danko, pp. 1.11–1.17. University of Tennessee, Knoxville, TN.

Chandrasekaran, P. & Dexter, S. C. (1993). Mechanism of potential ennoblement on passive metals by seawater biofilms. In *Corrosion 93*, Paper no. 493. NACE, Houston, TX.

Characklis, W. G. & Marshall, K. C. (1990). *Biofilms*. John Wiley & Sons, New York.

Corpe, W. A. (1980). Microbial surface components involved in adsorption of microorganisms onto surfaces. In *Adsorption of Microorganisms to Surfaces*, ed. G. Bitton & K. Marshall, pp. 105–44. John Wiley, New York.

Costerton, J. W. & Geesey, G. G. (1986). The microbial ecology of surface colonization and of subsequent corrosion. In *Biologically Induced Corrosion*, ed. S. C. Dexter, pp. 223–32. NACE, Houston, TX.

Crisp, D. J. (1984). Overview of research on marine invertebrate larvae, 1940–1980.

In *Marine Biodeterioration*, ed. J. D. Costlow & R. C. Tipper, pp. 103–26. Naval Institute Press, Annapolis, MD.

Dexter, S. C. (1985). Fouling and corrosion. In *Proceedings of a Conference on Condenser Biofouling Control – State-of-the-Art Symposium*, ed. W. Chow & Y. G. Massalli, EPRI CS-4339, pp. 2.28–2.39. Electric Power Research Institute, Palo Alto, CA.

Dexter, S. C. (1987a). Biological effects. In *The Metals Handbook*, 9th edn, vol. 13 *Corrosion*, pp. 41–3. American Society for Metals, Metals Park OH.

Dexter, S. C. (1987b). Localized biological corrosion. In *The Metals Handbook*, 9th edn, vol. 13 *Corrosion*, pp. 114–22. American Society for Metals, Metal Park OH.

Dexter, S. C. (1988). Laboratory solutions for studying corrosion of aluminum alloys in seawater. In *The Use of Synthetic Environments for Corrosion Testing*, ed. P. Francis & T. Lee, STP 970, pp. 217–34. ASTM, Philadelphia.

Dexter, S. (1989). Effect of seawater biofilms on corrosion potential and oxygen reduction of stainless steel. [Reply to Discussion]. *Corrosion*, 45, 787–9.

Dexter, S. C. (1993). Role of microfouling organisms in marine corrosion. *Biofouling*, 7, 97–127.

Dexter, S. C., Chandrasekaran, P., Zhang, H.-J. & Wood, S. (1993). Microbial corrosion in marine environments: effect of microfouling organisms on corrosion of passive metals. In *Proceedings of a Conference on Biocorrosion and Biofouling*, ed. H. Videla, Z. Lewandowski & R. Lutey, pp. 171–80. Buckman Laboratories Int., Memphis, TN.

Dexter, S. C. & Culberson, C. (1980). Global variability of natural seawater. *Materials Performance*, 19(9), 16–28.

Dexter, S. C. & Gao, G. Y. (1988). Effect of seawater biofilms on corrosion potential and oxygen reduction of stainless steel. *Corrosion*, 44, 717–23.

Dexter, S. C. & Lin, S.-H. (1991). Effect of marine bacteria on calcareous deposition. *Materials Performance*, 30(4), 16–21.

Dexter, S. C. & Lin, S.-H. (1992). Calculation of seawater pH at polarized metal surfaces in the presence of surface films. *Corrosion*, 48, 50–60.

Dexter, S. C., Lucas, K. E. & Gao, G. Y. (1986). Role of marine bacteria in crevice corrosion initiation. In *Biologically Induced Corrosion*, ed. S. C. Dexter, pp. 144–53. NACE, Houston, TX.

Dexter, S. C. & Zhang, H.-J. (1990). Effect of biofilms on corrosion potential of stainless alloys in estuarine waters. *Proceedings of the 11th International Corrosion Congress*, Florence, Italy, pp. 4.333–4.340.

Dexter, S. C. & Zhang, H.-J. (1991). *Effect of Biofilms, Sunlight and Salinity on Corrosion Potential and Corrosion Initiation of Stainless Alloys*, EPRI NP-7275, Final Report on Project 2939-4, Electric Power Research Institute, Palo Alto, CA.

Edyvean, R. G. J., Thomas, C. J., Brook, R. and Austen, M. I. (1986). The use of biologically active environments for testing corrosion fatigue properties of offshore structural steels. In *Biologically Induced Corrosion*, ed. S. C, Dexter, pp. 254–67. NACE, Houston, TX.

Fletcher, M., Latham, M. J., Lynch, J. M. & Rutter, P. R. (1980). The characteristics of interfaces and their role in microbial attachment. In *Microbial Adhesion to*

Surfaces, ed. R. Berkeley, J. Lynch, J. Melling, P. Rutter & B. Vincent, pp. 67–78. Ellis Horwood Ltd, Chichester.

Fontana, M. G. (1986). *Corrosion Engineering*, 3rd edn, McGraw-Hill Book Co., New York.

Gallagher, P., Malpus, R. E. & Shone, E. B. (1988). Corrosion of stainless steels in natural, transported and artificial seawater. *British Corrosion Journal*, 23, 229–33.

Gaudy, A. & Gaudy, E. (1980). *Microbiology for Environmental Scientists and Engineers*, McGraw-Hill Book Co., New York.

Gottschalk, G. (1986). *Bacterial Metabolism*, 2nd edn, Springer-Verlag.

Hamilton, W. A. & Maxwell, S. (1986). Biological and corrosion activity of SRB in natural biofilms. In *Biologically Induced Corrosion*, ed. S. C. Dexter, pp. 131–6. NACE, Houston, TX.

Holthe, R., Bardal, E. & Gartland, P. O. (1989). Time dependence of cathodic properties of materials in seawater. *Materials Performance*, 28(6), 16–23.

Iverson, W. P. (1968). Corrosion of iron and formation of iron phosphide by *Desulfovibrio desulfuricans*. *Nature*, 217, 1265–7.

Johnsen, R. & Bardal, E. (1985). Cathodic properties of different stainless steels in natural seawater. *Corrosion*, 41, 296–304.

Johnsen, R. & Bardal, E. (1986). The effect of microbiological slime layer on stainless steel in natural seawater. In *Corrosion 86*, Paper no. 227. NACE, Houston, TX.

Kain, R. M. & Lee, T. S. (1985). Recent developments in test methods for investigation crevice corrosion. In *Laboratory Corrosion Tests and Standards*, ed. G. Haynes & R. Baboian, ASTM STP 866, pp. 299–323. American Society for Testing and Materials, Philadelphia, PA.

Kester, D. R. (1978). Dissolved gasses other than CO_2. In *Chemical Oceanography*, 2nd edn, vol. 1, ed. J. P. Riley & G. Skirrow, pp. 497–556. Academic Press, New York.

Kobrin, G. (1986). Reflections on microbiologically induced corrosion of stainless steels. In *Biologically Induced Corrosion*, ed. S. C. Dexter, pp. 33–46. NACE, Houston, TX.

LaQue, F. L. (1975). *Marine Corrosion*. John Wiley & Sons, New York.

Lewandowski, Z., Lee, W. C. & Characklis, W. G. (1988). Dissolved oxygen and pH microelectrode measurements at water immersed metal surfaces. *Corrosion 88*, Paper no. 93. NACE, Houston, TX.

Lin, S.-H. & Dexter, S. C. (1987). Effects of temperature and magnesium ions on cathodic protection. In *Proceedings of the 6th International Offshore Mechanics and Arctic Engineering Symposium*, vol. 3, pp. 431–8. ASME, New York.

Lin, S.-H. & Dexter, S. C. (1988). Effects of temperature and magnesium ions on calcareous deposition. *Corrosion*, 44, 615–22.

Little, B., Ray, R., Wagner, P., Lewandowski, Z., Lee, W., Characklis, W. & Mansfeld, F. (1991). Impact of biofouling on the electrochemical behavior of 304 stainless steel in natural seawater. *Biofouling*, 3, 45–59.

Little, B., Walch, M., Wagner, P., Gerchakov, S. M. & Mitchell, R. (1984). The impact of extreme obligate thermophilic bacteria on corrosion processes. In

Proceedings of the 6th International Congress on Marine Corrosion and Fouling. Athens, Greece, pp. 511–20.

Loeb, G. I. & Neihof, R. A. (1975). Marine conditioning films. In *Applied Chemistry at Protein Interfaces*, ed. R. Baier, pp. 319–35. Advances in Chemistry Series 145, American Chemical Society, Washington, DC.

Mansfeld, F., Tsai, R., Shih, H., Little, B., Ray, R. & Wagner, P. (1992). Results of exposure of stainless steels and titanium to natural seawater. *Corrosion Science*, 33, 445–56.

Mollica, A. (1992). Biofilm and corrosion on active-passive alloys in seawater. *International Biodeterioration and Biodegradation*, 29, 213–29.

Mollica, A. & Trevis, A. (1976). Corrélation entre la formation de la pellicule primaire et la modification de la cathodique sur des aciers inoxydables: expérimentes en eau de mer aux vitesses de 0.3 à 5.2 m/s. In *Proceedings of the 4th International Congress on Marine Corrosion and Fouling*, Juan-les-Antibes, France, pp. 351–65.

Mollica, A., Trevis, A., Traverso, E., Ventura, G., De Carolis, G. & Dellepiane, R. (1989). Cathodic performance of stainless steels in natural seawater as a function of microorganisms settlement and temperature. *Corrosion*, 45, 48–56.

Money, K. L. & Kain, R. M. (1988). Synthetic versus natural environments for corrosion testing. In *The Use of Synthetic Environments for Corrosion Testing*, ed. P. Francis & T. Lee, STP 970, pp. 205–16. American Society for Testing and Materials, Philadelphia.

Motoda, S., Suzuki, Y., Shinohara, T. & Tsujikawa, S. (1990). The effect of marine fouling on the ennoblement of electrode potential for stainless steels. *Corrosion Science*, 31, 515–20.

Pope, D. H. (1986). *A Study of Microbiologically Influenced Corrosion in Nuclear Power Plants and a Practical Guide for Countermeasures*. EPRI NP-4582, Electric Power Research Institute, Palo Alto, CA.

Pope, D. H., Duquette, D., Wayner, P. C. Jr & Johannes, A. H. (1984). *Microbiologically Influenced Corrosion: A State-of-the-Art Review*. MTI Publ. No. 13, Materials Technology Institute of the Chemical Process Industries, Inc., Columbus, OH.

Pope, D. H. & Stoecker, J. G. (1986). Microbiologically influenced corrosion. In *Process Industries Corrosion – The Theory and Practice*, ed. B. J. Moniz & W. I. Pollock, pp. 227–41. NACE, Houston, TX.

Pope, D. H. & Zintel, T. P. (1988). Methods for investigation of under-deposit microbiologically influenced corrosion. In *Corrosion 88*, Paper no. 249. NACE, Houston, TX.

Pope, D. H., Zintel, T. P., Kuruvilla, A. K. & Siebert, O. W. (1988). Organic acid corrosion of carbon steel. In *Corrosion 88*, Paper no. 79. NACE, Houston, TX.

Pourbaix, M. (1974). *Atlas of Electrochemical Equilibria in Aqueous Solutions*. NACE, Houston, TX.

Rowland, H. T. & Dexter, S. C. (1980). Effects of the seawater carbon dioxide system on the corrosion of aluminum. *Corrosion*, 36, 458–67.

Scotto, V. (1989). Electrochemical studies on biocorrosion of stainless steel in seawater. *EPRI Workshop on Microbial Induced Corrosion*, ed. G. Licina, pp. B.1–B.36. Electric Power Research Institute, Palo Alto, CA.

Scotto, V., DiCintio, R. & Marcenaro, G. (1985). The influence of marine aerobic microbial film on stainless steel corrosion behavior. *Corrosion Science*, 25, 185– 94.

Starkey, R. L. (1986). Anaerobic corrosion – perspectives about causes. In *Biologically Induced Corrosion*, ed. S. C. Dexter, pp. 3–7. NACE, Houston, TX.

Tatnall, R. E. (1981). Case histories: bacteria induced corrosion. *Materials Performance*, 20, 41–8.

Tatnall, R. E. (1986). Experimental methods in biocorrosion. In *Biologically Induced Corrosion*, ed. S. C. Dexter, pp. 246–53. NACE, Houston, TX.

Tiller, A. K. (1986). A review of the European research effort on microbial corrosion between 1950 and 1984. In *Biologically Induced Corrosion*, ed. S. C. Dexter, pp. 8–29. NACE, Houston, TX.

Zhang, H.-J. & Dexter, S. C. (1992). Effect of marine biofilms on crevice corrosion of stainless alloys. In *Corrosion 92*, Paper no. 400. NACE, Houston, TX.

6

The influence of marine macrofouling on corrosion

ROBERT G. J. EDYVEAN

Introduction

Marine fouling, in its fullest macroscopic extent, is a complex community of plants, animals and microorganisms that considerably alters and influences the immediate surrounding environment. While this community is highly variable throughout the world's oceans, the major groups of components and their effects are similar. The settlement of living organisms on to solid surfaces in the sea bestows several advantages to growth nutrition and reproduction; hence competition for space is intense and the marine fouling community is dynamic, always changing, with organisms growing, dying and regenerating on both macroscopic and microscopic scales. This intense biological activity results in many changes to the substratum, metal being of interest in this case, not least as a physical barrier to the bulk physical and chemical components of the seawater. These environmental effects are discussed in particular relation to corrosion.

Corrosion

The loss of metal by corrosion occurs as a result of modifications to the atomic bonding of the metal, allowing atoms at the surface to react with the environment. A metal is a lattice of positively charged metal ions surrounded and held by negatively charged electrons. Atoms at the surface are less strongly bonded than those deeper in the metal lattice and, under suitable conditions, can dissolve into an electrolyte. The presence of the electrolyte, an ionically conductive solution, is imperative to the corrosion process. However, metal atoms can dissolve into the electrolyte only as positively charged ions, thus creating excess electrons at the metal surface. These electrons cannot 'dissolve' and must take part in a separate reaction. Therefore, for corrosion to take place, electrons must be able to move away from the site of metal ion dissolution (known as the anode) to another site on the metal surface (known as the cathode) where they can take part in an 'electron sink' reaction.

The anodic (oxidation) reaction is usually straight forward, represented by the equation:

$$M_{(solid)} \rightarrow M^+ + e^-$$

The cathodic (reduction) reaction that removes electrons from the metal can be more complex and depends on the nature of the electrolyte. The main reaction is the reduction of oxygen:

$$O_2 + 2H_2O + 4e^- \rightarrow 4OH^-$$

However, in anaerobic (oxygen free) or acid electrolytes the reaction switches to the reduction of hydrogen:

$$2H^+ + 2e^- \rightarrow H_2$$

Hydrogen reduction is a much slower overall reaction than oxygen reduction (except in acid conditions) and this explains why corrosion is usually much less in anaerobic than in aerobic environments.

The cathodic reaction tends to be the rate-determining step in the overall corrosion reaction and also determines the sites of anodic and cathodic activity. For example, an area on the surface that experiences higher oxygen availability than an adjacent one tends to be cathodic, forcing the area with lower oxygen availability to be anodic. In uniform corrosion these anodic and cathodic sites are microscopic and constantly changing as the physical and chemical conditions change. The differences in conditions may be due to the slightly different surface characteristics of the individual grains or to slight differences in the electrolyte. The microscopic scale of reaction and the constant changing produces a metal dissolution which is uniform over the whole surface.

As corrosion is an electrochemical process, involving the movement of charged entities, it can be measured as an electrical current. Such measurements can be directly related to corrosion and can provide useful monitoring of the corrosion process.

The electrolyte is the most important factor in the corrosion reaction. Without the electrolyte, usually water, there can be no corrosion, and the nature of the electrolyte will influence the nature and rate of corrosion by both its physical and chemical characteristics. The fact that living organisms attached to a metal surface can radically alter the electrolyte means that they can have a considerable influence on corrosion.

Fouling

Fouling has been defined as the undesirable formation of inorganic and/ or organic deposits on surfaces, which results in unsatisfactory equipment performance or reduces equipment lifetime. There are many examples of inorganic fouling, both detrital and chemical in origin. Biological fouling, however, is the accumulation and growth of living organisms and their associated organic and inorganic material on a surface. It is, in essence, an ecosystem of aquatic organisms.

On non-toxic substrata in open seawater, where there is adequate light and nutrients, the fouling community can develop to its fullest, macroscopic, extent. The ecology of such fouling has been reviewed in detail by Richmond & Seed (1991). However, the composition of the community is highly sensitive to the environment, especially artificial environments such as the hulls of ships, offshore oil and gas platforms, and cooling-water intakes. The fouling ecosystem can be divided into seven different components, the presence or absence of which in any particular situation will depend on the physical and chemical parameters of the environment. These components are:

1. *Organic molecules*: Mostly the polymeric extracellular products of living organisms.
2. *Bacteria*: Probably the most prolific, widespread and adaptable groups of fouling organisms, bacteria can survive almost impossibly adverse conditions.
3. *Microfungi*: Often an overlooked component of a fouling community.
4. *Protozoa*: Intimately associated with bacteria and fungi, protozoa are associated with more 'open' water systems (i.e. systems that are mostly water).

5. *Microalgae*: Second only to bacteria in numbers, microalgae generally have a requirement for light but some groups, notably the blue-green algae (Cyanobacteria) and some diatoms have highly adaptable modes of nutrition and can grow in very low or zero light levels.
6. *Macroalgae*: While there are a number of freshwater forms, macroalgae are essentially components of open seawater fouling communities (where they can reach many metres in length). Certain groups will occur in seawater inlets of coastal cooling water systems and some can thrive in brackish waters. However, macroalgae are essentially fouling organisms of open and offshore structures.
7. *Invertebrates*: Again essentially marine, but, not having the requirement for light, invertebrate animal fouling can be more widespread. For example, they can extend deep into coastal cooling water systems and other seawater-carrying pipework, as well as being prominent on offshore structures and ships.

In addition to these strictly fouling organisms are the interactive organisms that live in and on the fouling community but are not attached to the substratum.

Four main stages can be distinguished in the sequence of biological fouling of a surface.

1. Organic molecules are transported from the bulk fluid and adsorbed to the surface.
2. Bacteria colonize the surface and form a biofilm.
3. The biofilm develops to include protozoa, fungi and microalgae (depending on light availability).
4. Macroscopic organisms settle and develop on the surface (highly dependent on conditions).

Stage 1, the adsorption of organic molecules, will occur in any environment that contains dissolved organic material. The processes that take place on the surface are rapid and complex. As a consequence, microbial cells and the settling stages of larger organisms always attach to a 'conditioned' surface that is often radically different, physically and chemically, from the original substratum.

Stages 1 and 2, the adsorption of organic molecules and the settlement of bacteria, occur in almost any environment where there is an aqueous phase capable of supporting, or not directly toxic to, bacteria. A major role of the adsorbed organic layer on the surface, and extracellular organic molecules on the surface of bacteria, may be to bridge 'dead zones' of non-moving fluid at surfaces that would otherwise provide a barrier to attachment. The degree of initial coverage appears to depend on many physical and chemical conditions, but by no means all of a surface is covered and there may be repulsive forces or 'zones of influence' around individual settled bacteria preventing others from attaching. However, once the organisms are irreversibly attached to the surface, processes of reproduction and alteration to metabolism take place that result in the formation of bacterial colonies. These colonies are cells embedded in copious amounts of extracellular polymer and further alter the physical and chemical characteristics of the surface on which they are growing. The result is the formation of a (often macroscopic) biofilm.

Stages 1, 2 and 3, the adsorption of organic molecules, the settlement of bacteria and the development of the biofilm to include other groups of organisms, will occur in most water-dominated systems (i.e. those systems that carry water or some non-toxic mixture dominated by the water phase). Given suitable conditions, the bacterial biofilm soon attracts organic and inorganic debris, and is rapidly colonized by microalgae, fungi and protozoa. In seawater, where light is available, bacteria and diatoms (a group of microalgae) can be present in large numbers very soon after immersion of a non-toxic material (Hendey, 1951), and these produce a biofilm ('slime' in engineering parlance) that can reach 2 mm in thickness and contain around 30 million bacteria/g (Hendey, 1951) and 270 000 diatoms/cm^2 (Edyvean & Moss, 1986).

Stages 1, 2, 3 and 4, the adsorption of organic molecules, the settlement of bacteria, the development of the biofilm to include other groups of organisms and colonization by macroscopic organisms, occur primarily in seawater situations where no biocides are used. Colonization by macroscopic organisms reaches its maximum development on the external surfaces of static marine structures. The sequence of macrofouling of a surface in seawater is well documented (Anon., 1952; Edyvean et al., 1985; Richmond & Seed, 1991).

In engineering terms this community is often described as comprising 'soft fouling' algae (except the crustose algae) and invertebrates (such as soft corals, sponges, anemones, tunicates and hydroids) and 'hard fouling' (crustose algae, barnacles, mussels, tubeworms, etc.).

For reasons of safety, there has been extensive monitoring of the macrofouling of offshore structures in the North Sea and this has been summarized in several publications (Edyvean *et al.*, 1985; Terry & Picken, 1986; Edyvean, 1987). The composition, amount and rate of development of the fouling communities depends to an extent on the location (geographical, depth and aspect) of the platform and the season of its immersion (Forteath *et al.*, 1984). Distance from land seems to have little effect on the rate at which the structures are colonized, but does have some effect on the species diversity (Terry & Picken, 1986). Zonation of communities, characteristic of different depths, can be recognized, with the fouling consisting predominantly of mussels and algae from sea level to 20 m below mean low water; soft corals, anemones and hydroids dominate the depth range 20 to 80 m below mean low water and tubeworms, barnacles, tunicates, hydroids and soft corals dominating below 80 m. Very high growth rates are often encountered; for example, mussels can reach densities of over 1000 individuals/m² (Goldie, 1981) and grow to 9 cm in 4 years (Goodman & Ralph, 1981), whereas the large seaweeds (species of *Laminaria*) reach maximum densities of 140 individuals/m² (Asen, 1983), weights of 6–9 kg/m² and growth rates of up to 1.3 cm/day (Johnston, 1981).

Fouling organisms interact in an ecosystem, and if left alone establish a dynamic equilibrium or 'climax community'. This community may range from being dominated by bacteria and other microscopic organisms to macroscopic marine fouling.

The biofilm and its interfaces

The key to the alteration of conditions at a metal surface, especially conditions in the electrolyte, and hence the enhancement (or retardation) of corrosion, is the formation of the biofilm. A biofilm is the optimal community of fouling organisms in a given environment. It can consist of anything from a bacterial 'slime' to a macroscopic fouling community. However, the term 'biofilm' is usually recognized as applying to microorganisms and their products immediately adjacent to the substratum, whether as the sole component on a surface or growing under larger fouling organisms. This biofilm, predominantly bacterial but influenced by other organisms, can be imagined as a 'gel', 95% (w/v) or more water, made of an exopolysaccharide (polymers secreted outside the cell) matrix in which bacteria, other cells and inorganic detritus are suspended. The 'density' of the gel is not uniform and has been described as thick around bacterial colonies and thin in the interconnecting areas (Costerton, 1991). This allows considerable ease of movement of ions and other charged particles but controls larger compounds and particles and allows the microorganisms to exert considerable control over their environment.

On a freshly exposed surface the population of bacteria develops rapidly, often within 1 or 2 weeks and in some cases within hours of immersion, and this is followed by the production and accumulation of exopolymer. The mass of this exopolymer gel may far exceed that of the microorganisms and the biofilm can soon take on a macroscopic appearance. The exopolymer stabilizes and protects the microorganisms at the surface. Reproduction of the attached bacteria will create a 'colony'. A colony, being the offspring of one cell, has the same metabolic functions as the parent. This is an important factor in concentrating some chemical action at one site. However, if other cells, of different species, are forming colonies in the same area, then an 'aggregate' will form, and, if an aggregate contains species that interact, especially on an intimate metabolic level, a 'consortia' will have been formed.

In the next phase of biofilm development, protozoa, microscopic animals and, where light permits, microalgae colonize the surface. At the same time the settlement stages of macroscopic organisms arrive at the biofilm and begin to develop. In a suitable environment the macroscopic organisms develop to their full extent forming an often thick biological layer on the metal surface. Biofilms are thus structured assemblages of organisms surrounded by considerable extracellular material and containing complex and ever changing subcommunities. The macroscopic organisms provide diverse environments for the microscopic organisms. As the macrofouling community develops, this microscopic biofilm can change with aerobic organisms in the interstices of the macroscopic organisms and anaerobic (lacking oxygen) bacteria under them. The creation of sites of intense anaerobic activity in the shelter of larger fouling organisms is particularly important in 'open' seawater, where dissolved oxygen would usually be plentiful and the juxtaposition of such aerobic and anaerobic environments can create considerable dichotomies of chemical and physical conditions at the metal surface.

The conditions at the substratum will be quite different from that in the bulk phase or at an unfouled surface, and the activity of microorganisms within biofilms will result in a range of consequences. There is no longer a simple electrolyte system; it is now a three phase system – the metal substratum, the biofilm and the electrolyte. The interaction of all three phases results in concentration gradients and other localized effects. This new system influences processes such as heat transfer, reduction in fluid flow, drag effects and corrosion.

The simplest model of a biofouled system is where the structure is considered to be like a membrane adherent to the metal surface. Thus many of the assumptions on which much traditional corrosion theory is based (Arvia, 1986) are greatly modified. The biofilm forms a barrier or regulator to the exchange of ions between the metal surface and the aqueous environment and many reactions between the products of the bacteria and the metal will take place within the biofilm thickness. The high growth rates, varied metabolic products (many of them corrosive) and high surface to volume ratio of microorganisms allow them to interact very actively with the environment. Metal–solution interfaces can be changed to such a degree that corrosion rates can be accelerated by factors of 1000 to 100 000 (Costello, 1969).

The consequences of marine fouling

There are four ways in which marine fouling may affect marine structures: obscuring the substratum, increasing hydrodynamic loading, enhancing corrosion and enhancing corrosion fatigue.

Obscuring the substratum

This is a widespread problem caused by fouling, especially on offshore structures. The fouling has to be cleared before visual inspection and non-destructive testing of weld lines can be carried out. Even a small amount of fouling can obscure markings that divers use as reference points and also quite large areas of deterioration such as cracks and corrosion-pitted regions. The amount of time that has to be spent clearing fouling considerably increases the costs and risks involved (Ingram, 1978; Oldfield, 1981).

Hydrodynamic loading

The effects of wave, wind and storm action, particularly on fixed marine structures, are severe (Heaf, 1981) and any enhancement of loading could be very detrimental. On an offshore oil platform, the first 30 m of the structure below the water line carries some 70% of the total loading due to wave action (Heaf, 1981), and the presence of fouling, especially large algae that can dominate this zone (e.g. the kelp seaweeds in the North Sea), will considerably enhance this loading by increasing both the diameter and roughness of tubular members of the structure. Both of these factors increase the drag coefficient and hence the drag forces on the structure (Kingsbury, 1981; Wolfram & Theophanatos, 1985). It has been calculated that a layer of fouling 150 mm thick will increase the loading by 42.5% and the fatigue damage by 62% (Heaf, 1981). Heaf also calculated that this would decrease the fatigue life (the predicted life to failure) by 54%. Minor structural failures have already been reported for which the reduction of fatigue life by marine fouling has been blamed (Anon., 1978) and even microbiological 'slimes' are enough to modify the drag characteristics to some extent (Freeman, 1977).

The effects of large fouling seaweeds on drag forces have been investigated by Young and Norton. Figure 6.1 shows the effect of increasing water velocity on the drag created by seaweeds attached to a tubular structure. In Fig. 6.1(a) the drag is shown to increase as water velocity increases. However, the calculated drag coefficient decreases (Fig. 6.1(b)). This is due to the 'streamlining' effect of the change of profile of the fronds of the seaweeds as water velocity increases (Young, 1987). Figure 6.2 indicates how dramatically drag increases as the amount of algal fouling increases. Studies summarized by Vaux (1988) and shown in Fig. 6.3 indicate that the overall force coefficient on tubular structures can be increased by the presence of fouling by a factor of up to 3.

Corrosion

The two main influences of fouling on corrosion oppose each other: retardation or promotion of metal ions leaving the surface. Retardation, often, though rather loosely, termed passivation, is a loss of chemical reactivity of the metal and may be due to a barrier effect of fouling cover. There is evidence that uniform biofilms can substantially reduce corrosion (Bultman et al., 1977), but biofilms are rarely uniform and it is precisely this heterogeneity that causes corrosion.

Seawater is a well-known corrosive environment and any biological activity can enhance its aggressiveness in several ways (Sanders & Maxwell,

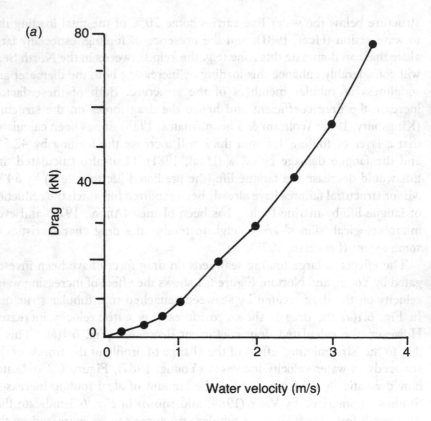

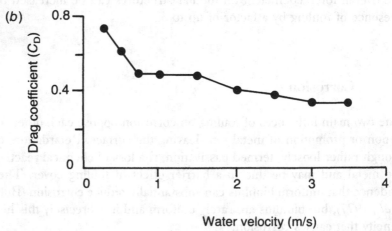

Fig. 6.1 (a) Drag effect on a large seaweed recorded at increasing water flow velocities and (b) the calculated drag coefficient. (From Young, 1987, with permission.)

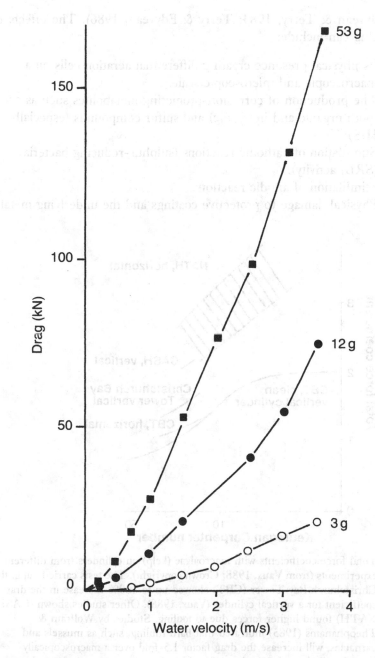

Fig. 6.2 Drag effect on seaweeds of increasing size recorded at increasing water flow velocities. (From Norton, 1991, with permission.)

1983; Edyvean & Terry, 1984; Terry & Edyvean, 1986). The effects of such fouling can include:

1. Its physical presence creating differential aeration cells on a macroscopic and microscopic scale.
2. The production of corrosion-promoting metabolites such as acids (both organic and inorganic) and sulfur compounds (especially H_2S).
3. Stimulation of cathodic reactions (sulphur-reducing bacteria (SRB) activity).
4. Stimulation of anodic reactions.
5. Physical damage to protective coatings and the underlying metal.

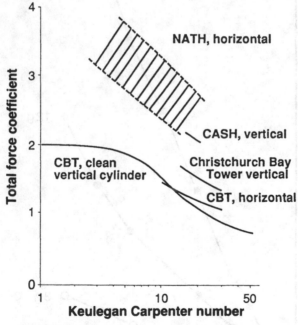

Fig. 6.3 Total force coefficients with macroalgae (kelp) on cylinders from different experiments (from Vaux, 1988; Crown copyright). The tests carried out at the Christchurch Bay Tower (CBT) showed up to 100% increase in the drag coefficient for a vertical cylinder (Vaux, 1988). Other studies shown (CASH, NATH) found higher forces due to fouling. Studies by Wolfram & Theophanatos (1985) indicated that hard fouling, such as mussels and barnacles, will increase the drag factor 1.5-fold over a macroscopically smooth cylinder, whereas large frondose algae up to several metres long can increase the loading by a factor of 3.

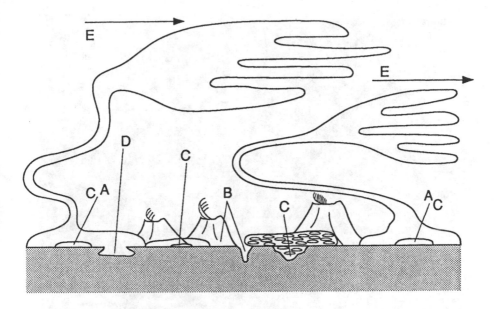

Fig. 6.4 Influences of marine fouling on offshore structures. A, areas of trapped water; B, oxygen concentration cells; C, sites for anaerobic bacteria; D, removal of bright metal; E, drag effects fatigue.

Figure 6.4 shows some of the influences of fouling on a metal in seawater. In areas of trapped water (A) and crevices (B, C) under either macrofouling or bacterial biofilms, considerable changes in pH, dissolved oxygen and ionic balance can occur. These changes can enhance corrosion by the formation of differential aeration, pH and chemical concentration cells. These cells permanently separate anodic and cathodic sites and thus concentrate metal loss to small areas. The result is severe localized corrosion by 'pitting'.

The main cause of such cells is variations in oxygen availability at the metal surface. Any area that remains consistently exposed to a lower level of oxygen than another area, yet has electrical contact with that other area, will act as an anode. This is due to the cathodic oxygen reduction reaction dominating at the more highly oxygenated site and 'forcing' the less oxygenated site to act as the anode. The strength of the reaction can be impressive; Miller *et al.* (1964) have measured potential differences of 60 mV between anodic sites under a biofilm and uncovered, cathodic, sites on aluminium.

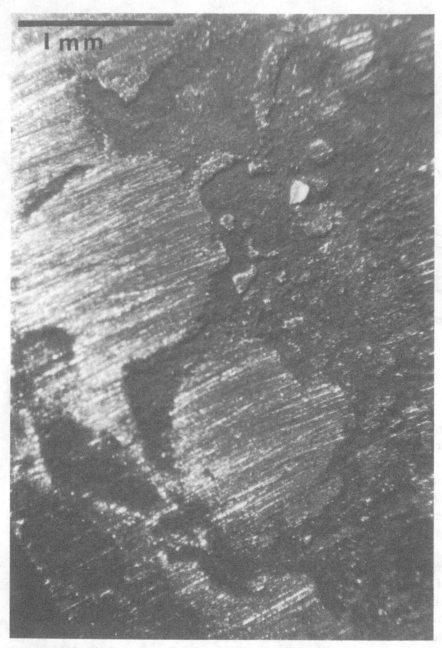

Fig. 6.5 Differential aeration corrosion of 50D steel around the bases of barnacles after 40 days of settlement (south coast of England).

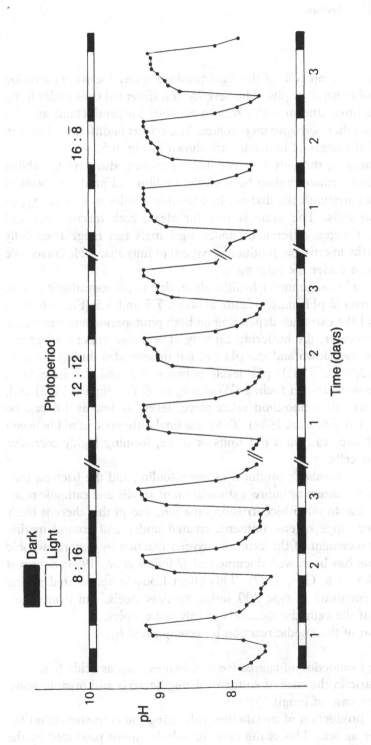

Fig. 6.6 pH changes under a growing fouling layer of young *Enteromorpha* (a green fouling alga) under varying photoperiods. Bars over numbers indicate dark periods. Illumination 40 µE/m² per s, temperature 20 °C.

Oxygen concentration cells of this kind produce severe localized corrosion in the form of crevices or pits. The severity of differential cells under living organisms is often due to active oxygen removal (or production) and the production of other corrosive metabolites. The effects of differential oxygen cells around the bases of barnacles are shown in Fig. 6.5.

Microorganisms, through their metabolic activities, also have the ability to alter the ionic concentration beneath the biofilm and produce chemical and pH concentration cells that act in a manner similar to that of oxygen concentration cells. The same is true for algae, both macroscopic and microscopic. Oxygen differences under algal mats can range from fully aerated (healthy microalgae producing oxygen) to fully anaerobic (anaerobic bacterial action under the algal mat).

The daily pH change under healthy algae, due to photosynthetic action, tends to be over 2 pH units, usually between 7.5 and 9.5 (Fig. 6.6) with the range and the extremes depending on both photoperiod and irradiance (Fig. 6.7). However, the buffering capacity of seawater under fouling can be rapidly broken down and the pH can fall to around 6 during the dark (Terry & Edyvean, 1981). pH levels between 4.5 and 7.5 have been measured beneath animal fouling (Woolmington & Davenport, 1983) and, if bacterial acid decomposition takes place, levels as low as 1.8 can be created (Terry & Edyvean, 1984). Thus, the total difference in pH between two adjacent sites can be 8 pH units or more, forming highly corrosive concentration cells.

Corrosion by metabolic products of macrofouling and the bacteria they harbour, and the direct or indirect stimulation of anodic and cathodic reactions, are similar to other biocorrosion situations except that there is likely to be a wider range of environments created under and around marine fouling. Enhancement of the cathodic oxygen reaction by general aerobic bacterial films has been well documented (Mollica *et al.*, 1984; Scotto *et al.*, 1985; Dexter & Gao, 1987). This effect leads to accelerated pitting and crevice corrosion of type 300 series stainless steels, and it increases the severity of the cathodic members of galvanic couples.

Stimulation of the anodic reaction is accomplished by:

1. The production of aggressive metabolites such as acids (e.g. sulfuric in the case of sulfur-oxidizing bacteria and organic acids in the case of fungi).
2. The production of metabolites enhancing the corrosive action of other anions. This is the case for sulfide anions produced by the

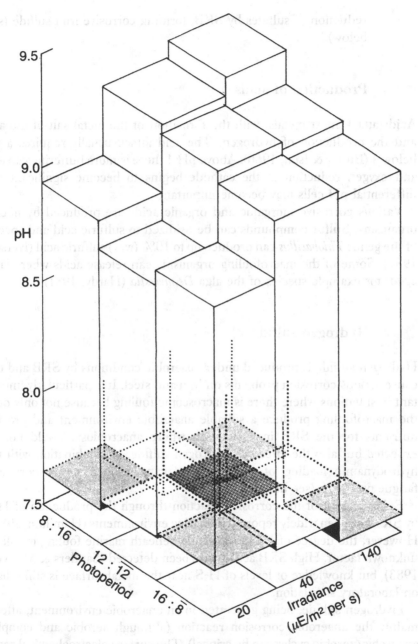

Fig. 6.7 The effect of photoperiod and illumination on the pH variation under a biofilm of the blue-green alga *Oscillatoria* sp. Bars over numbers indicate dark periods.

reduction of sulfates by SRB, forming corrosive iron sulfide (see below).

Production of acids

Acids attack most metals, with the formation of the metal salt of the acid and the production of hydrogen. The acid attack usually requires a pH below 4 (Butler & Ison, 1966). Above pH 4 there is more buffering capacity and oxygen reduction at the cathode begins to become significant and differential pH cells may become important.

Various corrosive inorganic and organic acids are produced by micro-organisms. Sulfur compounds can be oxidized to sulfuric acid and species of the genus *Thiobacillus* can produce up to 10% (w/v) sulfuric acid (Iverson, 1987). Some of the macrofouling organisms can release acids when damaged, for example species of the alga *Desmerestia* (Hardy, 1981).

Hydrogen sulfide

Hydrogen sulfide is produced under anaerobic conditions by SRB and can cause serious corrosion problems on iron and steel. It is particularly important in situations where there is macroscopic fouling because not only does the macrofouling produce a suitable anaerobic environment and provide nutrients for the SRB in a situation where anaerobiosis would not be expected but also the effects of hydrogen sulfide, in combination with the hydrodynamic loading of macrofouling, can produce severe corrosion fatigue problems (see below).

Enhancement of the corrosion reaction through the production of H_2S by SRB has been widely reported in marine environments (Hamilton, 1983). However, the degree of H_2S production beneath marine fouling is still an unknown factor. High SRB activity has been detected (Sanders & Maxwell, 1983), but knowledge of levels of H_2S near the metal surface is still reliant on laboratory simulation.

Hydrogen sulfide, being generated in an anaerobic environment, affects mainly the anaerobic corrosion reaction (although aerobic and complex anaerobic/aerobic cycles can be critical). The surface electrochemical reactions are thus (for a ferrous metal):

$Fe \rightarrow Fe^{2+} + 2e^-$ (Anode)

and

$2H^+ + 2e^- \rightarrow H_2$ (Cathode)

This cathodic reaction can be split into two components:

$H^+ + e^- \rightarrow H$

and

$H + H \rightarrow H_2$

the latter being the rate-limiting step in the overall reaction.

As the cathodic reaction in anaerobic conditions is far slower than its counterpart under aerobic conditions (oxygen reduction), the rate of corrosion in anaerobic environments is usually very slow. In fact a 'polarization' effect has been described in which hydrogen remains adsorbed on to the metal surface and acts as a barrier to further corrosion.

When hydrogen sulfide is present, the ferrous ions are presented with an alternative reactant and the basic corrosion reaction becomes:

$Fe^{2+} + H_2S \rightarrow FeS + 2H^+$

Although this reaction is a very simplified statement of the process, it does serve to show the two important components of hydrogen sulfide corrosion of ferrous metals, i.e. iron sulfide and hydrogen (the role of hydrogen is discussed in more detail in the next section).

One of the original explanations for the corrosive nature of anaerobic microorganisms was the Cathodic Depolarization Theory in which hydrogen, adsorbed on to cathodic surfaces under anaerobic conditions and hence acting as a barrier to further corrosion, is removed by SRB (which have suitable enzyme systems), thus promoting corrosion where these bacteria are active (Hamilton, 1986).

Apart from the direct effects of the sulfides themselves and of SRB there is also the possibility of the formation of highly corrosive elemental sulfur and the production of sulfuric acid by the reaction of hydrogen sulfide and oxygen. The importance of such anaerobic–aerobic transitions has been emphasized (Hardy & Bown, 1984), with a near 100-fold increase in corrosion when SRB cultures are periodically exposed to air (Hardy & Bown, 1984).

Corrosion fatigue

Some definitions need to be given here first:

> *Corrosion* is due to an aggressive environment.
>
> *Fracture* is due to excessive loading.
>
> *Fatigue* is due to a cyclic loading.
>
> *Stress corrosion* is due to the combined effects of an aggressive environment and loading.
>
> *Corrosion fatigue* is due to the combined effects of an aggressive environment and cyclic loading.

Corrosion fatigue is the combination of a corrosive environment and applied cyclic stress to produce failure of a metal by the development and growth of cracks. The effect of seawater provides just such a combination of corrosive environment (enhanced by fouling) and stress (wave action, also enhanced by fouling). Corrosion fatigue can be very important because the effect of the main protection method for offshore structures, cathodic protection, is ambivalent, having been shown to be both detrimental and protective, depending on conditions (Austen & Walker, 1984).

The rate of crack growth under corrosion fatigue conditions is controlled by the rate of dissolution of the metal at the crack tip and hydrogen embrittlement (Bristoll & Roeleveld, 1978). Hydrogen embrittlement involves the entry of atomic hydrogen into a metal, rendering it brittle and more susceptible to cracking under stress. Marine fouling can thus enhance corrosion fatigue, in addition to hydrodynamic loading, by providing the conditions and the organic sulfur compounds for the production of hydrogen sulfide by the SRB. H_2S is particularly aggressive in corrosion fatigue as the sulfide ions both stimulate anodic dissolution and prevent the combination of hydrogen atoms to form the gaseous molecule, thus making more hydrogen available for embrittlement. Dramatic increases in crack growth rates in constructional steels have been demonstrated in H_2S-saturated environments (Bristoll & Roeleveld, 1978; Vosikovsky & Rivard, 1982; Austen & Walker, 1984), producing crack growth rates of anything from 20 to 571 times the rate found in air (Austen & Walker, 1984), compared to 4 to 10 times the rate for seawater with no H_2S. However, H_2S-saturated (around 3000 to 3500 p.p.m.) conditions are unlikely to be produced by any biological means, although more recent work has shown that significant enhancement of crack growth rates can be found at levels of H_2S produced

by SRB (Thomas *et al.*, 1988). Thomas *et al.* (1988), using seawater environments in which the H_2S was biologically generated, have found crack growth
rates of 5 to 11 times those in fresh seawater at H_2S levels of 70 to
100 p.p.m. and up to 25 times that found in fresh seawater at higher (400–
500 p.p.m.) levels and, whereas very few data are available on levels of
biologically produced H_2S under marine fouling, levels of 50–100 p.p.m.
are easily generated.

However, it is probably a combination of temperature, nutrient availability
and suitable areas for H_2S production that are the greatest parameters
limiting this enhancement of corrosion fatigue by SRB activity. Anaerobic
environments coinciding with high nutrient levels (e.g. under marine fouling) will be limited and transitory due to the exhaustion of nutrients and
the dynamic nature of the system. However, it is important for the potential
problem to be considered and to remember that the SRB are likely to be
found in dynamic ecological associations with other species, which may
themselves be promoting corrosion, leading to pitting and the initiation of
cracks. Fatigue consists of three stages: crack initiation, crack growth and
final fracture. While processes such as differential aeration and the production of adhesive metabolites leads to crevice and pitting corrosion, which
in turn may initiate fatigue cracks, it has to be assumed that the presence
of flaws in structures (especially in welds) will considerably reduce the
(sometimes long) initiation time. Thus, if a site of H_2S generation (a crack
growth promoting bacterial metabolite) coincides with a pre-existing flaw,
crack growth could proceed very rapidly.

Prevention and cure

The literature on the control and prevention of biological corrosion produces two traditional maxims: prevention is better than cure, and cleanliness
is paramount.

In order to prevent or control biological corrosion one or more of the
following methods are used (Tiller, 1988):

1. Biocides or biostats (to control the biological activity).
2. Cathodic protection or corrosion inhibitors (to control the
   corrosion).
3. Upgrading the material (to overcome the problem).
4. The use of non-metallic materials (to avoid the problem).

5. The use of protecting coatings and wrappings (to distance the problem from the metal).

To these can be added, in the case of macrofouling, physical removal methods. All these methods have their place but are subject to various constraints and problems and none can be guaranteed to be successful.

On external surfaces, exposed to open water, the use of biocides is limited to antifouling systems. Antifouling coatings include retrofitted 'wraps' containing copper mesh. Recently there has been an increased interest in antifouling coatings, both paints and systems such as copper mesh mounted on a neoprene backing. These 'retrofit' systems are expensive and tend to be used only where essential, for example in the splash zones. Antifouling coatings are difficult to maintain due to the lack of periodic dry docking, but paints and other antifouling systems are being developed for use in sensitive areas. However, there are reports that show coatings (especially paints and coal tar epoxy coatings) to be broken down and damaged by both macro- and microfouling (Edyvean et al., 1985). Barnacles and other macroscopic marine fouling will quickly destroy paints (Edyvean & Terry, 1983, 1984). Other reports indicate that corrosive metabolites produced on the coating surface can diffuse through some coatings and cause corrosion and disbondment underneath (Stranger Johannessen, 1987).

In terms of macrofouling, maintaining a clean system usually entails the physical removal of the fouling. This ranges from 'pigging' of pipelines, or forcing soft cleaning balls through heat exchangers, to regular removal of fouling of offshore structures by divers using water jets or other cleaning methods (Bain, 1981; Partridge, 1981). The latter is often a legal and insurance requirement on offshore oil and gas platforms and entails considerable cost and risk to personnel. With all cleaning operations on fixed open water structures there is a problem of access. The superstructure can be accessed with scaffolding and the submerged areas with divers or remote machinery. There has, until recently, been considerable difficulty in gaining access to the 'splash zone' area of greatest fouling and corrosion potential. New access systems are being developed to overcome the problems and allow protected access to these areas (N. Thompson, personal communication).

Other antifouling measures that have been considered include the use of current-driven plastic discs rotating around the tubular members of the structure to prevent growth and the application of 'easy clean' or antifouling coatings.

Cathodic protection essentially utilizes the electrochemistry of the corrosion reaction to prevent metal ions leaving a surface. The principle of cathodic protection is to eliminate the anodic sites on a structure, i.e. to make the whole structure a cathode in the reaction. This can be achieved either by an impressed current, providing electrons and hence supporting the cathodic reactions on the metal to be protected, or by 'sacrificial anodes', which, as their name implies, are pieces of a metal or alloy more base (and therefore anodic to the metal to be protected) that are connected to it in a galvanic cell. To protect steel in seawater, alloys of zinc, aluminium or magnesium are used (Ashworth & Booker, 1986). Cathodic protection is often used in conjunction with coatings. However, the presence of marine macrofouling can cause physical damage to protecting coatings and the underlying metal and provide conditions in which microorganisms capable of enhancing corrosion can thrive (Edyvean et al., 1985; Terry & Edyvean, 1986). It has even been known for bright metal to be removed when hold-fasts of large kelp seaweeds are pulled away from metal substrata (L. A. Terry, personal communication).

Cathodic protection alters the chemistry at the metal surface resulting, amongst other changes, in a high localized pH due to the creation of hydroxyl ions. The effects of cathodic protection on marine fouling, and the ability of cathodic protection to operate effectively in the presence of marine fouling, are contradictory. Littauer & Jennings (1968) have shown a retardation of biofouling in seawater using pulsed cathodic polarization of steel, and work in the early 1950s investigated the possibility of using cathodic currents as an antifouling measure for marine vessels (Preiser & Silverstein, 1950; Harvey & Streever, 1953). However, it is obvious from offshore structures with cathodic protection that fouling growth is not inhibited, both on the protected metal and, often, on sacrificial anodes.

The influence of cathodic protection on bacterial fouling, especially in the early stages of exposure and settlement where there is high current demand, is less well defined, with studies showing both increased (Gordon et al., 1981) and decreased (Dahr et al., 1982) numbers with cathodic protection. It seems that the nature of both the bacteria and the metal substratum are important in determining their response to cathodic protection. More recent studies have shown aerobic bacteria to be reduced in numbers (Maines et al., 1991), while anaerobic SRB are increased in numbers (Guezennec, 1991) and as active on cathodically protected as on freely corroding steel (Sanders & Hamilton, 1986). This could be of considerable importance in relation to corrosion fatigue influenced by marine fouling. The macroscopic fouling provides an environment for anaerobic bacteria, especially SRB, to become active. The SRB produce hydrogen sulfide, which, in turn, increases hydrogen effects in the metal and the rate of fatigue crack growth.

There have been reports of surface pitting corrosion due to the presence of SRB under marine fouling, even when cathodic protection is applied (Tischuk, 1984; Eidsa & Risberg, 1986). This is due to the difficulty in achieving uniform protection over a complex structure and the extra cathodic current demand due to the presence of SRB. In effect, areas where SRB are active under marine fouling are underprotected.

Neither is cathodic protection necessarily protective against corrosion fatigue. Again the research evidence is inconclusive but several studies have indicated that, because of the possibility of hydrogen being generated by cathodic protection, cathodic protection itself is actually detrimental to corrosion fatigue.

The high pH generated by the oxygen reduction reaction at the metal surface under cathodic protection conditions can lead to the solubility product of calcium and magnesium compounds in the seawater being exceeded and precipitating a 'calcareous scale'. Studies have shown significant microfouling activity and macrofouling settlement at the same time as calcareous scale deposition (Moss, 1981), especially over a relatively long time scale (weeks rather than days or hours). Edyvean (1984) found microalgal fouling and the development of macrofouling settlement stages to be rapid on protected steel and to influence the deposition chemistry of the calcareous scale, altering its physico-chemical and crystallographic nature. As the scale forms a protective barrier and reduces current demand, its alteration can influence the performance and economics of the cathodic protection system. The calcareous scale also produces an ideal inert surface for the settlement of macrofouling organisms.

Conclusions

The main effects of marine fouling are those of producing unpredicted environments at the metal surface, localizing adverse conditions and localizing environments. In recent years large industries have become more aware of the problems and there have been a greater number of publications and conferences on the subject. While there is a limit to the speed of generation of new data and explanations and therefore some danger of too frequent conferences, the increased exposure should enable more personnel involved in design and maintenance of equipment to become familiar with the problem and its solutions.

References

Anon. (1952). *Marine Fouling and its Prevention*. Woods Hole Oceanographic Institute, US Naval Institute, Annapolis.

Anon. (1978). Fouling, corrosion problems need research. *Ocean Industry*, August, 312–14.

Arvia, A. J. (1986). Electrochemical approach of Metal/Solution interface in biodeterioration. In *Proceedings of Argentine–USA Workshop on Biodeterioration*, CONICET-NSF, ed. S. C. Dexter & H. A. Videla, pp. 5–15. Aquatec Quimica, Sao Paulo.

Asen, P. A. (1983). Fouling of a North Sea Platform. Unpublished paper C1 005 presented at the XIth International Seaweed Symposium, 19–25 June 1983, Qingdao, China.

Ashworth, V. & Booker, C. J. L. (1986). *Cathodic Protection*. Ellis Horwood, Chichester.

Austen, I. M. & Walker, E. F. (1984). Corrosion fatigue crack propagation in steels under simulated offshore conditions. In *Fatigue '84, Proceedings of the 2nd International Conference on Fatigue Thresholds*, vol. 3, ed. C. J. Beevers, pp. 1457–71.

Bain, D. C. (1981). Trends in water jetting removal techniques. In *Marine Fouling of Offshore Structures*, vol. II. Society for Underwater Technology, London.

Bristoll, P. & Roeleveld, J. A. (1978). Fatigue of offshore structures: effect of seawater on crack propagation in structural steel. European offshore steels research project seminar. Preprints vol. 2, paper 18, pp. 439–58. Welding Institute, Cambridge.

Bultman, J. D., Southwell, C. R. & Hummer, C. W. (1977). Biocorrosion of structural steels in seawater. *Reviews on Coatings and Corrosion*, **2**, 187–214.

Butler, G. & Ison, H. C. K. (1966). *Corrosion and its Prevention in Waters*. Leonard Hill, London.

Costello, J. A. (1969). The corrosion of metals by microorganisms: a literature survey. *International Biodeterioration*, **5**, 101–18.

Costerton, W. (1991). The role of biofilms in microbial corrosion. In *Microbial Corrosion*, vol. II, ed. C. A. C. Sequeira, B. A. K. Tiller, pp. 25–32. Elsevier Applied Science, London and New York.

Dahr, H. P., Howell, D. W. & Bockris, J. O'M. (1982). The use of in situ chemical reduction of oxygen in the diminution of adsorbed bacteria on metals in seawater. *Journal of the Electrochemical Society*, **129**, 2178–82.

Dexter, S. C. & Gao, G. Y. (1987). Effect of seawater biofilms on corrosion potential and oxygen reduction of stainless steel. In *Corrosion 87*, Paper no. 377. NACE, Houston, TX.

Edyvean, R. G. J. (1984) Interactions between biofouling and the deposit formed on cathodically protected steel in seawater. In *Proceedings of the 6th International Congress on Marine Corrosion and Fouling*, Athens, Greece, pp. 469–83. COIPM.

Edyvean, R. G. J. (1987). Biodeterioration problems of North Sea oil and gas production – a review. *International Biodeterioration*, **23**, 199–231.

Edyvean, R. G. J. (1988). Algal–bacterial interactions and their effects on corrosion and corrosion-fatigue. In *Microbial Corrosion*, ed. C. A. C. Sequeira & A. K. Tiller, vol. I, pp. 40–52. Elsevier Applied Science, London and New York.

Edyvean, R. G. J. & Moss, B. L. (1986). Microalgal communities on protected steel substrata in seawater. *Estuarine Coastal and Shelf Science*, **22**, 509–27.

Edyvean, R. G. J. & Terry, L. A. (1983). Polarization studies of 50D steel in cultures of marine algae. *International Biodeterioration Bulletin*, **19**, 1–11.

Edyvean, R. G. J. & Terry, L. A. (1984). The effects of marine fouling on the corrosion of offshore structures. In *UK Corrosion 84*, pp. 195–8. Institute of Corrosion Science and Technology, Leighton Buzzard.

Edyvean, R. G. J., Terry, L. A. & Picken, G. B. (1985). Marine fouling and its effects on offshore structures in the North Sea – a review. *International Biodeterioration*, **21**, 277–84.

Eidsa, G. & Risberg, E. (1986). Sampling for the investigation of sulfate reducing bacteria and corrosion on offshore structures. In *Biologically Induced Corrosion*, ed. S. C. Dexter, pp. 109–13. NACE, Houston, TX.

Forteath, G. N. R., Picken, G. B. & Ralph, R. (1984). Patterns of macrofouling on steel platforms in the central and northern North Sea. In *Corrosion and Marine Growth on Offshore Structures*, ed. J. R. Lewis & A. D. Mercer, pp. 10–22. Ellis Horwood, Chichester.

Freeman, J. H. (1977). The marine fouling of fixed offshore installations. *Department of Energy Offshore Technology Paper* no. OTP 1.

Goldie, B. P. F. (1981). Assessment of marine fouling on gas platform 'WE'. In *Marine Fouling of Offshore Structures*, vol. II, Society of Underwater Technology, London.

Goodman, K. S. & Ralph, R. (1981). Animal fouling on the Forties platforms. In *Marine Fouling of Offshore Structures*, vol. I, Society for Underwater Technology, London.

Gordon, A. S., Gerchakov, S. M. & Udey, L. R. (1981). The effect of polarisation on the attachment of marine bacteria to copper and platinum surfaces. *Canadian Journal of Microbiology*, **27**, 698–703.

Guezennec, J. (1991). Influence of cathodic protection of mild steel on the growth of sulphate reducing bacteria at 35 °C in marine sediments. *Biofouling*, **3**, 339–48.

Hamilton, W. A. (1983). The sulfate-reducing bacteria: their physiology and consequent ecology. In *Microbial Corrosion*, pp. 1–5. The Metals Society, London.

Hamilton, W. A. (1986). The sulfate reducing bacteria and anaerobic corrosion. *Annual Review of Microbiology*, **39**, 195–217.

Hardy, F. G. (1981). Fouling on North Sea platforms. *Botanica Marina*, **24**, 173–6.

Hardy, J. A. & Bown, J. L. (1984). Sulphate-reducing bacteria: their contribution to the corrosion process. *Corrosion*, 40, 650–4.

Harvey, H. F. & Streever, O. J. (1953). Electrolytic corrosion inhibiting and cleaning with energized anodes. *Transactions of the Society of Naval Architects and Marine Engineers*, 61, 431–63.

Heaf, N. J. (1981). The effect of marine growth on the performance of fixed offshore platforms in the North Sea. In *Marine Fouling of Offshore Platforms*, vol. 1, Society for Underwater Technology, London.

Hendey, N. I. (1951). Littorial diatoms of Chichester Harbour with special reference to fouling. *Journal of the Royal Microscopical Society*, 71, 1–86.

Ingram, T. L. C. (1978). The maintenance of offshore structures. *Offshore*, 37, 32–5.

Iverson, W. P. (1987). Microbial corrosion of metals. *Advances in Applied Microbiology*, 32, 1–36.

Johnston, C. S. (1981). Forecasting growth patterns – kelp as an example. In *Marine Fouling of Offshore Structures*, vol. I. Society for Underwater Technology, London.

Kingsbury, R. W. S. M. (1981). Marine fouling of North Sea installations. In *Marine Fouling of Offshore Structures*, vol. I. Society for Underwater Technology, London.

Littauer, E. & Jennings, D. M. (1968). The prevention of marine fouling by electrical currents. In *Proceedings of the 2nd International Congress on Marine Corrosion and Fouling*, Athens, Greece, pp. 527–36. COIPM.

Maines, A. D., Evans, L. V. & Edyvean, R. G. J. (1992). Interaction between microbial fouling and cathodic protection scale. In *Microbial Corrosion*, vol. 3, ed. C. A. C. Sequeira & A. K. Tiller, pp. 213–20. Institute of Materials.

Miller, R. V., Herron, W. C., Krighen's, A. G., Cameron, J. L. & Terry, B. M. (1964). Microorganisms cause corrosion in aircraft fuel tanks. *Materials Protection*, 3, 60–7.

Mollica, A., Trevis, A., Traversso, E., Ventura, G., Scotto, V., Alabisio, G., Marcenaro, G., Montini, U., de Carolis, G. & Dellepiane, R. (1984). Interaction between biofouling and oxygen reduction rate on stainless steel in seawater. In *Proceedings of the 6th International Congress on Marine Corrosion and Fouling*, Athens, pp. 269–81.

Moss, B. L. (1981). Marine algae fouling offshore structures in the North Sea. Unpublished Paper presented at a conference on Marine Fouling of Offshore Structures, 19–20 May. Society for Underwater Technology, London.

Norton, T. A. (1991). Conflicting constraints on the form of intertidal algae. *British Phycological Journal*, 26, 203–18.

Oldfield, D. G. (1981). Scale of the (marine fouling) problem in UK waters. In *Marine Fouling of Offshore Structures*, vol. II, Society of Underwater Technology, London.

Partridge, D. J. (1981). Mechanical methods of removing marine fouling. In *Marine Fouling of Offshore Structures*, vol. II, Society for Underwater Technology, London.

Preiser, H. S. & Silverstein, B. L. (1950). Marine applications of cathodic protection and the electrocoating process. *Journal of the American Society of Naval Engineers*, 62, 881–905.

Richmond, M. D. & Seed, R. (1991). A review of marine macrofouling communities with special reference to animal fouling. *Biofouling*, 3, 151–68.

Sanders, P. F. & Hamilton, W. A. (1986). Biological and corrosion activities of sulfate-reducing bacteria in industrial processing plant. In *Biologically Induced Corrosion*, ed. S. C. Dexter, pp. 47–68. NACE, Houston, TX.

Sanders, P. F. & Maxwell, S. (1983). Microfouling, macrofouling and corrosion of metal test specimens in seawater. In *Microbial Corrosion*, Book 303, pp. 74–83. The Metals Society, London.

Scotto, V., Di Cintio, R. & Marcenaro, G. (1985). The influence of marine aerobic microbial film on stainless steel corrosion behaviour. *Corrosion Science*, 25, 185–94.

Stranger Johannessen, M. (1987). Microbial deterioration of corrosion protective coatings. In *Microbial Problems in the Offshore Oil Industry*, ed. E. C. Hill, J. L. Shennan & R. J. Watkinson, pp. 57–62. John Wiley & Sons, New York.

Terry, L. A. & Edyvean, R. G. J. (1981). Microalgae and corrosion. *Botanica Marina*, 24, 177–83.

Terry, L. A. & Edyvean, R. G. J. (1984). Influences of microalgae on corrosion of structural steel. In *Corrosion and Marine Growth of Offshore Structures*, ed. J. R. Lewis & A. D. Mercer, pp. 38–44. Ellis Horwood, Chichester.

Terry, L. A. & Edyvean, R. G. J. (1986). Recent investigations into the effects of algae on corrosion. In *Algal Biofouling*, ed. L. V. Evans & K. D. Hoagland, pp. 211–30. Elsevier, Amsterdam.

Terry, L. A. & Picken, G. B. (1986). Algal fouling in the North Sea. In *Algal Biofouling*, ed. L. V. Evans & K. D. Hoagland, pp. 179–92. Elsevier, Amsterdam.

Thomas, C. J., Edyvean, R. G. J. & Brook, R. (1988). Biologically enhanced corrosion-fatigue. *Biofouling*, 1, 65–77.

Tiller, A. K. (1988). The impact of microbially induced corrosion on engineering alloys. In *Microbial Corrosion*, vol. I, ed. C. A. C. Sequeira & A. K. Tiller, pp. 3–12. Elsevier Publishers, London and New York.

Tischuk, J. L. (1984). Operation and maintenance of impressed current cathodic protection systems. In *Corrosion and Marine Growth on Offshore Structures*, ed. J. R. Lewis & A. D. Mercer, pp. 61–8. Ellis Horwood, Chichester.

Vaux, R. (1988). Kelp adds to wave loading. *Offshore Research Focus*, No. 62, p. 12.

Vosikovsky, O. & Rivard, A. (1982). The effect of hydrogen sulphide in crude oil on fatigue crack growth in a pipeline steel. *Corrosion*, 38, 19–22.

Wolfram, J. & Theophanatos, A. (1985). The effects of marine fouling on the fluid loading of cylinders: some experimental results. In *Proceedings of the 17th Offshore Technology Conference*, Houston, May, pp. 517–26.

Woolmington, A. D. & Davenport, J. (1983). pH and pO_2 levels beneath marine macrofouling organisms. *Journal of Experimental Marine Biology and Ecology*, 66, 113–24.

Young, C. P. L. (1987). The mechanical properties of seaweed thalli. Ph.D. thesis, University of Liverpool.

7

Chemical and physicochemical aspects of metal biofilms

H. HENRICH PARADIES

Introduction

The first mention of the term 'biofilm' in the scientific literature was perhaps that of O'Connell (1941), describing the characteristics of microbial deposits in water circuits. A continuation of that work (Hadley, 1948) described the corrosion of metals and steel alloys by microorganisms in aqueous and oil environments. However, the first serious study of biofilms was performed by Zobell (1943), who studied a two-step process for microbial colonization, the initial reversible step of adherence of the cell to the surface and the subsequent irreversible binding of the cell. In addition, Zobell suggested the possibility of macromolecular conditioning by films that can modify surfaces prior to microbial colonization. Since that time, research in this area has been slow, principally because of difficulties in surface-sensitive methods, including physicochemical studies such as intrinsic viscosity, other hydrodynamic experiments and conformational studies, wettability and hydrophobicity. Surface charge and wettability of macromolecules are governed by pH, ionic strength, ionic charge of the molecules in solution and the pK_a values of the ionizable groups within the surface layer. These factors influence microbial colonization and adhesion.

Biofilms in biology, biotechnology and corrosion

It is well established that biopolymers, not only proteins or oligopeptides and polysaccharides, contain cation and anion exchange sites. The cation-binding, ionizable groups found in these biopolymers are carboxyl, organic phosphate and organic sulfate and to some extent hydroxyl groups in stereochemical conformational states in carbohydrates. Carboxylic acid groups are widely distributed in biopolymers, being found mostly as side-chain constituents of proteins, i.e. aspartic acid or glutamic acid residues, the uronic, neuraminic and muraminic acids and related substituted monosaccharides or polysaccharides. Phosphodiester links impart strong negative charges to the nucleic acid backbone, and both diester and monoester groupings are found in bacterial polysaccharides and in closely related macromolecules. Lipoprotein and lipopolysaccharides also contain in some cases phosphodiester as part of the lipid moiety. Sulfate esterified to a carboxylate hydroxyl group is common in algal polysaccharides and is capable of providing certain amounts of negative charge density. Phenolic hydroxyl can also provide weak negative charge depending on pH and also binding potential for cations.

Anion exchange on biopolymers, especially on biofilms, takes place on a variety of organic nitrogen-based groups, mainly in polypeptides. In proteins, amino (α-amino group of the lysine), partial imidazole (histidine) and guanidino (arginine) groups are common centres of cationic charge.

Exopolymers, which are polysaccharides found outside the microbial cell wall and membranes, are common products of microbial cells that are widely used to enhance oil recovery. Polysaccharides produced from microorganisms have certain advantages over those products produced synthetically with respect to production costs and chemical yields. These polymers used in tertiary oil recovery improve water flooding and micellar polymer operations. The role of the polymer is to reduce the flow capacity of the solution in the rock system. Xanthan, a bacterial exopolysaccharide from *Xanthomonas campestris*, has been shown to produce higher viscosity and lower sensitivity to saline than synthetic polymers. The effectiveness of an exopolysaccharide depends on the salinity, pH, temperature, cations, especially those of Fe^{2+}, Co^{2+}, Ni^{2+}, Cu^{2+} and complexes thereof, viscosity and other characteristics of the oil field. The use of xanthan as a drilling mud has been applied by Exxon since 1979.

Apart from xanthan, a new biopolymer within the class of exopolymers is produced by *Acinetobacter calcoaceticus*; it belongs to the lipoheteropolysaccharide type to which fatty acid esters have been attributed. The polysaccharide polymer is composed of galactosamine and aminouronic acid, and contains many hydrophilic groups. The lipophilic nature of the exopolymer is due to the presence of 2- and 3-hydroxydodecanoic acid esters. The relative molecular mass of this particular polymer is about one million and the surface area occupied by this molecule is greater than $50\,000\ \text{\AA}^2$ ($1\ \text{\AA} = 0.1\ \text{nm}$).

Recently, it has been discovered that extracellular polymers produced by bacteria are involved in severe copper corrosion processes observed in water supplies and pipes in large buildings and hospitals (Fischer et al., 1987, 1988a, 1991; Paradies et al., 1988, 1990). It is now well accepted that these exopolymers, which can anchor sessile bacteria to metallic surfaces, can bind copper ions with high affinity (Jolley et al., 1987; Mittelman & Geesey, 1987). It is well known that microbial films of different chemical composition and thickness can develop on every type of metallic surface as well as on synthetic polymers with different chemical compositions, e.g. polyvinyl or urethane residues in contact with aqueous environments. The metabolic reactions carried out by various types of microorganisms residing in or on the biofilm can promote severe corrosion (Paradies et al., 1991).

Solution experiments and spectroscopic studies have provided direct evidence for the formation of multimolecular surface complexes or surface precipitates on solid oxides as well as on clean metal surfaces. For example, the effect of surface oxide layers on the oxidation behaviour of imidazole-treated copper has been studied by Yoshida & Ishida (1984) by means of Fourier transform reflection–absorption spectroscopy. Their results implicated the formation of multinuclear surface complexes of undecylimidazole and oxides. The difference in morphology and orientation of the undecylimidazole on the copper oxide surface is due to the reactivity of the imidazole and substrate surface, deposition rate of the imidazole, and evaporation rate of solvent from the solution placed on the surface. Other evidence of multinuclear metal ion complexes at solid–water interfaces was obtained from X-ray absorption spectroscopy experiments by Chistholm-Brause et al. (1990). These authors describe an X-ray absorption spectroscopy study of divalent cobalt (Co(II)) complexes sorbed onto three different solids, γ-Al_2O_3, rutile (TiO_2) and kaolinite ($Al_2Si_2O_5(OH)_4$). They found direct evidence for the presence of multinuclear sorption complexes at surface coverages below one monolayer of Co(II) atoms. These spectroscopic studies reveal distinct differences in the number of coordinating atoms and interatomic distances in the surface complexes formed on each of the solids at the same sorption density. According to Chistholm-Brause *et al.* (1990), the results suggest that different oxide and clay surfaces influence the structure and properties of aqueous surface complexes. This correlates with the observations for dissolution of copper and complexation to adhering biofilms during microbially induced corrosion processes (Paradies *et al.*, 1991). Therefore, the inorganic or organic surfaces seem to influence the structure and properties of aqueous metal–surface complexes and have to be accounted for in models of metal ion sorption involved in any corrosion process.

It has been reported by Daniels *et al.* (1987) that anaerobic bacteria can produce methane from carbon dioxide by using either elemental iron or iron in steel as the sole source of electrons in the reduction process. This is an example of direct interaction of microorganisms with a metal surface. Such methanogenic bacteria could play a significant part in the corrosion of buried metal objects or metals in oxygen-free environments. In this particular case the iron is oxidized by cathodic depolarization, in which electrons from the metal combine with protons from water to produce ferrous iron and hydrogen gas. The thermodynamically unfavourable iron oxidation is catalysed by the bacteria continually consuming the hydrogen gas that is released from the metal surface.

Vali & Kirschvink (1989) reported well-preserved magneto fossils (fossil remains of bacterial magneto sources) that show the same crystal structures as those found in magneto sources from extant bacteria, whereas others in these same preparations display a wide range of dissolution, corrosion and aggregation effects. These magneto fossils are found in various deep-sea sediments. They have been linked to the preservation of stable natural remnant magnetization.

Corrosion processes involving microorganisms in oil wells and municipal sewerage systems have been reported by Tatnall (1981), Costerton *et al.* (1978), Ford *et al.* (1989*a*,*b*) and Characklis (1980). In addition there have been recent publications of relevant symposia edited by Mittelman & Geesey (1987) and by Sequeira & Tiller (1988, 1993) and a comprehensive review of biofilms by Characklis & Marshall (1989).

Biofilms either are formed by bacteria and secreted into the aqueous solution or are formed after bacteria attach to and replicate on a surface. Exopolymers elaborated by the adherent microorganisms anchor the cells to the surface and to each other. For these reasons the term 'biofilm' is not so precisely defined as is usual in chemistry or physical chemistry, i.e. as a homogeneous thin film.

Biofilms show great heterogeneity in composition and physical structure, e.g. gelation, porosity, macromolecular conformation, sintering and fractal geometry of the inorganic and organic macromolecules involved (Paradies *et al.*, 1992). In order to gain information about the mechanism of (bio)film adherence to a surface, the mechanism of dissolution of metals, biomimetic or micellar catalysis at the interface, or how the interface is structured, it appears necessary to delineate the chemical composition of the different building blocks of such a (bio)film. Other studies include possible inter-actions of cells and biofilms with surfaces, as well as structural differences between 'soluble' and 'insoluble' (bio)films. Biofilms show quite minimal solution properties: (a) the ability to flow freely, with a tenuous gel structure at rest, the aqueous solution being transparent, but forming colloidal aggre-gates; (b) formation of a tenuous gel structure with the capability of holding particles in suspension over a long period of time. This is defined as a 'soluble' biofilm, whereas the 'insoluble' biofilm is irreversibly precipitated from an aqueous solution. The structure and specificity of the molecular receptor units of proteins and enzymes depend strongly on the dimensions and orientation of the receptor sites, which in turn depend on the shape and conformation of the host molecule. However, the surfaces of solids provide an extended framework of rigid binding sites whose geometry is fixed.

Metal–biofilm interactions

The deposition of a simple film depends in part on charge separation and the consequent formation of an electrochemical double layer on both the adsorbing surface and the adsorbed macromolecules. However, in most practical systems the interfacial region of metal and biofilm is modified by the presence of microorganisms and their metabolic products. Charge separation can occur by two main mechanisms:

1. Dissociation of ionizable groups, e.g. $-OH$, $-COOH$, $-NH_2$, $-SO_3H$. Thus, with oxidic material, i.e. CuO, Ag_2CO_3, NiO as well as silica or alumina, dissociation of surface OH can occur, and the surface may become positively or negatively charged depending on the pH, i.e.:

$$- M - \overset{+}{O}H_2 \overset{-H^+}{\rightleftharpoons} - M - OH \rightleftharpoons - MO^- + H_2O \qquad (7.1)$$

The biofilm will influence these equilibria and charge neutralization will not be the only mechanism whereby 'biofilm ions' (as a polyelectrolyte) may be adsorbed. For instance, with many hydrophobic surfaces (i.e. clean metal surface having no oxides or hydroxides as thin films on the metal surface), adsorption may take place through the hydrophobic bonding to the lipophilic moiety of the polysaccharide chain.

Neutral relevant macromolecules can be adsorbed on charged or uncharged metal surfaces. Various conditions may occur, depending on the nature of the surface and the biomacromolecules. If the surface is charged then adsorption of the biological macromolecule will cause a redistribution of the counterion charge. This normally leads to an outward shift in the Stern potential, where the zeta potential decreases. Therefore, on any hydrophilic surface adsorption of the exopolysaccharide (biofilm) can take place by strong hydrogen bonding between amino, carboxyl, or thiol groups, peptide units and ether bridges, as well as other polar groups on various surfaces including biological surfaces (cell membranes) or metal surfaces. This will also lead to a redistribution of charge in the double layer. In addition the polysaccharides, consisting of several flexible sequences, may adopt various conformations at the metal–liquid interface.

2. Three main types of interparticle interaction forces can be distinguished: (a) double layer, (b) steric and (c) van der Waals'.

(a) Double-layer interaction occurs between particles with an electrical double layer. The double layers existing in solution extend to a distance of $1/K_{DH}$ (the double-layer thickness), K_{DH} being the Debye-Hückel parameter, which depends on electrolyte concentration and valency ($1/K_{DH} = 3.04/$(salt concentration in mol/l)$^{1/2}$ Å for 1 : 1 electrolytes).

(b) Steric interactions occur when the particles have adsorbed layers of exopolymers or other biomacromolecules. For instance, when two particles with an adsorbed layer approach each other to a separation distance that is less than 2Δ, interference of the chains occurs. Repulsive effects in part of the biomacromolecule can arise also from a loss of configurational entropy of the flexible segments on the approach of another surface, metal or metal colloids, as well as a coiled macromolecule. As a result, the volume available for the adsorbed flexible chains on the metal surface becomes restricted, leading to a loss of configurational entropy. This effect is referred to as the volume restriction effect.

(c) The last type of interaction, which is universal in all disperse systems, is the van der Waals' attraction, comprising dipole–dipole, dipole–induced dipole, and dispersion interactions. The London (dispersion) attractions are of particular importance for colloidal particles, since the attraction between molecules (including colloidal metal oxides, hydroxides and carbonates) is additive. The attractive force between these particles in a dispersion varies with distance as a power law. These forces are very important for the adhesiveness of cells. The major forces of attraction between cells and substrate have been found to be attractive van der Waals' forces and plurivalent cation bridging.

Chemical composition of biofilms

When addressing the chemical composition and physical structure of biofilms we need to consider polysaccharides, lipids, lipoproteins, fatty acids with saturated long-chain alkyl chains (C_{17}–C_{19}), proteins and glycoproteins. Some microorganisms produce surface-active compounds, extra- or intracellular, when grown in media with hydrocarbons as a carbon source. These compounds, found in biofilms also, can modify the interfacial and surface conditions. These biosurfactants include: glycolipids (tetralose lipids, rhamnose lipids, sepharose lipids and polysaccharide lipids) produced by *Nocardia, Arthrobacter* and *Mycobacterium*; amino acid-lipids (lipopeptides) produced by *Bacillus, Streptomyces, Corynebacterium*; and phospholipids and fatty acids, especially hydroxy-fatty acids or α-alkyl-β-hydroxy-fatty acids produced by *Pseudomonas, Acinetobacter, Micrococcus* and *Candida*. The hydrophilic parts of these molecules are carbohydrates, amino acids, cyclic peptides, phosphates, carboxylic acids and primary or secondary (chiral) alcohols.

Inorganic materials found in the biofilm include silica, the most notable examples being the diatoms and certain sponges. In addition complex inorganic structures between silicates and aluminium and other cations, e.g. Ni^{2+}, Fe^{2+}, Cu^{2+}, Na^+, K^+, Mg^{2+} including the colloidal forms of silica, are of some relevance in forming polymeric, inorganic films. It is necessary to characterize these polymeric molecules in more detail, especially their potential for involvement in film formation and corrosion processes, adherence, particle size distribution, etc.

Biofilms of mainly organic composition

The main class of organic compounds associated with biofilm bacteria is considered to be the polysaccharides. The basic units are hexoses in the pyranose form although pentose sugars are also important. The vast majority of bacterial polysaccharides are heteroglycans composed of oligosaccharide repeating units (Aspinall, 1987). Among these heteropolysaccharides are extracellular, cellular and lipopolysaccharides all of which may have importance in metal–biofilm interactions. Peptidoglycan is an important component of bacterial cell walls and is composed of polysaccharide chains with alternating N-acetylmuramic acid and N-acetylglucosamine units cross-linked through some of their carbonyl groups via oligopeptide chains (Fig. 7.1). There is extensive scope in such a structure for ion binding and binding through different physicochemical interactions with metal surfaces (Lederer, 1971). Furthermore, the alternating L- and D-amino acid sequence of the peptidoglycan tetrapeptide furnishes structural strength (D-, L-heteropolymers) and allows amino acid R-groups to align on one side of the peptide chains.

Biofilms containing fatty acid residues
Biofilms produced by *Pseudomonas aeruginosa* (strain 44T1) have glycolipidic structure. This was observed experimentally by fast atom bombardment–mass spectroscopy (FAB–MS) of biofilm from a severe microbially induced corrosion process on copper surfaces (Paradies *et al.*, 1991*d*). Generally, mycolic acids are observed in *Corynebacteria*, *Nocardia* and *Mycobacteria*, which produce characteristic types of mycolic acids having chain lengths of C_{32}–C_{36} (corynemycolic acid; Fig. 7.2), about C_{50} (*Nocardia*) and up to C_{90}.

Biofilms consisting of polysaccharides; mainly algal biofilms
Algae are producers of hetero- and homopolysaccharides that are also food reserves, e.g. glycogen, starch, laminaron. However, many polysaccharides are cell wall and protective extracellular materials. These latter include neutral cellulose, mannans, xylans, flucoidans and a variety of acid-sulfated

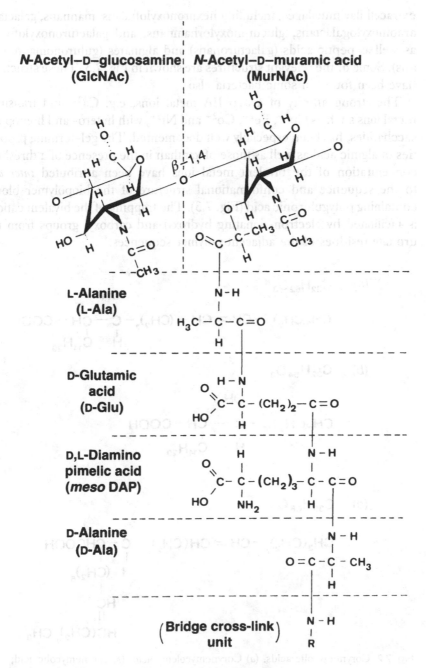

N-Acetyl–D–glucosamine
(GlcNAc)

N-Acetyl–D–muramic acid
(MurNAc)

β–1,4

L-Alanine
(L-Ala)

$H_3C-C-C=O$

D-Glutamic
acid
(D-Glu)

$C-C-(CH_2)_2-C=O$

D,L-Diamino
pimelic acid
(*meso* DAP)

$C-C-(CH_2)_3-C-C=O$

D-Alanine
(D-Ala)

$O=C-C-CH_3$

$\left(\begin{array}{c}\textbf{Bridge cross-link}\\\textbf{unit}\end{array}\right)$

Fig. 7.1 General structure of the peptidoglycan repeating unit.

extracellular mucilages, including hexuronoxylofucans, mannans, galactans, arabinoxylogalactans, glucuronoxylorhamnans, and galacturonoxylofucans as well as peptic acids (galacturonans) and alginates (guluronomannuronans). Some of the relevant structures are shown in Fig. 7.3. These structures have been found in some bacteria also.

The strong affinity of group IIA metal ions, e.g. Ca^{2+} and transition metal ions such as Cu^{2+}, Fe^{2+}, Co^{2+} and Ni^{2+}, with hetero- and homopolysaccharides, has been especially well documented. The gel-forming properties of alginic acid as well as those of xanthan in the presence of a threshold concentration of the bivalent metal ions have been attributed *inter alia* to the sequence and conformational structure of the biopolymer blocks containing polyguluronic acid (Fig. 7.3). The trapping of the bivalent cations is facilitated by electron-donating hydroxyl and carboxyl groups from the uronate residues of the adjacent polymer sequences.

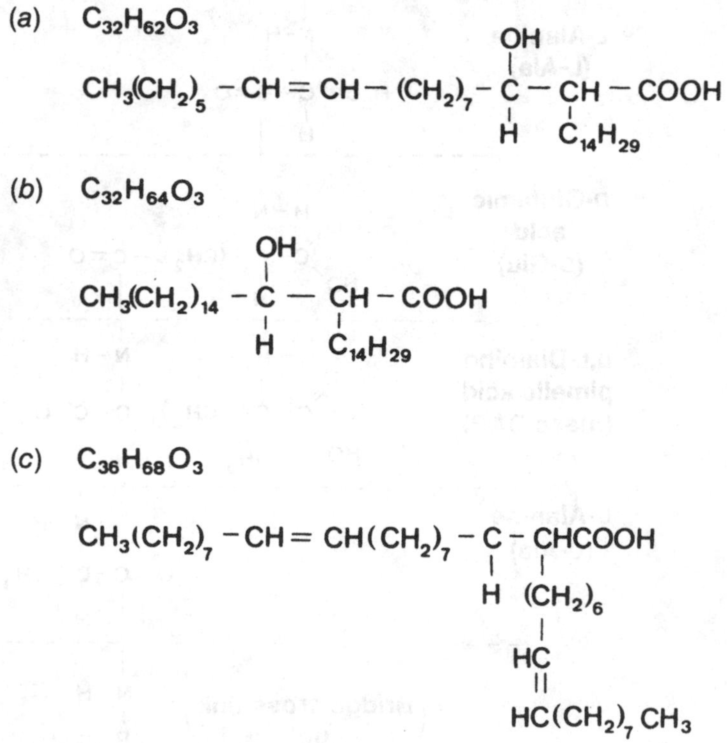

(a) $C_{32}H_{62}O_3$

$$CH_3(CH_2)_5 - CH = CH - (CH_2)_7 - \underset{\underset{H}{|}}{\overset{\overset{OH}{|}}{C}} - \underset{\underset{C_{14}H_{29}}{|}}{CH} - COOH$$

(b) $C_{32}H_{64}O_3$

$$CH_3(CH_2)_{14} - \underset{\underset{H}{|}}{\overset{\overset{OH}{|}}{C}} - \underset{\underset{C_{14}H_{29}}{|}}{CH} - COOH$$

(c) $C_{36}H_{68}O_3$

$$CH_3(CH_2)_7 - CH = CH(CH_2)_7 - \underset{\underset{H}{|}}{C} - \underset{\underset{(CH_2)_6}{|}}{CHCOOH}$$

$$\underset{\underset{HC(CH_2)_7 CH_3}{||}}{HC}$$

Fig. 7.2 Corynemycolic acids. (*a*) Corynemycolenic acid; (*b*) corynemycolic acid; (*c*) corynemycoladiremic acid. (According to Lederer, 1971.)

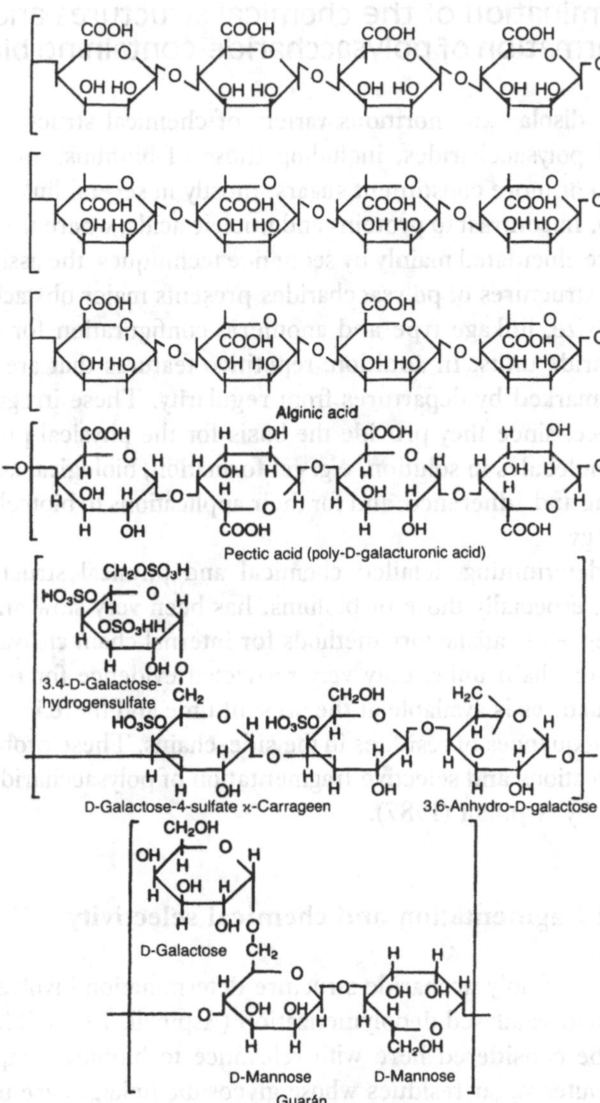

Alginic acid

Pectic acid (poly-D-galacturonic acid)

3.4-D-Galactose-
hydrogensulfate

D-Galactose-4-sulfate x-Carrageen   3,6-Anhydro-D-galactose

D-Galactose   CH₂

D-Mannose   D-Mannose
Guarán

D-Galactose 3,6-Anhydro-L-galactose

Fig. 7.3 Hetero- and homopolysaccharide structures produced partially from algae, extracellular materials and extracellular mucilages, e.g. alginic acid and peptic acid.

Determination of the chemical structures and conformation of polysaccharide-containing biofilms

Polysaccharides display an enormous variety of chemical structures. The vast majority of polysaccharides, including those of biofilms, are heteroglycans with two or more constituent sugars, mostly in several linkage types (Aspinall, 1983). In contrast to proteins and nucleic acids, where the chemical structures are elucidated mainly by sequence techniques, the assignment of the chemical structures of polysaccharides presents major obstacles with respect to ring size, linkage type and anomeric configuration for each of the monosaccharide units. In addition, repetitive features that are usually present can be marked by departures from regularity. These irregularities are of importance, since they provide the basis for the physical properties of these macromolecules in solution, e.g. gel formation, biological activities, metal ion binding and adherence, and for their applications to biotechnology and pharmacology.

Progress in determining detailed chemical and physical structures of polysaccharides, especially those of biofilms, has been very slow and difficult. In the absence of satisfactory methods for internal chain cleavage with retention of outer-chain units, only very restricted evidence for regularity of backbone structures is available at the present time and there is even less on the detailed sequences of residues in the side-chains. These problems of chemical modifications and selective fragmentation of polysaccharides have been addressed by Aspinall (1987).

Partial fragmentation and chemical selectivity

Classical methods of polysaccharide structure determination involve partial hydrolysis and acid-catalysed depolymerization (Aspinall, 1983). The polysaccharides to be considered here with relevance to biofilm composition contain mainly outer sugar residues whose glycosidic linkages are unstable to acid hydrolysis. Therefore, stepwise degradations by acid or more specific enzymic attack by glycosidase or exoglyconase results in complete loss of the outer residues. However, this procedure works at the expense of the loss of considerable information on attachment of the cleaved units. Endoglycanases with high biological activities and specificity are very rarely available. Accordingly, chemical techniques that apply modifications to functional groups already present or introduced through specific structural modifications are more common than are enzymic methods. Such degradation can be achieved by nitrous acid deamination of equatorially orientated 2-amino-2-deoxy-D-glycopyranosides and D-galactopyranosides with 2,5-anhydrohexose formation accompanied by glycoside cleavage (Aspinall, 1983). This method has been successfully applied to elucidate the structure of a biofilm produced on copper pipes in the County Hospital, Hellersen, Germany.

Another successfully applied approach is the base-catalysed degradation of esterified uronic acid residues or degradation at carbonyl groups that have been formed by oxidation of specific hydroxyl groups. This yields limited information if further degradation takes place at exposed reducing sugar residues because the hydroxyl groups are not protected by methylation. A new method for controlled depolymerization of glycuronans with retention of recognizable fragments from uronic acid residues has been developed by Aspinall & Rossell (1978). This chemical degradation seems very promising for determining the structural elements of biofilms, particularly in combination with enzymic techniques (H. H. Paradies, unpublished data).

Another method involving structural modification and selective cleavage is based on a decarboxylation–acetoxylation mechanism (Aspinall, 1987). In this case methylated glucosiduronic acids are treated with lead tetraacetate in boiling benzene. The degree of reaction can be monitored by the disappearance of carboxyl groups and by chemical analysis for the absence of uronic acid components in the modified polysaccharide. Identification of the modified and fragmented polysaccharides after separation and purification can readily be performed by FAB–MS. Exposed hydroxyl residues in the liberated oligosaccharides can be identified also by trideuteromethylation. The structures of the oligosaccharide derivatives can be established by ^{1}H-nuclear magnetic resonance (NMR), ^{13}C-NMR spectroscopy and mass spectroscopy, and from the methylated sugar after conversion into partially methylated alditol acetates for gas–liquid chromatography–mass spectrometry (GLC–MS) analysis after hydrolysis, reduction and acetylation.

Pectins, structurally related exudate gums including xanthans, present similar problems as described for glucuronomanans because they contain interior glycuronan chains. Moreover, there are even further variations in the arrangement of sugar residues, so that the backbone chains range from 4-linked α-D-galacturonans to rhamnogalacturonans with alternate 4-linked α-D-galacturonic acid and 2-linked α-L-rhamnopyranose residues.

The side-chains may be attached to one another or to other backbones by three residues or polysaccharide subunits with multiple residues of D-galactose and/or L-arabinose (see Aspinall, 1987). Hexa-5-enose degradation has been applied to exudate gums whose backbone structures are at opposite ends of the galacturonan-rhamnogalacturonan (Aspinall et al., 1963). Iodination of the carboxyl-reduced methylated glycan and subsequent treatment with zinc dust, followed by reduction and acetylation, yields two hexenitol-terminated oligosaccharides (Fig. 7.4), which can easily be detected and characterized by FAB–MS.

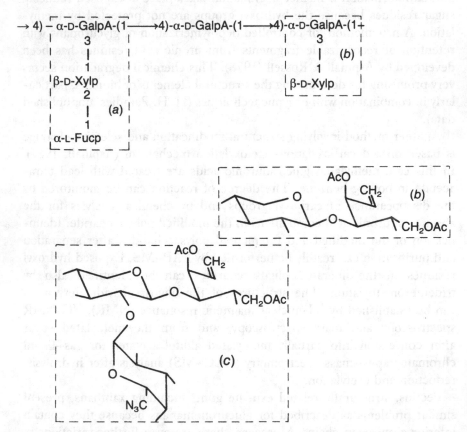

Fig. 7.4 A possible model for hex-5-enose degradation of carboxylic-reduced methylated oligosaccharide units as acids with: (a) NH₃, Pb(OAc)₄, t-BuOH, HCOOH, NaBH₄; (b) NaOH, Pb(OAc)₄; (c) LiAlH₄, PPH₃ (triphenylphosphine), 9-borobicyclo(3.3.1)nonane.

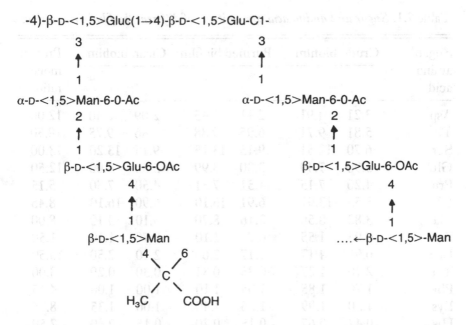

Fig. 7.5 Primary structure of xanthan, showing the repeating units in the acetic form. Acid hydrolysis yielded 4,6-O(S)-(1-carboxyethylidene)-β-D-mannopyranose and 4,6-O(R)-(1-carboxyethylidene)-β-D-mannopyranose.

A case history: determination of the chemical composition of a biofilm involved in a severe copper corrosion process

The organic nature of this particular biofilm having been established by extraction of xanthan (Fischer *et al.*, 1988*a*,*b*,*c*) (see Fig. 7.5), parts of the polysaccharide film were found to contain different amounts of other materials, e.g. pyruvate, L-amino acids and α-hydroxy acids having different chirality (Paradies *et al.*, 1992), along with neuraminic acid and galactosamine. Crude and purified ('clean') biofilm samples were obtained directly from the corroded copper pipes. The 'clean' biofilm did not contain any inorganic materials. It was extensively washed with ethanol–water mixtures and subsequently lyophilized. No phosphate was found in this material. Further purification of the 'clean' biofilm involved an extraction with chloroform/ether for the removal of possible lipids that might adhere non-specifically to the biofilm. The extraction was followed by extensive

Table 7.1. *Sugar and amino acid compositions of different 'biofilm' preparations*

Sugar/ amino acid	Crude biofilm		Purified biofilm		Clean biofilm		Protein molar ratio
Asp	3.21	4.91	2.11	2.45	2.09	2.40	12.00
Thr	5.81	9.71	6.95	9.88	6.86	9.75	8.50
Ser	6.70	12.51	9.15	13.15	9.15	13.20	13.00
Glu	5.90	7.49	3.30	3.99	3.30	4.00	12.50
Pro	4.20	7.15	4.51	7.31	4.50	7.30	5.15
Gly	5.55	13.91	6.91	16.10	6.90	16.10	8.45
Ala	3.82	8.50	3.16	8.70	3.10	3.10	8.00
Ile	0.95	1.55	0.75	1.10	0.70	1.10	1.50
Leu	0.95	4.17	2.17	2.60	2.10	2.50	10.50
Tyr	2.10	1.27	0.35	0.31	0.30	0.29	3.00
Phe	1.70	1.85	1.05	1.10	1.00	1.00	4.15
Lys	1.50	1.99	1.06	1.40	1.00	1.35	8.75
His	0.47	0.67	0.15	0.20	0.15	0.20	2.50
Arg	2.60	2.74	2.14	2.10	2.15	2.10	3.15
GalNAc	18.00	14.50	19.80	14.85	20.00	14.99	—
NANA	28.00	14.50	26.00	14.80	25.00	14.99	—
aa/dioside[a]	—	6.00	—	—	—	—	—

Note: The valine peak appeared to be contaminated with hexosamine material, and could not be separated quantitatively.
[a]Dioside is the sum of the concentrations of N-acetylneuraminic acid (NANA) and N-acetylgalactosamine

dialysis against distilled water. Exogenous proteins of unknown origin were removed by extraction with chloroform/isopropanol and with acetic acid, as normally performed for extraction of ribosomal proteins (Franz & Paradies, 1976). The quantitative sugar and amino contents of the biofilm and 'clean' biofilm are listed in Table 7.1.

Table 7.2 lists glycopeptides obtained by the action of pronase on the crude biofilm after dialysis of N-acetylgalactosamine and N-acetylneuramic acid, identified and measured by FAB–MS. The increase in the total sugar content of the remaining glycopeptides of the two biofilms

Table 7.2. *Amino sugars, amino acids and free α-NH₂ groups (μmol/mg original material) in the biofilm before and after pronase digestion and dialysis, respectively*

	Crude biofilm	Pronase digested clean biofilm	
		Before dialysis	After dialysis
A. Crude biofilm			
GalNac	0.91	0.91	0.91
NANA	0.85	0.85	0.84
α-NH₂	0.45	2.51	0.39
Amino acids	4.15	5.00	2.36
		Molar ratio	
aa/dioside	5.50	3.95	3.00
B. Clean biofilm			
GalNac	0.75	0.75	0.75
NANA	0.80	0.81	0.81
α-NH₂	0.45	2.51	0.39
Amino acids	3.15	5.00	2.40
		Molar ratio	
aa/dioside	4.00	3.91	3.01

Note: For abbreviations, see Table 7.1.

(Table 7.2) indicates that almost 40% of the amino acids present have disappeared through dialysis. The amino acid : disaccharide molar ratio drops from 4.6 to 2.9. This is possible only if further attack of pronase on the peptide chain is inhibited by neighbouring glycosidic prosthetic groups.

SDS–polyacrylamide gel electrophoresis (PAGE) of total glycopeptide indicates that the mixture is heterogeneous with respect to electrophoretic mobilities. At least four to six fractions are readily detected after staining with Coomassie Blue or by absorption at 210–230 nm. However, as shown in Table 7.3, sugar and amino acid contents of these fractions do not vary to a great extent. After purification of the fractions, the following main conclusion can be drawn:

Table 7.3. *Sugar and amino acid composition of pronase-digested and dialysed clean biofilm. Fractions I to IV were obtained by SDS-polyacrylamide gel electrophoresis. For calculating the molar ratios, GalNAc was taken as 14.8 to facilitate comparison with Table 7.1*

	Total glycopeptide fraction content		Glycopeptide (molar ratio)			
	(%)	(Molar ratio)	I	II	III	IV
Asp	1.05	1.05	1.40	—	1.40	1.54
Thr	7.01	8.00	11.51	8.70	9.15	10.50
Ser	6.45	8.10	10.71	8.80	9.20	10.45
Glu	2.90	2.71	2.55	2.10	2.92	2.10
Pro	4.31	5.15	8.20	5.30	3.20	3.70
Gly	4.00	8.10	12.00	9.20	14.60	10.00
Ala	2.78	4.20	7.00	3.75	5.70	5.50
Val	2.92	2.95	1.00	2.22	1.50	3.10
Ile	—	—	—	—	—	—
Leu	1.07	1.12	—	—	—	—
Tyr	—	—	—	—	—	—
Phe	—	—	—	—	—	—
Lys	—	—	—	—	—	—
His	—	—	—	—	—	—
Arg	—	—	—	—	—	—
GalNAc	24.20	14.50	14.50	14.60	14.60	14.70
NANA	33.50	14.60	14.70	15.00	15.10	14.90
aa/dioside	—	3.00	3.50	3.15	3.21	3.15

Note: For abbreviations, see Table 7.1.

1. In no case is the total content of dicarboxylic amino acid sufficient to account for the individual linkages between –COOH of these amino acids and the disaccharides that may constitute the prosthetic groups. The percentage of β-hydroxyamino acids, e.g. serine and threonine, increases with respect to the total peptide fraction. Their total amount is far greater than that which would

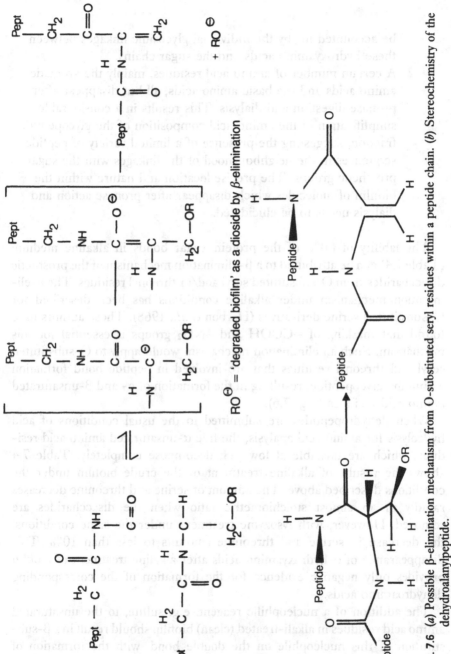

Fig. 7.6 (a) Possible β-elimination mechanism from O-substituted seryl residues within a peptide chain. (b) Stereochemistry of the dehydroalanylpeptide.

be accounted for by the individual glycosidic linkages between these hydroxyamino acids and the sugar chains.

2. A certain number of amino acid residues, mainly the aromatic amino acids and the basic amino acids, all but disappear after pronase digestion and dialysis. This results in a considerable simplification of the amino acid composition of the glycopeptide fraction, suggesting the presence of a limited variety of peptide sequences in the neighbourhood of the linkages with the sugar prosthetic groups. The precise location and nature within the biofilm of molecules which disappear after pronase action and dialysis needs to be elucidated.

The lability of 80% of the protein–sugar bonds in alkaline medium (Table 7.4) can be attributed to a β-elimination mechanism of the prosthetic disaccharides from O-substituted seryl and/or threonyl residues. The β-elimination mechanism under alkaline conditions has been described for O-substituted serine derivatives (Harbon *et al.*, 1968). These authors have found that masking of –COOH and –NH₂ groups is essential for this mechanism. Such an elimination mechanism would apply to O-substituted seryl and threonyl residues that are involved in peptide bond formation within the glycopeptide, resulting in the formation of α- and β-unsaturated amino acid residues (Fig. 7.6).

When dehydropeptides are submitted to the usual conditions of acid hydrolysis for amino acid analysis, the free α-unsaturated amino acid residues, which are unstable at low pH, decompose completely. Table 7.4 shows the results of alkaline treatment of the crude biofilm under the conditions described above. The amount of serine and threonine decreases rapidly in an almost stoichiometric ratio when the disaccharides are removed. However, with lysozyme treatment under the same conditions, the decrease in serine and threonine amounts to less than 10%. This disappearance of α-hydroxyamino acids after alkaline treatment of biofilm provides only negative evidence for the formation of the corresponding dehydroamino acids.

The addition of a nucleophilic reagent, e.g. sulfite, to the unsaturated amino acid residues in alkali-treated (clean) biofilm should result in a β-substitution of this nucleophile on the double bond, with the formation of cysteic acid from substituted serine and α-amino-β-sulfonylbutyric acid from threonine. Table 7.4 shows the results, in addition to the specific decrease of serine and threonine, of alkali treatment of the biofilm. The

Table 7.4. *Sugar and amino acid composition of the clean biofilm after alkali treatment and Na$_2$SO$_3$ addition. For calculation of the molar ratios alanine (Ala) was equated to 8.0 as in Table 7.1*

	Clean biofilm		Alkali-treated clean biofilm		Alkali-treated + Na$_2$SO$_3$ + clean biofilm	
	(%)	(Molar ratio)	(%)	(Molar ratio)	(%)	(Molar ratio)
Cys-SO$_3$	—	—	—	—	4.00	3.75
Asp	1.32	1.90	1.10	1.48	1.10	1.30
Thr	6.21	9.55	1.60	2.26	1.65	2.15
Ser	6.31	10.91	2.40	4.00	3.15	4.60
Glu	3.43	4.16	2.80	3.75	3.80	4.00
Pro	4.37	6.79	6.50	7.00	6.00	5.75
Gly	5.70	13.61	6.50	14.15	4.55	12.50
Ala	3.71	8.00	4.60	8.00	4.60	8.00
Cys-S-S	0.20	0.21	—	—	—	—
Val	2.60	4.10	2.40	3.51	2.27	3.00
Ile	0.71	1.00	0.50	0.60	0.51	0.65
Leu	1.42	2.30	1.87	2.70	1.50	2.06
Tyr	0.12	0.15	0.11	0.11	0.13	0.12
Phe	1.01	1.10	0.96	1.10	0.85	0.81
Lys	0.51	0.60	0.25	0.31	0.65	0.70
His	0.13	0.15	0.13	0.15	0.09	0.15
Arg	2.80	2.40	2.18	2.15	0.64	0.60
GalNAc	18.90	15.00	3.00	2.60	3.10	2.60
NANA	27.10	14.90	5.20	2.61	5.10	2.60

Table 7.5. *Specific determination of pyruvate, α-oxobutyric acid and quinoxalinols derived from the clean biofilm*

Quinoxalinol derivative	Standard solution (1 mol/3 ml)	Clean biofilm (2 mg/2 ml)	Quinoxalinol or oxalinol (mol/10 mg)	α-Hydroxy amino acids destroyed (%)
Pyruvate	1.150	0.950	4.25	98 (Ser)
α-Oxobutyric acid	1.215	1.045	4.31	100 (Thr)

acidic compounds like cysteic acid and α-amino-β-sulfonylbutyric acid are eluted. A ratio of 2.5×10^{-6} M of cysteic acid to 10 mg biofilm (clean) was determined. The total yield of the sulfonylated amino acids as compared to the total amount of serine and threonine residues destroyed is very low (about 20%); this value is of the same order of magnitude as the yield for the serine residue in substituted chymotrypsin. According to high performance liquid chromatography analysis the sulfonylated derivative contains a mixture of cysteic acid and α-amino-β-sulfamylbutyric acids.

Quantitative estimation of α-oxo-acids, derived from dehydroamino acid residues

It is known that acid hydrolysis under mild conditions converts α-amino-acyl residues into pyruvic acid in a quantitative way. It can be inferred that the homologous α-amino-crotonyl residues should, under identical conditions, yield α-oxobutyric acid. An estimation of both α-oxo-acids, performed by three different methods, should yield two independent values for each α-oxo-acid. Alkali-treated biofilm was subjected to acid hydrolysis in 0.1–3 M HCl for 60 min at 100 °C, followed by determination of the *total* α-oxo-acids formed through the phenylhydrazine reaction, and by spectrophotometric assay of pyruvic acid (Paradies *et al.*, 1994*a*). A maximum value for both reactions is reached after hydrolysis with 3 M HCl. Under these conditions, total α-oxo-acids formed account for 75% of total β-OH α-amino acids destroyed, and the specific assay for pyruvic acid shows that 85% of the serine lost is recovered as the corresponding

Table 7.6. *Quantitative estimation of DNFB-amino acids after performic oxidation and alkaline H_2O_2 (Na_2O_2)-treated clean biofilm and crude biofilm*

DNFB-amino acids	Clean biofilm		Crude biofilm	
	+KOH	−KOH	+KOH	−KOH
Gly	0.51	0.50	0.51	0.04
Ala	0.12	0.015	0.12	0.01
Val	0.095	0.0091	0.095	0.00
Ser + Thr	0.07	0.01	0.07	0.02

Note: DNFB, dinitrofluorobenzene.

α-oxo-acid. The value for α-oxo-butyric acid is calculated by subtraction and corresponds to 60.5% of the threonine residues destroyed. However, both phenylhydrazine reaction and pyruvic acid determination do not work if the biofilm is not treated with either alkali or Na_2O_2, respectively (Table 7.5).

The recovery of pyruvic acid and α-oxo-butyric acids from substituted serine and threonine residues is quantitative. These results, together with the finding that the glycine content remains constant in the biofilm–KOH samples, indicate that the elimination reaction at the threonine residue proceeds entirely through the dehydropeptide. Another quite unexpected result is the selective splitting of the peptide link between the −COOH group of S-substituted seryl and threonyl residues. Table 7.6 reveals the α-NH₂ terminal amino acids obtained under these specified conditions. Dinitrofluorobenzene (DNFB)-linked amino acids identified include glycine, alanine and valine; DNFB-glycine accounts for 65% of the total DNFB-amino acids formed.

These results suggest that the peptide sequences in the vicinity of the O-substituted hydroxy-amino acids may be (or are) to a large extent repetitive. Accordingly the experimental evidence leaves little doubt that the biofilm found in corroded copper pipes at the County Hospital, Hellersen, has O-glycosidic bonds that are very alkali labile and sensitive to OH⁻ with respect to the linkages between sugars (diosides) and amino acids. Furthermore, the stoichiometry, the relation between the prosthetic groups liberated, and that between the two α-oxo-acids determined by two independent measurements, can be considered as evidence that no other types of linkage responsible for the alkali lability are present. A very interesting result of the chemical analysis of the biofilm is that serine and threonine participate in the O-glycosidic link-ages in equimolar ratio. However, about 20% of the glycosidic linkages are not alkali labile and these still remain to be elucidated.

Occurrence and complexation of α-keto-acids

α-Keto-acids, e.g. pyruvic acid, phenylpyruvic acid and (p-hydroxy-phenyl)pyruvic acid, are biologically important metabolic products (Meister, 1965). The keto–enol tautomerism of the free acids and salts has been inves-tigated by infrared (IR) and Raman spectroscopy quite extensively (Hanai *et al.*, 1989). Whereas the salts of these α-keto-acids, e.g. Li^+, Na^+, K^+ and Ca^{2+}, are well characterized, no experiments have been undertaken to investi-gate the complexation of α-keto-acids with Cu^{2+} (Cu^{1+}), Ni^{2+}, Fe^{2+} or Cr^{3+}. According to the IR spectra and Raman bands, the alkali salts do not have the enol structure, though the absence of the $C{=}O$ stretching band has to be explained. However, this is entirely different for Cu^{2+} complexes of pyruvic acid, phenylpyruvic acid and (p-hydroxyphenyl)pyruvic acid. A strong keto band appears at 1709 cm^{-1}, whilst the broad band at 3000 cm^{-1} (normally seen in the alkali salts in the hydrated state) disappears completely. Such a drastic spectral change cannot be explained in terms of simple removal of the water molecules. Interestingly, the same bands are obtained upon binding of Cu^{2+} to xanthan (Fig. 7.5), which contains approximately two-thirds of the side-chain pyruvate as a covalently linked (chiral) acetal residue. Such spec-tral differences have also been reported for pyruvic acid salts (Jencks & Carriuolo, 1958; Long & George, 1960).

From the results it can be concluded that the lithium, sodium and potass-ium salts of pyruvic acids, as well as those of xanthan, have the structural moiety $-CH_2-C(OH)_2-$. Furthermore, the NMR spectra of these 'hydrates' are almost identical with that of anhydrous pyruvic acid or phenylpyruvic acid sodium salts in heavy water. The same results are obtained for the sodium, potassium and lithium salts of xanthan. The proton signal of $CH_2{-}CO$ is observed at 4.10 p.p.m. and that for $CH_2{-}C(OH)_2$ at 3.08 p.p.m. From the relative intensities of these signals, the content of the keto form of the pyruvic acids is determined to be 91%. For xanthan no keto forms are detectable, in accordance with the chemical primary structure. The signals of the unbound pyruvic acid and pyruvic acid deriva-tives, respectively, gradually diminish due to dehydration. These results show clearly that, whereas the hydration of the $C{=}O$ group occurs in the solid state, depending on the metal ion involved, the keto form is more stable in aqueous solution irrespective of the metal cation (H. H. Paradies, unpublished data). In a biofilm recently obtained from severe microbial corrosion damage (Fischer *et al.*, 1987, 1992), considerable amounts of bound and unbound pyruvic acid were found. The keto–enol tautomerism of these components is of considerable importance with respect to metal ion binding. In aqueous solution the metal cation is surrounded by water molecules, and no longer has any influence on the anion, so that the keto form becomes predominant for metal binding.

Determination and characterization of glycolipids as biofilm components

The biofilm, or more specifically the extracellular material having a high surface activity, has been isolated from *Pseudomonas* cultures in the presence of copper foils, and compared with that obtained from culture broths. After extraction with chloroform–methanol (2 : 1, v/v), drying and purifying on silica gel 60, the structures were determined by positive FAB–MS analysis (Thies *et al.*, 1994). The glycolipid-containing samples were dispersed in glycerol, thioglycerol or diethanolamine as the probe matrix. The mass spectra obtained by the FAB technique are shown in Fig. 7.7 for β[β(2-O-α-L-rhamnopyranoxyloxy)decanoyl]decanoic acid (glycolipid A). The signals at m/z 527, 549 and 1076 are in agreement with $(M + Na)^+$, $(M + 2Na - H)^+$ and $(2M + 3Na - H))^+$. The sequence signals shown in Fig. 7.7 can be assigned to the fragments indicated, yielding two units of β-hydroxydecanoic acid and one rhamnose molecule. However, Fig. 7.8, which shows the FAB spectrum of β[β(2-O-α-L-rhamnopyranosyloxy-α-L-rhamnopyranosyloxy)-decanoyloxy]decanoic acid (glycolipid B) with diethanolamine as probe matrix, indicates the presence of two molecules of rhamnose and two units of β-hydroxydecanoic acid. The structures of glycolipids A and B are shown in Figs. 7.9 and 7.10, respectively. Apparently, FAB–MS is a straightforward technique for direct analysis of trace amounts of components for biofilm analysis of chemical composition, relative molecular mass determination of building blocks and selective physical fragmentation of polysaccharide chains.

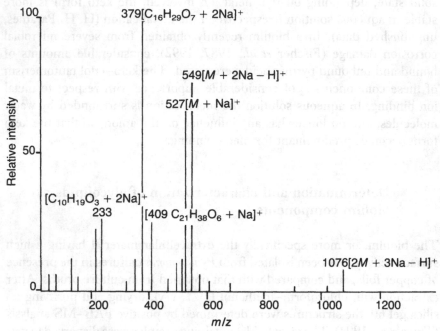

Fig. 7.7 FAB–MS spectrum of glycolipid A.

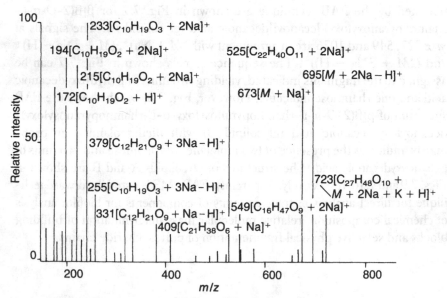

Fig. 7.8 FAB–MS spectrum of glycolipid B.

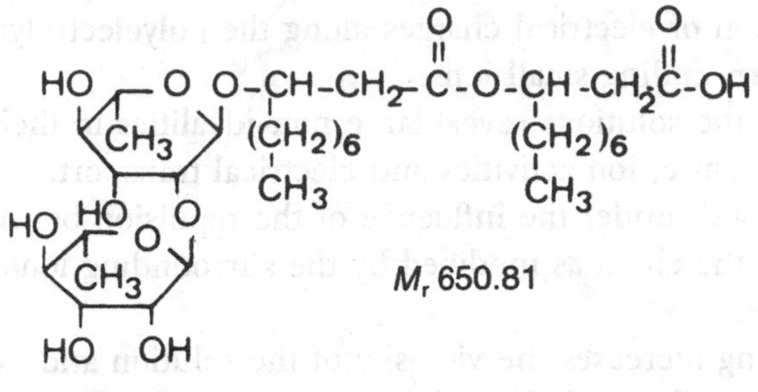

Fig. 7.9 Molecular structure of glycolipid A.

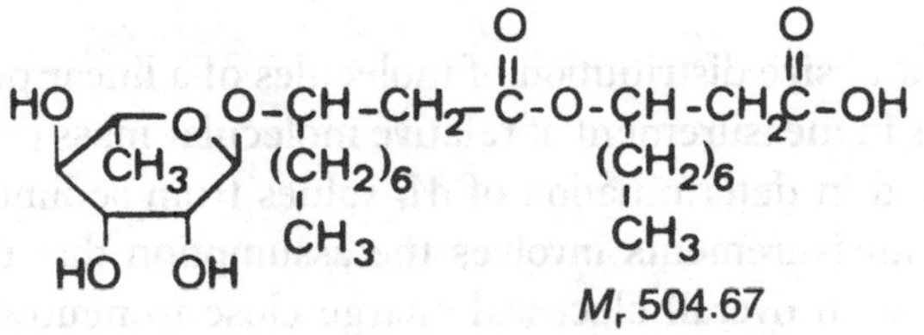

Fig. 7.10 Molecular structure of glycolipid B.

Polysaccharide conformation in solution

A detailed account of polysaccharide conformations and kinetics has been given by Goodall & Norton (1987); a review of the secondary and tertiary structure of polysaccharides in gels and solution has been published by Rees & Welsh (1977), and by Rees (1977). Ogston (1981) discussed the effect of concentration on the configuration of chain polymers, including polysaccharides, in binary and tertiary systems, providing the theoretical framework for experimental designs for reasonable studies of this class of macromolecules in solution. However, there are no detailed structural investigations on biofilm (polysaccharide) interactions on metal surfaces at a molecular level in the scientific literature, especially for salt-induced gelation, thixotrophy, wettability and spreading.

According to Overbeck (1976) the properties of linear polyelectrolytes, e.g. biofilms, can be related qualitatively as follows:

1. There is strong electrical interaction between the high concentration of electrical charges along the polyelectrolyte chain and the surrounding small ions.
2. Therefore, the solutions reveal large non-idealities in their osmotic pressure, ion activities and electrical transport.
3. The coils swell under the influence of the repulsion between the charges on the chain as modified by the surrounding ionic atmospheres.
4. This swelling increases the viscosity of the solution and expresses itself in the swelling polyelectrolyte gels. Models for these situations were presented by Scatchard *et al.* (1950) and Manning (1969, 1978).

The charge, shape and size distribution of molecules of a linear polyelectrolyte cause problems in measurement of relative molecular mass (M_r). The general formula applied in determination of M_r values from sedimentation viscosity and dialysis measurements involves the assumption that the particles under study have an overall electrical charge close to neutrality and maintain a globular shape approximately that of a sphere. This formula has doubtful validity for linear polyelectrolytes.

Hydrodynamic behaviour of polysaccharides in solution

Hydrodynamic techniques, e.g. sedimentation (analytical ultra-centrifugation), static and dynamic light-scattering and viscosimetry, have been applied to characterize macromolecules in solution as random coils, rods, ellipsoids, worm-like chains or globular particles. Preliminary measurements on hydrolysed biofilms obtained from copper pipes (Fischer *et al.*, 1987) reveal fractions of $M_r < 10^5$, mainly containing structural fractions of xanthan (H. H. Paradies, unpublished data). By small-angle X-ray-scattering experiments it has been found that these fractions in solution behave as rigid rods, rather than the worm-like chains with a persistence length of 400 Å demonstrated by Sato *et al.* (1984) for native non-degraded xanthan. A value for the native biofilm of 450 Å has been calculated for the polysaccharide involved in the corrosion of copper pipes (Fischer *et al.*, 1987). However, this biofilm contains peptide units in addition to the pyruvate residues (Fig. 7.10). In addition, it has been reported by Muller *et al.* (1986) that a xanthan with a high pyruvate content gives monomers in aqueous solution, and it was suggested that a xanthan sample may be either single- or double-stranded depending on how it has been treated after the fermentation step or during purification. However, cation activity measurements, conductivity, and increased ion association on ordering, as monitored according to the Manning theory, are more consistent with monomers than with dimers as measured by light-scattering experiments (Goodall & Norton, 1987).

Detailed studies of the kinetics of primary conformational ordering in xanthan have uncovered a 'two-state all-or-none' process in which blocks of helix residues grow within a single chain (Norton *et al.*, 1984). Both conformational equilibria and kinetics reveal that ordering can be intramolecular, and that helix and coil regions can be present in equilibrium within one single chain.

It has been found by Norton *et al.* (1984) and Goodall & Norton (1987) that the rate constant increases sharply when T is decreasing and approaching the melting temperature (T_m^0) for a salt-free xanthan solution, revealing a changeover from nucleation to growth control in accordance with the statistical process. So far a salt-free solution of xanthan, at T_m^0, contains blocks having an average of 30 helix residues alternating with blocks of the same length of coil residues. Each chain of the average of 10^3 residues, $\bar{n}_w = 10^3$, therefore contains on the average 16–18 ordered and approximately 17–18 disordered regions, where the extra disordered region results from the extra entropy of the ends of the chains. A comparison of the hydrodynamic data of xanthan with the results obtained for the native biofilm is needed for modelling metal–biofilm interactions.

Studies on salt effects and aggregation and gelation of biofilms in the presence or absence of metal surfaces or metal colloids (including colloidal metal hydroxides, carbonates, polymeric halides; Paradies *et al.*, 1988) would help us to understand the links between primary structure, solution conformation, aggregation and gelation processes. Preliminary measurements of a biofilm containing peptide units are summarized in Table 7.7.

Structural aspects of metal biofilms: physical properties, flocculation, deterioration of metal surfaces

The mechanical performances of assemblies or of composite materials depend on the quality of adhesion of the different constituent elements. With solids, e.g. metals, physical chemistry distinguishes more or less

Table 7.7. *Physicochemical properties of a biofilm[a] containing peptide units*

	Quantity	Technique
M_r	$2.5 \ (\pm 0.4) \times 10^6$	Light-scattering
$<R_g>$	450 ± 45 Å	Light-scattering
$<R_g>$	430 ± 30 Å	Small-angle X-ray scattering
M_r	$2.40 \ (\pm 0.4) \times 10^6$	Small-angle X-ray scattering
A_2	$3.5 \pm 10 - 4$ ml/mol per g^2	Light-scattering
$[\eta]$	175 ± 5 ml/g	Viscosimetry
R_H	390 ± 50 Å	Inelastic light-scattering
R_H	410 ± 50 Å	Viscosimetry
$\left(\dfrac{\partial n}{\partial c}\right)_{T_1 P_1 \mu}$	0.144 ml/g	Refractive index increment

Note: [a]The biofilm was obtained by peeling off the copper surface, removing inorganic material, and dissolving it at pH 7.0 (20 °C) in 4 M guanidinium chloride (H. H. Paradies, unpublished data). M_r is the average relative molecular mass; $<R_g>$ is the weight-average radius of gyration, A_2 is the second virial coefficient; $[\eta]$ is the intrinsic viscosity of the macromolecule; R_H is the hydrodynamic radius of the macromolecule in solution (Tanford, 1961; Franz & Paradies, 1976; Paradies, 1989).

arbitrarily between two types of surface; surfaces with low energy in the range of <50 mJ/m^2 (synthetic polymers) and surfaces of high energy usually >100 mJ/m^2, i.e. metals, minerals and glasses. Therefore, it is especially interesting to study the association of materials of these two different types because these associations are relevant to biofilm-coated metals and particularly to adhesion of a biofilm to a metal surface.

The variety of approaches to the study of adhesion processes is emphasized by the fact that quite a few theoretical models of adhesion phenomena have been developed. Mechanical and specific adhesion types have been distinguished. The mechanical model is based on the assumption that adhesion is the result of an anchoring of the polymer in the pores of channels of the substrate, i.e. metal or metal oxides. However, it seems now well accepted that molecular interactions between these materials in contact are largely responsible for their adhesion.

With relevance to metal–biofilm interactions, two aspects of the adhesion

Table 7.8. *Contact angle (θ) measurements (± 3°) between three liquids and interfacial biofilm surfaces*

Liquids	Free surface θ (deg.)	Interfacial surface (biofilm) θ (deg.)	Interfacial surface (Cu) θ (deg.)
CH_2I_2	35	39	25
Toluene	37	42	28
H_2O	85	83	70

between a biopolymer (or bacteria) and a high energy surface have to be stressed:

1. The formation during contact between a biofilm and a high energy substrate of an interfacial layer.
2. The modification, during interfacial contact, of the surface properties of the biofilm. This modification leads to the formation of a new interfacial surface different from the free surface of the biofilm.

Surface characteristics can be explored by contact-angle measurements (see Adamson, 1982). To determine the surface energy of the solid (metal, metal oxide), the contact angle between the liquid and the solid is measured. The surface energy is composed of the dispersive component and the polar component. These are important parameters for characterizing any surface.

For the low energy surface (e.g. metal surface coated with biofilm), the contact angle (θ of the solid (metal) is determined with a series of liquids with known surface energies (Schultz & Carré, 1982). In order to achieve some idea of the interfacial behaviour of the biofilm (Fischer *et al.*, 1988*b*) when coming into contact with a copper surface, contact-angle measurements have been performed (Paradies *et al.*, 1991). The inner and outer surfaces of the biofilm and the free site in contact with the copper surface have been analysed, with the addition of suitable liquids (CH_2I_2 and H_2O) with high and low surface polarity respectively. Table 7.8 shows the contact angles observed.

According to Fig. 7.11 there is an increase in the contact angle of the interfacial surfaces with time after detachment of the biofilm. After approximately 5 h the values of the contact angles reach those found on the free metal surface, normally:

θ (toluene) = 38°

θ (H$_2$O) = 81°

Having established the *in vitro* adhesion of a biofilm to the copper surface, the components of the surface energy of the biofilm faces can be computed from the contact-angle measurements. These are given in Table 7.9. The values do not change with the nature of the solvent used, nor with solution concentration, nor with the thickness of the biofilm formed.

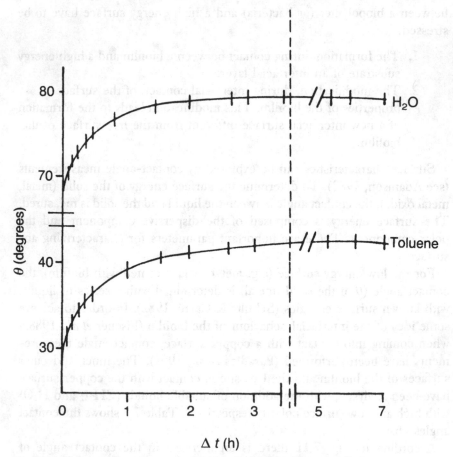

Fig. 7.11 Changes of contact angle (θ) with time in the presence of toluene or water.

Table 7.9. *Surface-energy components of a copper biofilm (mJ/m²) at 20 °C*

	γ_S^D	γ_S^P	γ_S
Free surface (air)	42.5	5	48.0
Interfacial surface biofilm	39.2	5	43.0
Interfacial surface Cu ($t = 0$)	48.0	7	54.5
Interfacial surface Cu ($t = 8$ h)	39.3	2.5	42.5

Note: γ^D is the dispersive component of the surface energy of the solid having the subscript S; γ_S is the total surface energy of the solid having the dispersive component γ_S^D and a polar component γ_S^P. The most general equation between the contact angle and the surface characteristics of the solid and the liquid given by:

$$\cos \theta_i = (\gamma_S^D)^{1/2} \times \frac{(\gamma_L^D)^{1/2}}{\gamma_L} + I_i^P - 1 + \frac{\pi_a}{\gamma_L}$$

where θ is the contact angle between the liquid and the copper surface in the presence of the liquid vapour, π_a is the spreading pressure, and I_i^P is the liquid–solid polar interaction energy. The subscript L stands for liquid.

It can be concluded from these results that:

The surface energy of the biofilm-coated copper surface that is in contact with a low energy surface, e.g. biofilms of different composition (xylans, xanthans etc.), is identical with the energy of the free surface.

However, the surface energy of the biofilm in contact with a high energy surface (copper) is higher than the energy of the free surface. This particular increase of the surface energy of the biofilm is accompanied by a decrease of the biofilm/copper interfacial energy. This variation can be attributed to a particular orientation or conformation and density of the polysaccharide chains in contact with copper (H. H. Paradies, unpublished data).

The interfacial surface of the biofilm after separation from the copper surface seems to be in a metastable state. As a consequence, its surface energy evolves slowly with time, at ambient temperature, towards a value corresponding to that of the free surface.

A particular behaviour of a thin biofilm is the tendency to peel off the copper surface upon drying, or to roll up after detachment from copper. This could relate to a thermodynamic imbalance between the two sides of the biofilm. This behaviour is reversed if the copper surface is partly oxidized.

The observed phenomena can be related to surface energies of composite materials also, especially to high energy surfaces. The polymers present surface properties that are quite different from those of the free surface. Of course, this phenomenon also predicts the performance of composite systems from the surface properties of the materials to be associated.

Metal oxides as surface oxides: interactions with water and biofilms

Passive films can grow on many metals homogeneously, laterally as well as normal to the surface. The growth of oxides depends strongly on the electronic properties and ionic conductivity of the inner layers. An inner layer of Fe_3O_4 is a good electronic conductor so that the potential drop that is manifested on oxide growth is located in the outer layer. The passivity of such oxide films is of considerable interest for analysing oxide growth quantitatively.

Copper forms passive layers at pH 6.0–7.0 and pH 7.5 in aqueous solutions of low ionic strength. Four different oxide species have been discovered and distinguished by their kinetic and capacitive behaviour: the oxide CuO_x, which is representative of monomolecular copper oxide, formed in short periods or at low potential; the oxides Cu_2O and CuO at intermediate potentials and longer polarization times; and a non-defined oxidation product $CuO_y.zH_2O$ at high potentials (Strehblow & Speckmann, 1984; Speckmann et al., 1985). Speckmann and colleagues explored the oxide formation by surface-sensitive techniques and electrochemical methods and concluded that the formation of CuO_x, Cu_2O and CuO take place homogeneously all over the surface to give almost constant thickness. The reaction occurred possibly by an islet mechanism for the duplex film as well as for the CuO_x film. The CuO_x film has been characterized further by Paradies *et al.* (1991) by means of EXAF spectroscopy (see below). Two structures were found (Fig. 7.12). One oxide has an adamantane-like arrangement and the other one a cubane structure, both being formed in the presence of oxygen dissolved in aqueous solutions at pH 7.5–8.0. Whereas the adamantane structure can be stabilized in the presence of a biofilm or alginic acid, the cubane structure of Cu_3O_4 has been discovered on the surface of $Cu^{\pm 0}$ at acidic pH (pH 5.5) and disproportionates into Cu_2O and CuO. Colloidal Cu_3O_4 has been observed in the cubane form in the presence of anionic amphiphiles (H. H. Paradies, unpublished data) at neutral pH. Whether these copper oxides are intermediates in the microbially induced copper corrosion processes (Fischer *et al.*, 1987) has not yet been verified. However, they can be produced in the presence of a biofilm on copper surfaces.

Surface oxide–water interaction

Au *et al.* (1979) studied Cu(111)–O(1s) spectra and discovered that there was enhanced bonding in molecularly adsorbed water compared with water absorption on the clean Cu(111) surface. This was reflected in an increase in the temperature of water desorption from Cu(111) (150 K) to about 200 K. Furthermore, there was a shift in the O(1s) binding energy from 533 eV (characteristic of $H_2O_{(ads)}$) to about 531.4 eV. The latter has been suggested to be characteristic of strongly hydrogen-bonded water, which at higher temperature generates surface hydroxyl 1s. The hydroxyl surface coverage at 295 K is about 10–15%. When the preabsorbed oxygen coverage approaches $\theta = 1$, the activation effect becomes progressively less significant (H. H. Paradies, unpublished data).

Studies on the role of oxygen activation of adsorbed water have been performed by Carley *et al.* (1983) on nickel surfaces. They found that the greatest activity was associated with pre-adsorbed oxygen. By comparison, both the metal oxide overlayer formed at 295 K and the bulk nickel oxide were unreactive, unlike the case of copper (H. H. Paradies, unpublished data). The ability to induce surface hydroxylation by chemisorbed oxygen adatoms has been confirmed by studies of the oxide overlayers at lead and zinc simple crystal surfaces (Roberts, 1988).

A scheme based on the results obtained for copper surfaces in the presence of a reconstituted biofilm is shown in Fig. 7.13. This emphasizes the role of the hydrogen-bonded water surface oxygen complex in determining

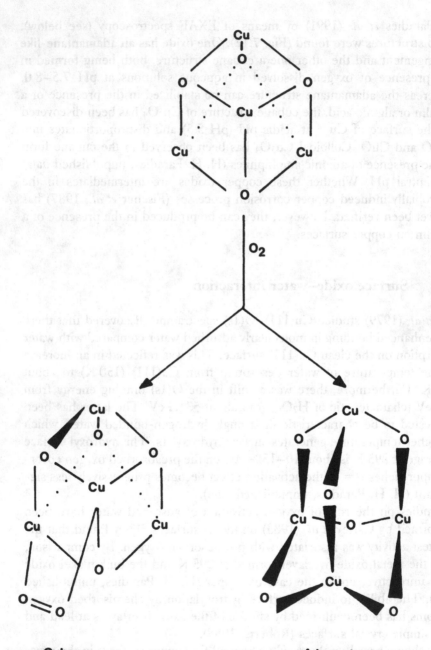

Cubane   **Adamantane**

Fig. 7.12 Possible molecular structures of copper oxides: cubane- and
adamantane-like structures in the presence of oxygen.

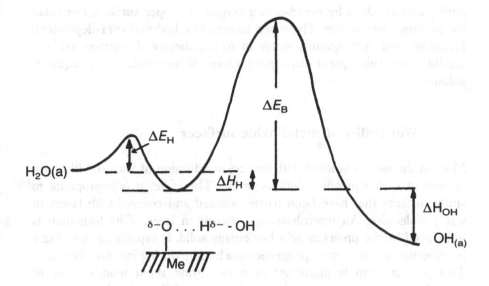

ΔE_H: Formation of H-bonded complex

ΔH_H: Stability of H-bonded complex

ΔE_B: Cleavage of complex

ΔH_{OH}: Stability of surface 'OH'

Fig. 7.13 Potential energy profile of surface oxygen-induced water interaction at a copper metal surface. For the Cu(111)–O surface the forward reaction is inhibited by the large E_B term, so that the reverse reaction (desorption) is preferred.

the reaction pathway. In addition the strength of complexation between the $O_{(ads)} \ldots HOH_{(ads)}$ and an amino acid residue (threonine) controls the occurrence of hydrogen abstraction with cleavage of the O—H bond leading to $\dot{O}H$ radicals and a second potentially reactive H_3O^+ (Paradies *et al.*, 1991*c*). Clearly it is the charge on the oxygen adatoms $O_{(ads)}$ and the amino acid residues (threonine or serine, as well as a hydroxyl group of one of the major residues) that is important.

The kinetics of this replacement reaction can be thought of as an acid–base reaction. The thermodynamic driving force for the replacement of surface oxygen by the hydroxyl from the biofilm arises from the formation of water or hydronium ions that desorb. Activation of N—H bonds from amino acid residues by preadsorbed oxygen at copper surfaces can occur by the same mechanism. Hydrogen abstraction, hydroxyl (pH-dependent) formation and consequently water or hydroxylamine desorption are also feasible, with subsequent disproportionation of hydroxylamine in aqueous solution.

Wettability of metal oxide surfaces

Most of the metals studied with respect to adhesion of bacterial films are in contact with aqueous solutions or air. Therefore, it is appropriate to study surfaces that have been partly oxidized and covered with layers of water molecules. An interphase or a transition layer, if its formation is influenced by the presence of a low energy solid, is capable of inducing a modification of the surface properties of a biofilm during interfacial contact. This phenomenon is important as it can bring about modifications of the adhesion energy and of the performance of the assembly or of the composite. As mentioned, it is impossible to predict these modifications from the surface energies of the materials which are in contact (see pp. 229–30).

However, by determination of the contact angle of the metal oxide surfaces and the surface energies of the oxide, the biofilm and the interfacial surface (opposed to the free surface, which is in contact with air, water or the lumen in general) can be determined. The biofilm is a representative of a surface with low energy ($\gamma_L = 21.5$ mJ/m^2), and CuO has a surface energy of $\gamma_S = 210$ mJ/m^2 (H. H. Paradies, unpublished data). The different sites of the biofilm, the free sites and the sites that were in contact with the CuO surface have been analysed with the help of representative liquids as shown previously (see p. 228 and Fig. 7.16). The components of the surface energy of the biofilm faces, calculated from contact-angle measurements, reveal that the values γ_S^D and γ_S (50 mJ/m^2 and 48.5 mJ/m^2, respectively) do not change with the nature of the solvent applied, nor with the solution concentration, nor with the thickness of the biofilm formed. From these results it can be concluded that the surface energy of the biofilm when in contact with a low energy surface (CuO) is almost identical with the energy of the free surface.

Flocculation of polysaccharides

One aspect of flocculation is biopolymer bridging, which has to be included in any consideration of microbial colonization. Bridging flocculation occurs because segments of a biopolymeric chain adsorb on different particles, thus linking the particles together. Adsorption is an essential step, and is required for several interactions between biopolymer segments and the particle surface.

Adsorption of a long-chain biopolymer at its surface usually involves the attachment of many segments, so that the affinity between an individual segment and the surface can be weak and yet the other polymeric segment chain can still be very strongly adsorbed. Polymer adsorption is often regarded as irreversible. The most important interactions are the following:

1. Ionic (electrostatic) interaction: in this case a polyelectrolyte adsorbs onto a surface bearing oppositely charged ionic groups. This always gives very strong adsorption and is an important mechanism in many practical instances, e.g. microbially induced corrosion.
2. Hydrophobic bonding: this is responsible for the adsorption of non-polar segments on hydrophobic surfaces.
3. Hydrogen bonding: this can take place when the surface and the biopolymer have suitable hydrogen-bonding sites. Hydroxyl groups or oxide surfaces can interact in this way with the α-amino, amide, secondary hydroxyl or carboxyl groups or peptide units present in the exopolymers. Amide, amino and peptide units have been shown to adsorb onto silica. When the silanol groups on the silica surface of glass are eliminated, these polymers can no longer adsorb.
4. Ion binding: with an ionic biopolymer and negatively charged surfaces, it is often discovered that a certain concentration of metal ion e.g. calcium or magnesium, is required to promote adsorption. These ions are known to bind quite strongly to carboxylate groups such as those on hydrolysed biofilms and may also serve as links between these groups and negative sites on the particle surfaces. The concentration, e.g. of calcium ions, needed to achieve this effect is of the order of $1-2$ mM, a level comparable to that found in waters of moderate hardness, so that differences in flocculation

behaviour in different types of water may be explained along these lines, especially in corrosion processes in large buildings and transmission lines.

5. Dipole–crystal field effects: in these a polar group on a biopolymer can interact with an electrostatic field at any crystal surface as in the case of biofilms adsorbing on metal oxides, fluorites or silica particles.

The various adsorption mechanisms discussed above depend on the nature of the biopolymer particle surface. In a mixed suspension, certain biopolymers may adsorb on one type of particle but not on others.

Flocculation by bridging

Typical polymeric flocculents can have molecular dimensions comparable to the size of colloidal particles (0.1–1 μm) and attachment of a biopolymer chain to several particles could explain the effectiveness of these materials as flocculents. One of the most important properties of flocs produced by biopolymers is that they can be considerably stronger than aggregates formed when particles are destabilized with simple salts or with specifically adsorbed counter-ions. Simply reducing or eliminating the electrical repulsion between particles causes them to be held together by van der Waals' forces, which may be rather weak and allow only fairly small aggregates to form. Normally aggregate size is limited by the degree of shear to which the suspension is subjected: the stronger the binding forces, the larger can be the aggregates under given shear conditions. Polymeric flocculents, e.g. insoluble biofilms, provide many links between particles, the strength of which is dependent on the carbon bonds along the polymeric backbone. This assumes that the adsorption is essentially irreversible. A single carbon bond in a polymer chain can be broken by an applied force in the region of 1–10 nN, which is much smaller than typical hydrodynamic forces between particles in agitated suspensions. This implies that several polymer bridges between particles would be needed to form flocs able to withstand moderate shear. This can easily be achieved in practice and large, strong flocs can be produced, especially with biopolymers of very high relative molecular mass. For very similar reasons, biopolymer flocculents can cause deposited particles to be attached strongly to substrates, especially to metals.

Effective bridging flocculation requires that the adsorbed bio-polymer extends far enough from the particle surface to attach to other particles, and that there is sufficient free surface available for adsorption of segments of these extended chains of the polysaccharide. When excess biopolymer is adsorbed, the particles can become destabilized, either because of surface saturation or by steric destabilization. This can be one explanation of the fact that an optimum dosage of flocculent is often found. At low concentrations there is insufficient biopolymer to provide adequate links between particles, and with larger amounts destabilization may occur.

Charged particles in water repel each other over a distance depending on the ionic strength of the solution. At low ionic strength, the electrical double layer around a charged biopolymer particle can be quite extensive (up to about 100 nm) and particles cannot approach each other very closely. For bridging flocculation to occur, the adsorbed polymer has to extend far enough from the surface to overcome electrical repulsion forces, implying that at low ionic strength biopolymers of quite high relative molecular mass would be needed. As ionic strength increases, the range of electrical repulsion is reduced, and low relative molecular mass polymers could be very effective. For discharge biopolymers, a concept of bridging through a repulsion barrier is supported by a number of experiments (Tanford, 1961).

The situation is considerably more complicated for charged electrolytes. The dimension of a polyelectrolyte chain in solution depends on ionic strength, since repulsion between charged segments along the chain is screened by counter-ions. At low ionic strength this screening is limited and polyelectrolyte chains adopt a rather extended configuration, which should make bridging flocculation more likely. At high salt concentration, screening of the charges gives a more compact configuration, reducing the chance of bridging contacts. However, increasing ionic strength also causes the range of interparticle repulsion to be reduced and may enhance the adsorption of electrolytes on similarly charged surfaces, both of which situations should increase the likelihood of bridging flocculation. These opposing effects of ionic strength could give an optimum salt concentration at which flocculation by polysaccharides is most pronounced.

An optimum charge density of electrolytes for bridging flocculation is fairly well established. Chain expansion can give improved flocculation, whereas reduced adsorption would have the opposite effect and the optimum degree of hydrolysis represents the best compromise between these two tendencies. Very similar results have been reported for flocculation by starches (Gregory, 1987). A limited degree of ionic character (approximately 30%) imparted by phosphate or sulfate groups is found to give optimum flocculation.

Charge neutralization

The only effective polymeric flocculants are polyelectrolytes with charge opposite to that of the particles. In water most particles are negatively charged and cationic polyelectrolytes are often necessary. However, there are many cases where negative particles can be flocculated by neutral or ionic polymers, especially inorganic polymers. With oppositely charged polyelectrolytes, e.g. exopolymers, it is likely that adsorption occurs, giving a rather flat configuration of the adsorbed chain because of the strong ionic interactions between the ionic groups of the polymer and charged sites of the particle surface. This would probably reduce the possibility of bridging contacts with other particles, especially with polyelectrolytes of low relative molecular mass. However, the adsorption of a cationic polyelectrolyte by a negatively charged particle would reduce the surface charge of the latter and this charge neutralization could be an important factor in destabilization of particles. Because of the strong interaction, adsorption of excess polyelectrolyte could occur, giving a positively charged surface and the possibility of restabilization of the particles for simple electrostatic reasons.

It may not be immediately apparent whether bridging or charge separation is an operative mechanism, especially in corrosion processes. There is a considerable amount of evidence suggesting that, for cationic polyelectrolytes and negative particles, charge neutralization plays a large part in the flocculation processes. The most direct evidence comes from measurements of electrophoretic mobility, and therefore from the zeta potential measurements of particles with added polyelectrolyte. With many different types of particle, including clays, cellulose fibres, silica, exopolymers, biofilms, glycans, proteins and bacteria, it has been found that the optimum flocculation dosage of cationic polyelectrolyte corresponds quite closely to the amount required to give a new electrophoretic mobility that neutralizes the particle charge (Tables 7.10 and 7.11).

Table 7.10. *Electrophoretic mobilities of different particles measured at pH 7.0 (25 °C) in 0.01 M NaCl*

Species	Biological characteristics	$10^8 \times$ mobility (m^2/s^1 per V)
Staphylococcus aureus	Methacillin sensitive	-1.00
	Methacillin resistant	-1.48
	Adapted to methacillin	-1.50
Streptococcus pyogenes	Type 26	-1.03
	Type 2M	-0.89
Human blood cells	Erythrocytes	-1.08
	Lymphocytes	-1.09
	Platelets	-0.85
Hamster kidney cells	Tumour	-1.51
	Tissue	-0.65
Chlorella	Alga	-1.75
Dunaliella	Alga	-1.80
Colloidal 'Au'	Substrates	-3.25
Colloidal 'Cu'	Of microbial origin	-2.90
Colloidal 'SiO$_2$'	Colonization	-3.01
	Colloidal	-2.55
Colloidal CuO$_x$	Inverse micelles	-3.05
	Alginate	-2.90

Although charge neutralization goes some way toward explaining the behaviour of cationic polyelectrolytes, especially polysaccharides, there are some effects of relative molecular mass and ionic strength that do not quite fit this simple picture (Gregory, 1982). These can be better explained by the electrostatic patch model (Kaspar, 1971; Gregory, 1982). Essentially these models apply to cases where the particles have a fairly low density of immobile surface charges and the adsorbing polyelectrolytes have a fairly high charge density. Under these conditions, it is not physically possible for each surface site to neutralize charged segments individually on the polymer chain, even though the particle may have adsorbed sufficient poly-electrolyte to achieve overall neutrality. We observe in this case patches of

Table 7.11. *Zeta-potentials and effective Hamaker constants of different particles in water (20 °C)*

Source	ζ-potential	$A_{131} \times 10^{16}$ (ergs)
Erythrocytes	−18	0.25
Lymphocytes	−14.3	1.25
Granulocytes	−12.5	2.51
Pseudomonas aeruginosa	−17.5	10.15
Escherichia coli, MRE 600	−18.5	1.25
Dunaliella	−25.0	16.5
Colloidal nanoparticles 'Cu'	−9.5	35.7

$\gamma_{3v} = 72.8$ erg/cm^2 (H$_2$O)
$\gamma_{3v} = 70.4$ erg/cm^2 (filtrate)
$A_{13}{}^1 = A_{11} + A_{33} - 2A_{13}; A_{13} = (A_{11} \times A_{33})^{1/2}$
$A_{131} = -12 \, \pi \, d^2_{131}, \Delta G^{adh}_{131} = 24 \, \Delta d^2_{131} \, \gamma_{13}$

Note: According to van Oss & Good (1992): Δ^{adh}_{131} is the free energy of adhesion at the minimum equilibrium distance d_{131}; γ_{13} is the interfacial tension, which is determined from the surface tension of the cells (γ_{1v} and of the liquid γ_{3v}) (Absolom & Neumann, 1987).

'excess positive charges', corresponding to adsorbed polyelectrolyte chains in a rather flat configuration, surrounded by areas of negative charges, representing the original particle surface. Particles having these 'patchy' or 'mosaic' types of surface charge distribution may interact in such a way that positive and negative patches come into contact, giving quite strong attachment.

The electrostatic patch concept seems to explain a number of features commonly observed in the flocculation of negative particles with cationic electrolytes. These include a rather small effect of increasing relative molecular mass and the effect of ionic strength on both the breadth of the flocculation dosage range and the rate of flocculation at optimum dosage (Gregory, 1982, 1987).

Both the adsorption and flocculation steps are essentially collision processes, the rates of which depend on transport phenomena. Their predominant transport mechanisms are diffusion or convection caused by fluid flow, the relative importance of each being determined by the size of particles and biopolymer molecules and the fluid motion. Normally there will be far more biopolymer molecules than other particles, and it might be thought that adsorption would be very rapid compared with the particle collision, and hence flocculation, rate. However, it will usually be necessary for a substantial fraction of the added biopolymer to be adsorbed before the particles are adequately destabilized. This applies to both bridging and charge-neutralization mechanisms.

Kinetic aspects of biopolymer flocculation

When a biopolymeric flocculent is added to a suspension, several processes are initiated, though the rates at which they significantly affect the flocculation will differ. The steps involved are:

1. Adsorption of the polymer particles.
2. Rearrangement of adsorbed chains to give an equilibrium configuration (conformational change).
3. Collisions between particles with adsorbed polymers to form aggregates, so-called flocs.
4. Break-up of flocs.
5. Mixing of the biopolymer molecules among the particles to give a uniform distribution.

These processes are not independent. For instance, if mixing is not achieved very rapidly then an uneven distribution of biopolymer may lead to local overdosing and restabilization of some of the particles. Biopolymers are often involved in corrosion processes when added as a rather dilute solution. At such concentrations droplets of the added solution can take time to disperse, and could act as 'nuclei' for floc formation. If mixing is very rapid, the biopolymer is instantaneously distributed among other particles and four rate processes can be considered (Fig. 7.14).

In the first case (Fig. 7.14(a)) sufficient biopolymer chains need to be adsorbed in order to provide bridges of adequate strength, and in the second (Fig. 7.14(b)) the particle charge has to be reduced sufficiently to overcome electrical repulsion. One important question in relation to corrosion processes is whether the necessary adsorption occurs in a time that is long or short compared with the average time between particle collisions. Assuming that the particle number concentration, N, remains constant throughout the processes and that the adsorption rate constant k_{abs} is independent of surface coverage (both questionable assumptions), then it is easy to show, according to Gregory (1982), that the time required for a fraction f of the polymer to absorb is:

$$t_a = -\frac{\ln(1-f)}{k_{abs} \times N} \tag{7.2}$$

This has to be compared with the average time between collisions or the time in which the number of particles in a flocculating dispersion is reduced to half of the initial value. This is given by:

$$t_f = 1/(k_d \times N_1) \tag{7.3}$$

In order to proceed we need to have estimates of the rate constants k_d and k_{abs}. In an unstirred dispersion these will depend on the diffusion

(a)

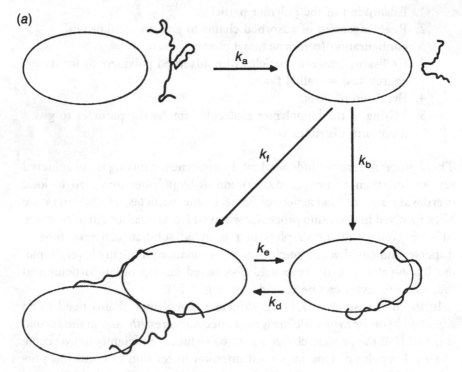

Fig. 7.14 (a) Kinetics (model) of biofilm adsorption and flocculation, having rate constants k_a, k_b, k_f, k_e and k_d.

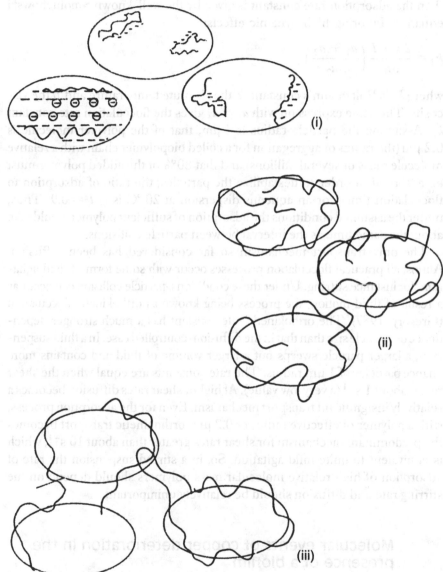

(*b*) Schematic modelling of an 'electrostatic-patch' interaction of negatively
charged biofilm particles with: (i) adsorbed anionic polyelectrolytes,
(ii) restabilization by adsorbed polymer, and (iii) bridging flocculation.

coefficients only, and hence on the size of the particles and polymer molecules. Assuming that both can be regarded as spheres, of radii a_1 and a_2, then the adsorption rate constant is given by the well-known Smoluchowski equation. Ignoring high dynamic effects:

$$k_\mathrm{d} = \frac{2\,k_\mathrm{B}LT}{3\eta}\left(\frac{a_1 + a_2}{a_1 a_2}\right)^2 \tag{7.4}$$

where k_B is Boltzmann's constant, T the absolute temperature and η the viscosity. The same expression with $a_1 = a_2$ gives the flocculation rate constant k_d. Assuming the particle radius is 1 μm, that of the polymer molecule is 0.2 μm (the radius of aggregation for a coiled biopolymer chain with a relative molecule mass of several millions) and that 80% of the added polymer must be adsorbed in order to destabilize the particles, the ratio of adsorption to flocculation times for an aqueous dispersion at 20 °C is $t_a/t_f \approx 0.9$. Thus, under the assumed conditions the adsorption of sufficient polymer would take about the same time as the interval between particle collisions.

The only transport mechanism so far considered has been diffusion. Almost all practical flocculation processes occur with some form of fluid agitation, for instance stirring. Under these conditions, particle collision can occur as a result of fluid motion, the process being known as orthokinetic flocculation (Gregory, 1987). The orthokinetic rate constant has a much stronger dependence on particle size than that in the diffusion-controlled case. In a fluid suspension, a larger particle sweeps out a larger volume of fluid and contains more chance particles of 1 μm radius. The rate constants are equal when the shear rate is about 1 s^{-1} (a very low value). At higher shear rates diffusion becomes a relatively insignificant transport mechanism. Even for the adsorption process, with a polymer of effective radius of 0.2 μm, orthokinetic transport becomes the predominant mechanism for shear rates greater than about 10 s^{-1}, which is equivalent to quite mild agitation. So, in a stirred suspension the rate of adsorption of high relative molecular mass polymers should depend on the stirring rate and diffusion should be relatively unimportant.

Molecular events of copper deterioration in the presence of a biofilm

A recent study of the deterioration of copper in an aqueous environment in the presence of a biofilm isolated from the surface of copper pipes from the County Hospital, Hellersen, showed that biofilm is capable of attacking copper surfaces. By application of surface-sensitive methods (e.g. X-ray photon spectroscopy, and surface-enhanced Raman scattering techniques, including extended adsorption fine-structure spectroscopy (Sham, 1986) of dissolved copper–biofilm complexes), it was possible to investigate some characteristics of this particular copper deterioration (Paradies et al., 1991; Paradies, 1994).

Extended X-ray absorption fine structure (EXAFS)

Knowledge of the molecular structures around the copper atoms in the biofilm, in the corrosion products, and of the copper surface beneath the biofilm are of importance in understanding the corrosion process. Analysis of the EXAFS can be useful for elucidation of specific copper sites under non-crystalline conditions. X-ray absorption spectroscopy (XAS) deals with the measurement and interpretation of the X-ray absorption coefficients of characteristic absorption edges of elements in different environments. The absorption coefficients often exhibit oscillations which extend to as much as 10^3 eV above the threshold. These are the experimental expressions for the EXAFS that make this technique ideal for studying short-range order in solution (Sham, 1986). Figure 7.15 shows the Fourier transforms, $\phi(R)$ versus R of the EXAF spectra of a copper foil (same material and purity as used for the copper pipes installed in the County Hospital, Hellersen), of the crystalline and non-crystalline material in the pits (mainly Cu_2O), the black material covering the surfaces of the pipe (mainly CuO according to the EXAFS) and the EXAF spectrum of the reconstituted biofilm. A phase shift has not been taken into consideration. It is obvious that the main portion of the EXAF spectrum obtained from the material from the pits is Cu_2O, since it is almost identical with preparations of pure Cu_2O. Similarly, the EXAF spectra of the black layers on the biofilm is due to CuO. Surprisingly, in both spectra there is no apparent interference of the biofilm with the spectra of Cu_2O or CuO. This is also seen in the Fourier transform of the spectra. Wet and reconstituted biofilms with copper salts of oxidation states $+1$ and $+2$ show a different Fourier transform of EXAFS, shown in Fig. 7.15. Figure 7.16 shows an EXAF spectrum of colloidal Cu^0 in the presence of imidazole at pH 8.0 in 0.01 M Tris buffer. The Fourier transform of the EXAFS of Fig. 7.16, which corresponds to a certain kind of 'radial distribution function' around the copper atom, including correction for phase shift, reveals two peaks: one at 1.97 Å and

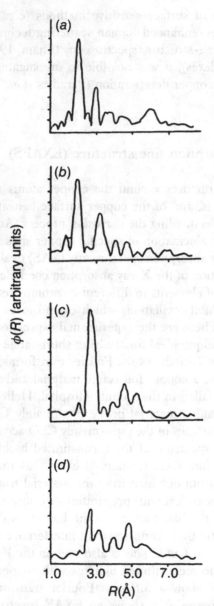

Fig. 7.15 Fourier transform of the EXAFS spectra of: (*a*) the non-crystalline material (CuO) on the surface of the biofilm; (*b*) the crystalline and non-crystalline material in the pits below the biofilm; (*c*) metallic copper of the same material that has been installed in the County Hospital, Hellersen; (*d*) the reconstituted biofilm with copper corrosion salts.

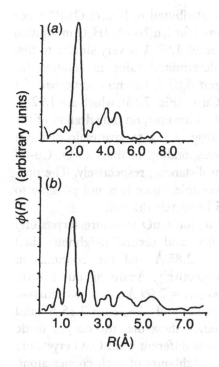

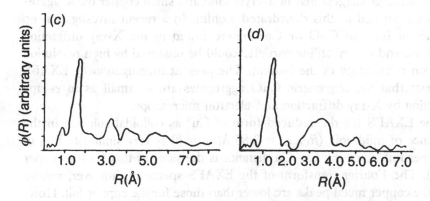

Fig. 7.16 Fourier transforms of the EXAFS spectra of: (a) colloidal $Cu^{\pm 0}$; (b) the
mechanically removed biofilm with the associated copper oxides and
hydroxides; (c) the 'reconstituted' biofilm with copper salts due to corrosion;
(d) and colloidal $Cu^{\pm 0}$ with adsorbed imidazole on the copper surface.

one at 3.05 Å. The former peak can be attributed to $[Cu(H_2O)_6]^{2+}$ since it is very similar to the EXAFS data obtained for $Cu(NO_3).3H_2O$ in solution containing $[Cu(H_2O)_6]^{2+}$ ions. The value of 1.97 Å is very similar to that reported in the solid state and the determined value in solution for $[Cu(H_2O)_6]^{2+}$. The second peak at about 3.05 Å has no counterpart for distances of Cu–O, Cu–Cu, Cu–N, or Cu_2O (Fig. 7.16), which are 1.92 Å, 2.58 Å and 2.25 Å (peptide), respectively. However, on dehydration of the specimen, the EXAFS spectra change (Fig. 7.15), to give main peaks at 1.92 Å, 2.28 Å, 2.58 Å and 4.85 Å corresponding to the Cu–O, Cu–N (peptide), Cu–Cu, CuO and/or Cu–Cu distances, respectively. The process of dehydration appears to be irreversible, since it is not possible to restore the EXAFS spectra of Fig. 7.15 upon rehydration.

The EXAFS parameters were fitted to the CuO structure (crystallite) determined by X-ray diffraction: the first and second neighbour shell distances, $R_{Cu-O} = 1.95$ Å and $R_{Cu-Cu} = 2.85$ Å and the coordination numbers $n_{Cu-O} = 4$ and $n_{Cu-Cu} = 8$, respectively. Analysing our spectra we found a neighbour shell distance of $R_{Cu-O} = 2.09$ Å and a coordination number $n_{Cu-O} = 2.8$ for the first peak and $R_{Cu-Cu} = 3.15$ Å and $n_{Cu-Cu} = 2.1$ for the second. These studies show that the copper oxide species existing in the dehydrated biofilm is different from CuO crystallite in the numbers of the first and second neighbours of each copper atom. These findings suggest that non-crystalline and small copper oxide aggregates are formed in this dehydrated biofilm. In a recent investigation no diffraction lines of CuO or Cu_2O were found in the X-ray diffraction spectrum and no crystalline particles could be observed by high resolution electron microscopy of the biofilm. The present investigation by EXAFS suggests that the oligomeric CuO aggregates are so small as to escape detection by X-ray diffraction and electron microscopy.

The EXAFS for the reduced form of Cu^0 as colloidal solution in the presence of imidazole ($R_{Cu-Cu} = 2.85$ Å, $n^c = 8$) is very similar to that of a copper foil, since the Cu–Cu distance is the same as that for the copper metal. The Fourier transform of the EXAFS spectrum, however, reveals that the copper metal peaks are lower than those for the copper foil. However, the distance 3.01 Å precludes this possibility of direct Cu–Cu bonding. At present it is not possible to assign the peaks in the EXAFS spectrum unequivocally, since curve-fitting procedures applied to known distances, specially for Cu–imidazole, were unsuccessful. For a more accurate representation of ligands coordinated to the metal sites, it is necessary to have reasonable curve fitting to obtain nearest neighbours, distances and coordination in solution. Qualitatively it can be said, in the light of the XPS results, that the broadened peak at 3.5–3.6 Å is probably due to backscattering from N-1 and C-5 of the imidazoles, which are the third shell of atoms in the imidazole group (Fig. 7.16). The peak at 20.8–21.1 nm can be assigned to a distance between Cu and N-3 of the imidazole (IM) system according to crystallographic analysis from Cu(IM)$_4$(ClO$_4$)$_2$ salts. At the present time it is not possible to distinguish Cu^{1+}–N$_3$ structures from Cu^{2+}–N$_3$ structures. However, upon oxygenation of the system Cu$^{\pm 0}$/ imidazole at pH 7.9 (20 °C), the EXAFS spectrum changes considerably. The large and broad peak at 3.51 Å is probably due to backscattering by a copper atom separated from another copper atom (absorbing) by 3.51 Å. The distance of 2.02 Å appears to be the distance Cu^{2+}–N$_3$, and the distance 1.93 Å seems to be the distance Cu–O found in the other EXAFS spectra (Fig. 7.15) and in the dehydrated state of the reconstituted biofilm. The Cu–Cu distance of 2.85 Å seen in the copper foil is surprising. Apparently, upon oxygenation the Cu has been oxidized completely to a Cu^{2+} species, coordinated by imidazole. Another Cu–O distance appeared at 1.93 Å. This is different from the Cu$_2$–O and Cu–O distance known from the crystalline structures. The possible involvement of a dioxygen complex, as observed in other systems (Karlin & Tyeklar, 1989), has not yet been investigated.

EXAFS of colloidal Cu^0 and imidazole (Fig. 7.16) may be compared with the spectra of a thin copper foil, CuO and Cu$_2$O, respectively. Although the main peak intensity is lower for the system Cu^0/imidazole at pH 8.0, when compared to the metal, the position of the peak coincides well with that of the copper foil. However, the radial distribution function is very different from that of the copper foil. Peaks were discovered at 2.05 Å, 12.58 Å and at 3.62 Å. The peak at 3.67 Å in the EXAFS is not seen in any of the other EXAFS obtained.

Surface-enhanced Raman spectroscopy (SERS)

Figure 7.17 shows a SERS and normal Raman spectra of the reconstituted Cu–biofilm, the biofilm, the crude Cu–biofilm and a surface-enhanced Raman scattering spectrum of 0.005 M imidazole on copper colloids. An astonishing feature is the adsorption band near 920 cm^{-1}. The surface enhancement factor for the particular band, the ratio of the Raman intensity for a single surface molecule with SERS to the intensity for a single molecule in solution, is estimated to be 1.5×10^4. The absence of the N–H vibration absorption bands at 855 and 750 cm^{-1} in the SERS spectrum seems to indicate deprotonation of imidazole. Similar results were obtained by using 0.005 M solutions of histidine, which is present in the biofilm in significant quantity. The new band, which appears at 345 cm^{-1} in the SERS spectrum, seems to be a Cu–N stretching and bending vibration absorption band (320–380 cm^{-1}). We may assign this band at 345 cm^{-1} in the SERS spectrum to the Cu–N vibration. Support for these findings comes from the infrared absorption frequencies in the middle and far infrared regions.

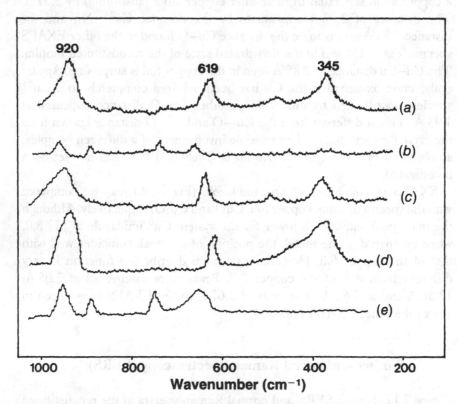

Fig. 7.17 Raman spectra of the various specimens studied: (*a*) surface-enhanced Raman scattering of the reconstituted copper biofilm with copper materials (mainly Cu$^{\pm 0}$); (*b*) the biofilm itself; (*c*) the crude copper biofilm without removing copper salts and copper materials (uncharacterized); (*d*) 0.005 M imidazole on copper colloids; (*e*) a normal Raman spectrum of imidazole (6.0 M).

X-ray photon spectroscopy (XPS)

The XPS spectrum (Fig. 7.18) of chemisorbed imidazole on a copper surface has some similarities to that of the biofilm with colloidal copper surfaces. The binding energy values of C(1s) were determined at 287.3, 285.8 and 286.5 eV respectively, those for N(1s) at 402.3 and 400.3 and for imidazole at 400.7 eV. However, a value for C(1s) of the chemisorbed imidazole on colloidal Cu^0 was found at 286.1 eV, corresponding to C-4 and C-5 of the imidazole, and a second was at 288.1 eV, which corresponds to C-2. For N(1s) a binding energy value of 400.0 eV (N-2 and N-3) was determined. The two nitrogens in the imidazole (N-1, 'pyrrole'; N-2, 'pyridine') have different environments. Therefore, it is not unexpected for XPS-spectrum of imidazole to reveal two binding energy values for N(1s) and three for C(1s). The XPS analysis for this system, imidazole and colloidal Cu^0, shows only one value of binding energy for N(1s) and two for C(1s), indicating the formation of an imidazole anion on the copper surface. The analysis of the Cu(2p) photoelectron lines shows two binding energy values, at 951.9 eV and 932.4 eV $(CU(2p)_{1/2}Cu(2p)_{3/2})$, and copper $L_3M_{4.5}M_{4.5}$ Auger lines are located at kinetic energies of 919.5 eV and 917.6 eV, respectively. The first value of the Auger line coincides with the kinetic energy of Cu^0 (919.4 eV) and the second with Cu^{+1} (917.4 eV). Evidently, Cu^{+1} gives a complex with imidazole, e.g. $Cu^+(C_3H_3N_2)^-$, on the surface of the colloidal $Cu^{\pm 0}$. This is consistent with the Raman results mentioned before.

The XPS spectra of the biofilm and Cu^{2+} salt that were obtained from the corrosion pits (Fig. 7.19) show energy bands at 400.0 eV (N(1s)), 918.9 eV, 919.5 eV and 917.4 eV, whereas the Cu(2p) photoelectron lines are located at 952.2 eV and 932.4 eV. The biofilm reconstituted with Cu^{1+} and Cu^{2+} salts at pH 7.5 and analysed by XPS reveals a shake-up structure and a shoulder on the copper $L_3M_{4.5}$ peak at 918.0 eV. This is a strong indication of Cu^{2+} oxidation state. In addition, looking at the binding energy of C(1s) (averaged) and N(1s) in the regions between 280–280 eV and 400–405 eV, respectively, one can detect binding energies of 285.5 eV and 402.5 eV. These can be assigned to C(1s) from C-4 and N-1 of the imidazole group of the histidine, which has been found in a fair amount in the biofilm. Note in Fig. 7.20 that the signal at 402.5 eV (N(1s)) is quite strong and clearly seen. In contrast, in the presence of $Cu^{\pm 0}$ in the colloidal state only the signal at 400.0 eV is observable (Fig. 7.19) due to deprotonation at N-1 of the imidazole. XPS spectra for the mechanically removed biofilms were

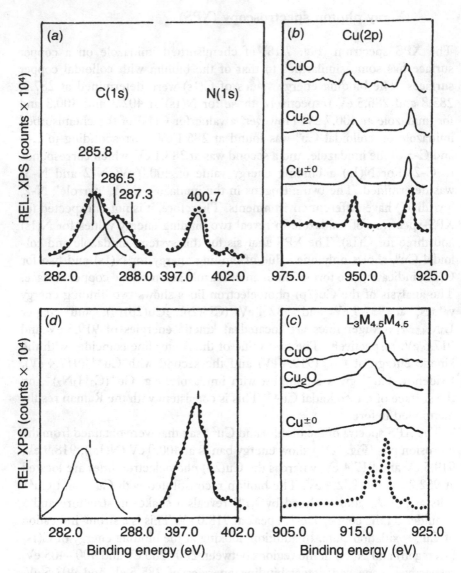

Fig. 7.18 XPS spectra of imidazole residues adsorbed onto a colloidal $Cu^{\pm 0}$ surface. The C(1s) band at 285.0 eV from the residual pump line oil contamination was used as the internal standard for spectral calibration. The Cu(2p) and the copper LMM Auger lines (. . .) are shown for imidazole copper also ((a)–(c)). Spectrum (d) shows the XPS results obtained in the presence of histidine instead of imidazole.

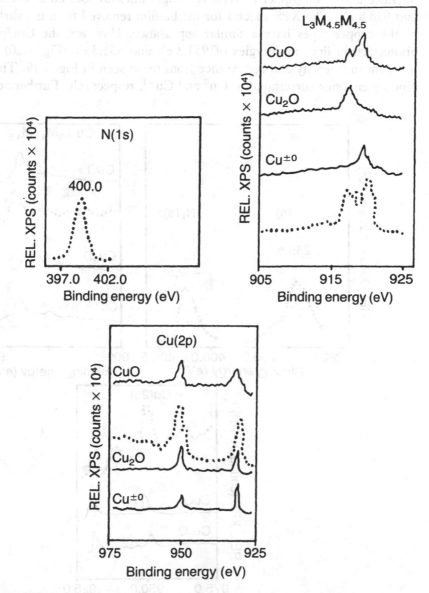

Fig. 7.19 XPS spectra of the mechanically removed ('native') biofilm (hydrated), in the presence of the copper corrosion products located at the interface biofilm–copper oxides or hydroxides–water (. . .).

obtained also. The copper $L_3M_{4.5}M_{4.5}$ Auger lines are located at 917.3 eV and 918.8 eV. The XPS spectra for the biofilm removed from the surface of the copper pipes have a similar appearance. However, the $Cu(2p)_{1/2}$ photoelectron lines at energies of 951.2 eV and 931.3 eV (Fig. 7.20) are different in intensity and appearance from those seen in Fig. 7.19. These binding energies correspond to Cu^0 and Cu^{+1}, respectively. Furthermore,

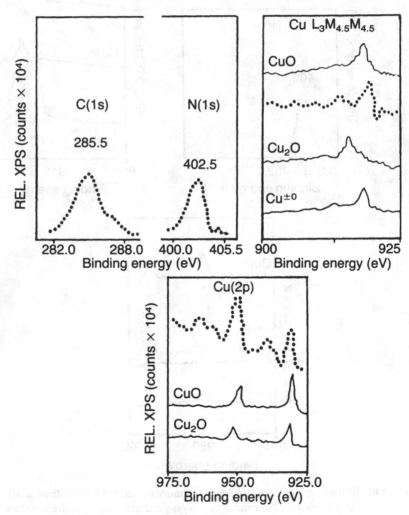

Fig. 7.20 XPS spectra of the biofilm and copper salts, and the reconstituted biofilm (. . .), showing the Cu(2p) photoelectron lines (binding energy) and the copper LMM Auger lines (kinetic energy).

looking at the binding energy level at 400.0–402.0 eV for N(1s), we discovered peaks at 400.0 eV and 288.1 eV (C(1s)). These correspond to the C-2 and N-1 and N-3 for the imidazole ring system. This indicates the presence of histidine and Cu^0 in the corrosion process when a microbial biofilm is involved. Table 7.12 lists the results of spectra obtained by XPS with respect to the complex formation of copper, copper salts and the biofilm from a mixture of colloidal $Cu^{\pm 0}$ and imidazole (or histidine at pH 8.0) and reconstituted biofilms.

Surfaces can form Cu^{2+} concentration cells with highly reactive exopolymers. One can extend the *in vitro* study to an *in vivo* situation with respect to adhesion, chemical composition and binding of Cu^{2+} to the *in vitro* exopolymer (biofilm). Apart from the chemical composition (Tables 7.1—7.6), very little information is available on the physical structure and solution behaviour of these biofilms. Furthermore, no information is available on the kinetics of sintering of gel films on metal surfaces.

The XPS experiments give the binding energy values for copper in both adsorbate and adsorbent (368.3 eV). Since the free path length of the photo-emitted electron in the energy range of interest is only a few ångströms, XPS analysis indicates that a very thin layer of chemisorbed material exists on the surface of the copper.

Tentative molecular mechanism of copper deterioration

Taking the chemical properties of imidazole and histidine, which has been found extensively in the biofilm, into consideration as well as the known structures of (imidazolato)-Cu(I) as a polymer, we can infer the following corrosion mechanism (Fig. 7.21).

The first step of the corrosion process may be the formation of a cuprous complex by ligation of the N-3 of imidazole with metallic copper (N-3 is the pyridine nitrogen, which has a large electronegativity; N-1 is the pyrrole nitrogen). In solutions at pH 7 or above, the unprotonated imidazole functions as a ligand through the two unpaired electrons on N-3. In this complex (step 1) the Cu atom and the amino group become reactive. When the solution is exposed to oxygen or hydroperoxide (which has been observed in corrosion products in the County Hospital, Hellersen) the $Cu^{\pm 0}$ is oxidized and imidazole will be protonated, resulting in the formation of (imidazolato)Cu(I) and H_2 pyrrole (step 2). Step 3 shows the formation of an infinite polymer consisting of (imidazolato)Cu(I), which forms a thin

Table 7.12. *XPS-photoelectron binding and Auger electron kinetic energy values (eV)*

Sample	Cu(2p)$_{1/2}$	Cu(2p)$_{1/2}$	Cu L$_3$M$_{4,5}$M$_{4,5}$		C(1s)	N(1s)
Biofilm + Cu^{2+}	951.9	932.4	919.6	917.5		
$Cu^{\pm 0}$	951.2	931.4	919.4			
Biofilm + Cu^{n+} salts	952.2	932.4	918.9	919.5		400.0
Biofilm, mechan.[a]	951.2	931.3	917.4	918.8	288.1	400.0
Imidazole					287.2(2) 285.8(4) 286.5(5)	402.3(1) 400.7(3)
Chemisorbed	951.9	932.4	917.2	917.6		
Imidazole + Cu^0	951.2	931.4	919.5		286.1(48) 288.1(2)	400.0(18)
Cu_2O	951.2	931.4	917.4			
CuO	952.4	932.0	918.6			
Biofilm + Cu^{2+}/Cu^{1+} reconstituted	951.2	931.3	918.0		285.5	402.5

Note: [a]Detached from copper surface.

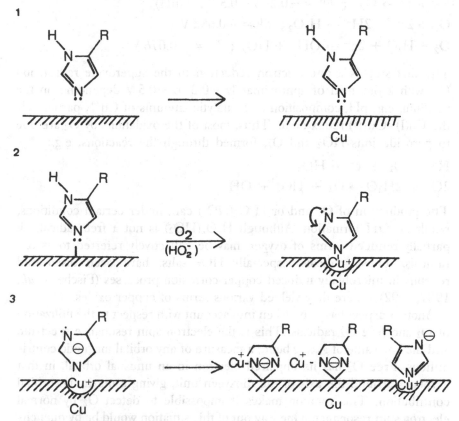

Fig. 7.21 Tentative model for the deterioration of copper due to microbially induced corrosion processes in the presence of a biofilm containing imidazole residues.

layer on the surface of the copper metal in addition to the biofilm, which has a thickness of at least 1000–5000 nm.

Cu(I) also reduces organic hydroperoxides. These hydroperoxides can attack metabolic products (e.g. pyruvate from microbial activity) by forming peracids, which are strong acids. These peracids or other hydroperoxides can oxidize Cu(I) to Cu(II). The latter has been found extensively on the biofilm surface, whereas Cu(I) is located more in the pits and at the interface of biofilm and metal surface.

Molecular oxygen is one of the major biological oxidizing agents, and a substrate for numerous enzymes and enzymic systems. Sequential univalent reduction of dioxygen yields superoxide (O_2^-), hydrogen peroxide (H_2O_2), hydroxyl radical ($^.OH$), and water:

$$O_2 + e^- \rightarrow O_2^- \; ; \; E^0 \approx -0.2 \text{ to } -0.5 \text{ V} \; ; \; f(\text{pH})$$
$$O_2 + 2e^- + 2H^+ \rightarrow H_2O_2 \; ; \; E^0 = +0.682 \text{ V}$$
$$O_2 + H_2O + 2e^- \rightarrow OH^- + HO_2^- \; ; \; E^0 = -0.076 \text{ V}$$

The first step is a one-electron reduction to the superoxide radical ion O_2^-, with a potential of approximately -0.2 to -0.5 V depending on the medium, e.g. pH, composition and catalytic amounts of Cu^{2+}, particularly the Cu(I)–Cu(II) redox cycle. Thus, most of the oxidations by O_2 are due to peroxide ions HO_2^- and O_2^-, formed through the reactions, e.g.:

$$H^+ + O_2 + e^- \rightarrow HO_2^-$$
$$2O_2 + 2H_2O \rightarrow O_2 + HO_2^- + OH^-$$

The production of O_2^- and/or $H_2O_2(HO_2^-)$ can, under certain conditions, result in $\cdot OH$ formation. Although $H_2O_2(HO_2^-)$ is not a free radical, all partially reduced forms of oxygen may be collectively referred to as oxy radicals. These radicals, especially HO_2^- salts, have been discovered recently in microbially induced copper corrosion processes (Fischer *et al.*, 1987, 1992), where they yielded various forms of copper oxides.

Another aspect has to be taken into account with respect to the utilization of O_2 and free O_2^+ radicals. This is the electron spin resonance spectrum and the low value of g_{max}, g being a measure of any orbital magnetic contributions. Free O_2^+ has its unpaired electron in an unusual orbital, in that it rotates around the axis of the dioxygen unit, giving a maximum orbital contribution. This rotation makes it impossible to detect O_2^+ by normal electron spin resonance. One way out of this situation would be by quenching this particular orbital rotation by various interactions, e.g. electron addition to normal O_2 dissolved in C_2H_2OH and frozen to 4 K in liquid helium. The key point would be selective hydrogen bonding or solvation by a type of alcohol that is confined to one plane, thereby preventing orbital motion. O_2^- in our 'CuO$_2$ polysaccharide gel' system has a g_{max} of 2.02, close to 2.00, and hence some sort of bonding that is stronger than normal solvation has to be involved. This is certainly due to bonding to a Cu centre:

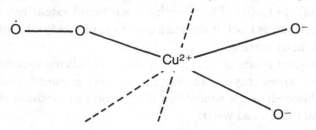

Free O_2^- radicals do not absorb infrared radiation, since the molecules have a high symmetry. However, the O—O bond in the Cu complex is asymmetric, therefore it is expected to absorb infrared.

General consideration of membrane processes involved in the microbial corrosion process

The existence and composition of the biofilm having been established, transport processes through this biofilm have to be considered. The biofilm can act as a membrane barrier. As known from many synthetic membrane systems, molecular transport entails the dissolution of components in the membrane matrix, i.e. biofilm, and their subsequent diffusional transfer through the biofilm itself. Though this has a certain volume, with flexible chain polymers like the biofilm described here the effects of free volume redistribution due to the mobility of matrix fragments (flexible sequents) may play a decisive role at the outer but not at the internal copper surface. This implies that for rigid chain polymers at temperatures below the glass-transition temperature, T_g, the higher efficiency of transmembrane particle transfer usually correlates with a pronounced structural disequilibrium of the polymer matrix.

A characteristic feature is the presence of certain submicrometre-deep cavities near the bulky substituents of the side-chain, i.e. the –OH, carboxylate-carboxy groups, covalently linked pyruvate, amides and polarized peptide units. For this reason, if transfer of the above type of particle through the membrane is achieved, introduction of the component sorption isotherm for the determination of surface particle concentrations should accompany the local values of the diffusional particle flux, $\mathcal{J}$, in the membrane:

$$\mathcal{J}(x_1 t) = -D \frac{\partial c(x_1 t)}{\partial x} \tag{7.5}$$

where $c(x, t)$ is the particle concentration in the biofilm, x is the coordinate normal to the membrane surface, and t is time.

Using simple assumptions concerning the type of isotherm (Henry's isotherm), the next expression for the steady-state flux of the passing particles follows:

$$\tilde{J} = \frac{\pi \, \Delta p}{d} \; ; \quad \pi \approx D \tag{7.6}$$

Superoxide ions, which have been detected also by electron spin resonance experiments, are readily formed from oxygen by electron addition. Free radicals can also be generated by certain microorganism–H_2O_2 systems according to:

$$microorganism + H_2O_2 \rightarrow microorganism \; (\ldots) + OH + OH^- \tag{7.7}$$

where the microorganism and the metal (Cu) surface act as a powerful electron donor, and H_2O_2 reacts by undergoing bond fission, the electron staying with one half to form the stable hydroxide ion, leaving the other as the highly reactive ˙OH radical.

However, it should be kept in mind that an atom or molecule that approaches the copper surface always experiences a net attractive potential. Under simple environmental conditions, i.e. one atom and 300 K in the presence of oxygen, nitrogen, water vapour and assorted hydrocarbons, metals are covered with a monolayer of adsorbate and multiple layers of adsorbate are often detectable. The constant presence of such adsorbate layers influences all chemical, mechanical, microbial and electronic surface properties. Adhesion, lubrication and the onset of chemical corrosion are a few of the possible surface processes that are controlled by the various properties of a monolayer of adsorbates on copper surfaces (Fischer et al., 1992).

The experimental evidence leaves little doubt that the biofilm found in copper corrosion processes at the County Hospital, Hellersen, has O-glycosidic bonds that are very alkali labile and sensitive to OH^- with respect to the linkages between sugars (diosides) and amino acids. Furthermore, the stoichiometric amounts as well as the relation that has been found between the prosthetic groups liberated, and between the two α-oxo-acids determined by two independent measurements, can be considered as evidence that no other types of linkage responsible for alkali lability are present. A very interesting result of the chemical analysis of the biofilm is that serine and threonine participate in the O-glycosidic linkages in equimolar ratio. However, about 20% of the glycosidic linkages are not alkali labile and their chemical nature remains to be elucidated.

Conclusion and future studies

Apart from microbial studies in terms of adhesion, metabolism and replication of microorganisms on a metal surface (Gaylarde & Beech, 1988; Beech & Gaylarde, 1989), it is certain that surface studies of metal solids require extensive surface-sensitive physical techniques. However, those studies are rather difficult to pursue. One part of the problem is the metal surface itself. In the near future techniques such as surface-extended absorption fine-structure spectroscopy using synchroton facilities, as well as surface studies of metals by total X-ray reflection, will contribute to our understanding of mechanisms of biofilm formation on metal surfaces.

Since X-rays in total reflection from a mirror surface penetrate very little into the mirror medium, peculiarities in the reflected intensity reveal structural peculiarities of the (metal) surface itself. Analysis of the reflected intensity can provide a new and fruitful technique for studying surface properties that involve variation of electron density with depth, e.g. corrosion, porosity, ageing or annealing, and interactions between biofilms and metal surfaces.

Recent studies on copper surfaces by total X-ray reflection at room temperature yield well-resolved spectra (H. H. Paradies, unpublished data). These curves can be explained by assuming that the copper that has been exposed to the atmosphere at room temperature has completely oxidized to about 160 Å depth. If oxidation is less deep, there probably exists some general reduction of density, i.e. porosity, and an electron density minimum just below an internal oxide seal. This seal, however, about 20–25 Å below the nominal surface plane, arrests further oxidation of more deeply lying loose-packed copper crystallites that have a huge surface area. These small crystallites in particular could well be the target for microbial adherence, since the 'crystallite' size may be almost as small as individual molecules – a liquid-like surface with essentially no intercrystalline spaces. Furthermore, the effect of the observed reflection trap ('seal') in the surface of the copper tubes can also be produced by the degree of close packing of Cu_2O crystallites, which gradually increase the depth of the trap. The 'crystalline' size may be first as small as individual molecules – a liquid-like surface with essentially no intercrystalline space. Also, in competing with oxidative processes, particularly in the presence of the biofilm, the liquid-like surface affects the density maximum, resulting in limited-depth intercrystalline adsorption of oils, residues of the biofilm, metabolic products, e.g. pyruvic acid, HO_2^-, or bacteria. Moreover, electrons that move from inside the copper (or oxide) surface to attack the oxygen (CO_2, HCO_3^-) or groups of the biofilm in a process similar to chemisorption result in an excess of electrons at the metal surface, e.g. n-type material (Thies *et al.*, 1994*a*).

Another interesting possibility in early biofilm deposition on such surfaces is that the copper crystallites may grow vertically and then 'bridge over', enclosing holes at the substrate. If, as the biofilm thickness increases, such vertical aggregation with subsequent lateral 'bridging over' continues to occur, enclosing holes that are much smaller than those adjacent to the substrate, in the long term the embedded holes will tend to collapse.

Whilst physical studies will eventually confirm the mechanism of adhesion between metal surfaces and inorganic/organic polymeric materials, it is essential to explore the chemical structure of the biofilm in more detail. It is very likely that new sequence techniques will have to be developed. The stereochemistry of certain groups arranged within the biopolymers has to be established in purified and homogeneous biofilms. In addition, conformational studies in solution will exploit different processes with respect to flocculation transition states, gelling and coacervation when biofilm materials come into contact with metal surfaces. Various physicochemical techniques, e.g. NMR, SERS, fluorescence techniques, contact-angle measurements as well as X-ray reflectivity experiments, may give some answers to the detailed structure of the biofilm and metal surfaces.

Molecular modelling as well as quantum mechanical calculations on known parts of the biofilm can yield valuable information about possible conformations, stability in solution and biofilm–solution interactions.

Another, yet unsolved, problem is the mechanism of interaction of a microorganism with a metal surface. It is necessary to gain an understanding of any recognition sites on the cells at a molecular level.

At present there are more questions than real experimental evidence for a discrete mechanism. However, the combination of surface-sensitive methods and molecular biological techniques together with carefully designed experiments using clearly defined parameters will yield the most promising results.

Recent developments

Despite the still unknown mechanisms of the deterioration of metal surfaces by microorganisms, two main steps of the microbial action are essential: (a) initial binding to surfaces, and (b) accumulation (or aggregation) of microorganisms at surfaces, accompanied by a production of exopolymeric substances. Recent experiments on the atypical salt regulating strain of *Xanthomonas comprestis* and *Pseudomonas aeruginosa* 44T1 indicate the presence of a protein of M_r 96 000 with a subunit stoichiometry of the α,β type, responsible for the biosynthesis of exopolymers (Hinze *et al.*, unpublished data). Expression of protein activity as assessed by the production of exopolymeric substances is strongly dependent on the nature of the surface (hydrophobic versus hydrophilic) and the source of the material, e.g. metal, glass or ceramics.

Physically solid surfaces covered with long-chain polymers that are grafted and irreversibly adsorbed onto the metal surface have important consequences with respect to adhesion, protection of the surface and finally, in preventing destruction of the foreign object by microorganisms, by 'walling off', covering or encapsulating the object. Therefore, the composition and organization of the biofilm layer will influence subsequent physical and chemical surface events. Therefore, it is essential to characterize the surface of any materials, e.g. metallic, non-metallic or biomaterials. In order to establish quantitative correlations between chemicals in the surface, particularly in metal–film interactions, acid–base thermodynamics, adhesion strength and locus-of-failure have to be demonstrated. Strong adhesive bonds between the biofilm and any metal surface require intimate interfacial contact to permit intermolecular interactions across the interface. The thermodynamic energy of adhesion, W_a, indicates the degree of intermolecular interaction. This is the sum of contributions from London–Lifshitz dispersion interactions (W_d) and Lewis acid–base (electron donor–acceptor) interactions (W_{ab}) between the molecules (Good & van Oss, 1992):

$$W_a = \gamma_1 + \gamma_2 - \gamma_{12} = W_d - W_{ab} \tag{7.4}$$

γ_1 and γ_2 being the surface free energies of the individual components and γ_{12} the interfacial free energy between metal surface and biofilm. It is primarily the acid–base component of the energy of adhesion that has the potential for enhancement, via surface modification of the metal surface, to increase (decrease) interfacial interactions by modulating adhesive bonds (Hinze *et al.*, 1994; Thies *et al.*, 1994*a*). This is also extremely important for bacterial adhesion to metallic surfaces.

The adhesion of *P. aeruginosa* 44T1 to copper or iron surfaces is driven by the balance between the surface energies of the polar and the dispersive components (γ_S^P and γ_S^D) of the solid metal surface, respectively, rather than by the total surface energy, γ_S, or by wettability by the metallic surface.

Therefore, polar interactions can appreciably reduce bacterial adhesion to metal surfaces, or increase it through interaction with a biofilm. This may provide a substantial economic incentive to evaluate counter measures to microbially influenced corrosion (Geesey *et al.*, 1986; Fischer *et al.*, 1994; Wagner *et al.*, 1994).

Membrane-mimetic behaviour of the biofilms has to be considered also (Paradies, 1986; Chamberlain *et al.*, 1994), particularly for generating toward the metal surface an H^+ gradient that depends on the pK_a of the biofilm, pH and the composition of the water. Another aspect is the production of metallic copper and copper oxide clusters as growing nanoparticles with fractal geometry due to micellar catalysis of the biofilm as observed in the presence of xanthan or alginate when used as artificial biofilms (Paradies *et al.*, 1994c). Considering the magnitude of the Donnan effect, the important parameter is the ratio of the concentration of charge from the biofilm (biopolymer) to the total concentration of ionic species present in solution oriented towards the metal surface. According to the Donnan ratio, R_D:

$$R_D = \frac{(Me^+)^1}{(Me^+)^2} = \frac{(X^-)^2}{(X^-)^1} \tag{7.8}$$

where Me^+ is the metal ion, X^- is Cl^- or HCO_3^- and 1 and 2 the different sites on the membrane. In the presence of salt, which is unequally distributed on both sites (1 and 2), this yields:

$$R_D - Z(\text{biofilm})/[S] - 1 = 0 \tag{7.9}$$

where Z is the charge and [S] the salt concentration.

In the case where Z (biofilm)/2[S] = 10, $R_D = 20$, so there is a 20-fold excess of Na^+ or H^+ on site (1) towards the metal and a 20-fold excess of Cl^- on site (2) towards the inner site of the biofilm membrane. This situation is achieved at rather low concentrations of salt, e.g. 10^{-2}–10^{-4} M NaCl. This is equivalent to a Donnan potential of $\phi_D = 75$ mV, as observed in laboratory experiments (Siedlarek *et al.*, 1994). Therefore the Donnan effect clearly deserves serious consideration, particularly where binding of ions to a macromolecule is studied by means of equilibrium dialysis, as emphasized by a recent study (Yang *et al.*, 1990).

The author thanks the International Copper Research Association, New York City, and the Ministry of Research and Technology, Bonn, Germany, for financial support and encouragement. Especially, I thank: my colleague Professor W. Fischer for introducing me to the field of corrosion science and for valuable discussions on biofilms; MEDICE, Inc., for support in conducting the FAB–MS analysis of the various biofilms; Mrs Kirsten Huschke for her patience in typing the manuscript; BCS for long lasting support; and Professor Dr S. B. Hanna (UMR), Department of Chemistry, for his support and hospitality. I thank also Dr Georg Cypher (ICA, New York) for his continuous interest in the subject, and many encouraging discussions about copper chemistry and physics. Special appreciation goes to Dr Christine Gaylarde for criticism, suggestions and patience during the editing process.

References

Absolom, D. R. & Neumann, A. W. (1987). Colloid and surface phenomena in immunology. In *Surface and Colloid Science*, vol. 14, ed. E. Matiyevic, pp. 215–64. Plenum Press, New York and London.

Adamson, A. W. (1982). *Physical Chemistry of Surfaces*. Wiley-Interscience, New York.

Aspinall, G. O. (ed.) (1983). *The Polysaccharides*, vols. 1–3. Academic Press, New York.

Aspinall, G. O. (1987). Chemical modification and selective fragmentation of polysaccharides. *Accounts of Chemical Research*, **20**, 114–20.

Aspinall, G. O., Charlson, A. J., Hirst, E. L. & Young, R. (1963). The location of L-rhamnopyranose residues in gum arabic. *Journal of the Chemical Society*, 1686–702.

Aspinall, G. O. & Rossell, K. G. (1978). Cleavage of glycopyranosiduronamide linkages in methylated polysaccharides. *Canadian Journal of Chemistry*, **56**, 685–90.

Au, C. T., Breza, J. & Roberts, M. W. (1979). Hydroxylation and dehydroxylation at Cu[1,1,1] surfaces. *Chemical and Physical Letters*, **66**, 340–3.

Beech, I. B. & Gaylarde, C. C. (1989). Adhesion of *D. desulfuricans* and *P. fluorescens* to mild steel surfaces. *Journal of Applied Bacteriology*, **67**, 201–7.

Carley, A. F., Rassias, S. & Roberts, M. W. (1983). The specificity of surface oxygen in the activation of water at metal surfaces. *Surface Science*, **135**, 35–51.

Chamberlain, A. H. L., Fischer, W. R., Hinze, U., Paradies, H. H., Sequeira, C. A. C., Siedlarek, H., Thies, M., Wagner, D. & Wardell, J. N. (1994). An interdisciplinary approach for microbially induced corrosion of copper. In *Microbial Corrosion*, vol. III, ed. C. A. C. Sequeira & A. K. Tiller. Elsevier Applied Science, London and New York, in press.

Characklis, W. G. (1980). *Biofilm Development and Destruction*. Final Report EPRI CS1554, Project RP902-1, Electric Power Research Institute, Palo Alto, CA.

Characklis, W. G. & Marshall, K. C. (1990). *Biofilms*. John Wiley and Sons, Inc., New York.

Chistholm-Brause, C. J., O'Day, P. A., Brown, G. E. Jr & Parks, G. A. (1990). Evidence for multinuclear metal–ion complexes at solid/water interfaces from X-ray absorption spectroscopy. *Nature*, **348**, 528–30.

Costerton, J. W., Geesey, G. G. & Cheng, K.-J. (1978). How bacteria stick. *Scientific American*, **238**, 86–95.

Daniels, L. D., Belay, N., Rayagopal, B. S. & Weimer, P. J. (1987). Bacterial methanogenesis and growth from CO_2 with elemental iron as the sole source of electrons. *Science*, **237**, 509–11.

Fischer, W., Haenßel, I. & Paradies, H. H. (1987). Gutachten: Schadensanalyse von Korrosionsshäden an Brauchwasserleitungen aus Kupferrohren im Kreiskrankenhaus Lüdenscheid/Hellersen, FRG. *Märkischer Kreis*, 17 March.

Fischer, W., Haenßel, I. & Paradies, H. H. (1988a). First results of microbial induced corrosion of copper pipes. In *Microbial Corrosion*, vol. I, ed. C. A. C. Sequeira & A. K. Tiller, pp. 300–28. Elsevier, Applied Science, London and New York.

Fischer, W., Haenßel, I. & Paradies, H. H. (1988b). The role of exopolymers on metallic surfaces. In *ACS Division Symposium, Colloid and Surface Science*, Toronto, abstract no. 241.

Fischer, W., Paradies, H. H., Haenßel, I., Angell, P. & Chamberlain. A. H. L. (1988c). Composition and structure of biofilms associated with copper in freshwater. *Eurocorrosion*, **1**, abstract no. 175.

Fischer, W., Paradies, H. H., Wagner, D. & Haenßel, I. (1992). Copper deterioration in a water distribution system of a county hospital in Germany caused by microbial induced corrosion. *Werkstoffe und Korrosion*, **43**, 56–62.

Fischer, W. R., Wagner, D. & Paradies, H. H. (1994). An evaluation of countermeasures to microbially influenced corrosion (MIC) in copper potable water supplies. In *Microbiologically Influenced Corrosion (MIC) Testing*, ASTM STP. 1232, ed. J. R. Kearns & B. Little, pp. 275–82. American Society for Testing and Materials, Philadelphia.

Ford, T. E., Maki, J. S. & Mitchell, R. (1987a). The role of metal-binding bacterial exopolymers in corrosion processes. In *Corrosion 87*, Paper No. 380. NACE, Houston, TX.

Ford, T. E., Walch, M. & Mitchell, R. (1987b). Corrosion of metals by thermophilic microorganisms. *Materials Performance*, **26**(2), 35–9.

Franz, A. & Paradies, H. H. (1976). Geometry of the ribosomal protein S4 in solution. *European Journal of Biochemistry*, **67**, 23–30.

Gaylarde, C. C. & Beech, I. B. (1988). Molecular basis of bacterial adhesion to metals. In *Microbial Corrosion*, vol. I, ed. C. A. C. Sequeira & A. K. Tiller, pp. 20–8. Elsevier Applied Science, London and New York.

Geesey, G. G., Mittelmann, M. W., Iwaoka, T. & Griffiths, P. R. (1986). Role of bacterial exopolymers in the deterioration of metabolic copper surfaces. *Materials Performance*, **25**, 37–40.

Good, R. J. & van Oss, C. J. (1992). The modern theory of contact angles and hydrogen bond components of surface energies. In *Modern Approaches to Wettability: Theory and Applications*, ed. M. E. Schrader & G. I. Loeb, pp. 1–27. Plenum Press, New York and London.

Goodall, D. M. & Norton, I. T. (1987). Polysaccharide conformation and kinetics. *Accounts of Chemical Research*, **20**, 59–65.

Gregory, J. (1982). The effect of polymers on dispersion properties. In *Flocculation by Polymers*, ed. Th. F. Tadros, pp. 301–11. Academic Press, London.

Gregory, I. (1987). Flocculation by polymers and polyelectrolytes. In *Solid/Liquid Dispersion*, ed. Th. F. Tadros, pp. 163–81. Academic Press, London.

Hadley, R. F. (1948). Corrosion by microorganisms in aqueous and soil environments. In *The Corrosion Handbook*, ed. H. H. Uhlig, pp. 466–81. John Wiley and Sons, Inc., New York.

Hanai, K., Kuwae, A., Kawai, S. & Ono, Y. (1989). Keto–enol tautomerism and vibrational spectra of phenylpyruvic acids. *Journal of Physical Chemistry*, **93**, 6013–15.

Harbon, S., Herman, G. & Clauser, H. (1968). Quantitative evaluation of O-glycosodic linkages between sugars and amino acids in ovine submaxillary gland mucoprotein. *European Journal of Biochemistry*, **4**, 265–72.

Hinze, U., Thies, M. & Paradies, H. H. (1994). Copper surface wettability and bacterial adhesion in biodeterioration of metallic copper. *Colloids and Surfaces*, in press.

Jencks, W. P. & Carriuolo, J. (1958). Structure of pyruvate in aqueous solution. *Nature*, **182**, 598–9.

Jolley, I. G., Geesey, G. G., Hawkins, M. R., Wright, R. B. & Wichlacz, P. L. (1987). Auger electron spectroscopy and X-ray photoelectron spectroscopy by gum arabic, bacterial culture supernatant and *Pseudomonas atlantica* exopolymer. *Surface and Interface Analysis*, **11**, 371–6.

Karlin, K. D. & Tyeklar, Z. (1989). Copper-dioxygen chemistry, a bioinorganic challenge. *Accounts of Chemical Research*, **22**, 241–8.

Kaspar, D. R. (1971). Theoretical and experimental investigations of the flocculation of charged particles in aqueous solutions by polyelectrolytes of opposite charge. Ph.D. thesis, California Institute of Technology.

Lederer, E. J. (1971). The mycobacterial cell wall. *Pure and Applied Chemistry*, **25**, 135–51.

Long, D. A. & George, W. O. (1960). Spectroscopic study of the pyruvate ion. *Transactions of the Faraday Society*, **56**, 1570–81.

Manning, G. S. (1969). Limiting laws and counterion condensation in polyelectrolyte solution. I. Colligative properties. *Journal of Chemical Physics*, **51**, 924–33.

Manning, G. S. (1978). The molecular theory of polyelectrolyte solutions with applications to the electrostatic properties of polynucleotides. *Quarterly Review of Biophysics*, **2**, 179–246.

Marshall, K. C. (1984). *Microbial Adhesion and Aggregation*. Springer-Verlag, Berlin.

Meister, A. (1965). *Biochemistry of the Amino Acids*, vol. II. Academic Press, New York.

Mittelmann, M. W. & Geesey, G. G. (1987). *Biological Fouling of Industrial Water Systems: A Problem Solving Approach*, Water Micro Associates, San Diego, CA.

Muller, G., Chauvetean, G. and Lecourtier, J. (1986). Salt-induced extension and dissociation of a native double-stranded Xanthan. *International Journal of Biological Macromolecules*, **8**, 306–10.

Norton, I. T., Goodall, D. M., Frangon, S. A., Morris, E. R. & Rees, D. A. (1984).

Mechanism and dynamics of conformational ordering in Xanthan polysaccharides. *Journal of Molecular Biology*, 175, 371–84.

O'Connell, W. J. Jr (1941). Characteristics of microbiological deposits in water circuits. *Proceedings of the American Petroleum Institute*, 23(III), 66–83.

Ogston, A. G. (1981). *Chemistry and Technology of Water Soluble Polymers*, ed. C. A. Finch. Plenum Publishing Corporation, New York.

Overbeck, J. Th. (1976). Polyelectrolytes, past, present and future. *Pure and Applied Chemistry*, 46, 91–101.

Paradies, H. H. (1986). Proton-transfer rates of sulfonamides in natural and fully synthetic membranes. *Journal of Physical Chemistry*, 90, 5956–60.

Paradies, H. H., Haenßel, I., Fischer, W. & Wagner, D. (1990). *Microbial Induced Corrosion on Copper Pipes*. INCRA Report no. 444, New York.

Paradies, H. H. (1994). Surface-enhanced Raman scattering, photoelectron X-ray spectroscopy and extended absorption fine structure spectroscopy of copper complexes of deteriorated copper surfaces. *Berichte der Bunsengesellschaft für Physikalische Chemie*, in press.

Paradies, H. H., Haenßel, I. & Fischer, W. (1988). Interfacial growth of microorganisms on copper surfaces. ACS-Division *Symposium, Colloid and Surface Science*, Toronto, abstract no. 245.

Paradies, H. H., Haenßel, I., Fischer, W. & Wagner, D. (1992). Microbial induced copper corrosion: a detailed chemical and physical analysis, I. *Werkstoffe und Korrosion*, 43, 496–507.

Paradies, H. H., Haenßel, I., Fischer, W. & Wagner, D. (1994a). Quantitative evaluation of O-glycosidic linkages between sugars and amino residues in biofilms due to corroding microorganisms on copper surfaces. II. *Journal of Organic Chemistry*, submitted for publication.

Paradies, H. H., Hinze, U. & Thies, M. (1994b). Donnan equilibria as observed on preparations of algenic acid. *Berichte der Bunsengesellschaft für Physikalische Chemie*, in press.

Paradies, H. H., Haenßel, I., Wagner, D. & Fischer, W. (1991). The role of exopolymers on copper surfaces. In *Microbial Induced Corrosion*, vol. II, ed. C.A.C. Sequeira & A. K. Tiller, pp. 163–88. Elsevier Applied Science, London and New York.

Rees, D. A. (1977). *Polysaccharide Shapes*. Chapman and Hall, London.

Rees, D. A. & Welsh, E. J. (1977). Sekundär- und Tertiärstruktur von Polysacchariden in Lösungen und Gelen. *Angewante Chemie*, 89, 228–39.

Roberts, M. W. (1988). Metal oxide overlayers and oxygen induced chemical reactivity studied by photoelectron spectroscopy. In *Surface and Near-Surface Chemistry of Oxide Materials*, ed. J. Nowotny & C.-C. Dufour, pp. 219–46. Elsevier Science Publishers B. V., Amsterdam.

Sato, T., Norisuye, T. & Fuyita, H. (1984). Multi-stranded helix of xanthan: dimensional and hydrodynamic properties in 0.1 M aqueous sodium chloride. *Macromolecules*, 17, 2696–700.

Scatchard, G., Scheinberg, I. H. & Armstrong, S. H. Jr (1950). Physical chemistry of protein solutions. *Journal of the American Chemical Society*, 72, 535–46.

Schultz, I. & Carré, A. (1982). The adhesion of polymers to high energy solids. In

Macromolecules, ed. H. Benoit & P. Rempp, pp. 289–304. Pergamon Press, New York and Frankfurt.

Sequeira, C. A. C. & Tiller, A. K. (eds.) (1988). *Microbial Corrosion*, vol. I. Elsevier Applied Science, London and New York.

Sequeira, C. A. C. & Tiller, A. K. (eds.) (1993). *Microbial Corrosion*, vol. III. Elsevier Applied Science, London and New York.

Sham, T. K. (1986). Application of X-ray absorption spectroscopy to the studies of structure and bonding of metal complexes in solution. *Accounts of Chemical Research*, 19, 99–104.

Siedlarek, H., Wagner, D., Fischer, W. R. & Paradies, H. H. (1994). A new approach to the understanding of microbiologically influenced corrosion of copper-ionic transport properties by biopolymers. *Corrosion Science*, in press.

Speckmann, H. D., Longrengel, M. M., Schultze, I. W. & Stenblow, H.-H. (1985). Growth and reduction of duplex oxide films on copper. *Berichte Bunsengesellschaft für Physikalische Chemie*, 89, 391–402.

Strehblow, H.-H. & Speckmann, H.-H. (1984). Corrosion and layer formation of passive copper in alkaline solution. *Werkstoffe und Korrosion*, 35, 512–17.

Tanford, C. (1961). *Physical Chemistry of Macromolecules*. Wiley, New York.

Tatnall, R. E. (1981). Fundamentals of bacteria induced corrosion. *Materials Performance*, 20, 32–8.

Thies, M., Hinze, U. & Paradies, H. H. (1994a). Physical behaviour of biopolymers as artificial models for biofilms in biodeterioration of copper. Solution and surface properties of biopolymers. In *Microbial Corrosion*, vol. III, ed. C. A. C. Sequeira & A. K. Tiller. Elsevier Applied Science, London and New York, in press.

Thies, M., Hinze, U. & Paradies, H. H. (1994b). Fractal geometry of flocculated colloid copper hydroxide sols. *Physical Reviews Letters*, in press.

Wagner, D., Fischer, W. R. & Paradies, H. H. (1994). Correlation of field and laboratory microbiologically influenced corrosion (MIC) data for a copper potable water installation. In *Microbiologically influenced Corrosion (MIC) Testing*, ASTM STP. 1232, ed. J. R. Kearns & B. Little, pp. 253–65. American Society for Testing and Materials, Philadelphia.

Vali, H. & Kirschvink, J. . (1989). Magneto fossil dissolution in a palaeomagnetically unstable deep sea sediment. *Nature*, 339, 203–4.

Yang, L. K., Harpt, N., Grasmick, D., Vuong, L. N. & Geesey, G. G. (1990). A two-phase model for determining the (?) constants for interactions between copper and alginic acid. *Journal of Physical Chemistry*, 94, 482–8.

Yoshida, S. & Ishida, H. (1984). The effect of surface oxide layers on the oxidative behaviour of imidazole-treated copper. *Journal of Materials Science*, 19, 2323–35.

Zobell, C. E. (1943). The effect of solid surfaces on bacterial activity. *Journal of Bacteriology*, 46, 39–56.

8

Monitoring techniques for biologically induced corrosion

ROGER A. KING

Introduction

Biological growths on engineering materials can affect the performance of the plant, structure or component. Typical problems raised by engineers are loss of heat transfer in heat exchangers, corrosion or deterioration of the material of construction, increased pumping costs, increased loading on structures from wave action, unacceptable odours, blockage of filters and spoilage of product. It has proved difficult to evaluate the economic cost of these effects as the costs are hidden in general maintenance budgets. Not surprisingly, in the absence of hard facts on the costs of adverse microbial activity many engineers dismissed such growth in plant or on structures as a minor irrelevance and nuisance but not a major cost item. This perception is, however, changing.

First, the costs of corrosion and fouling have been evaluated (Table 8.1). Corrosion has been generally estimated to cost around 3–4% of the Gross National Product (GNP) of a nation, though this varies depending on the degree and nature of the industrialization of the nation (Anon, 1971; Payer *et al.*, 1978). The contribution to this cost from microbiological deterioration has not been identified except for underground corrosion (Booth, 1964; Wakerley, 1979), where up to 50% of corrosion was claimed to result from microbial activity. Overall costs of adverse microbial growth in industry

Table 8.1. *Costs of corrosion in individual industries in the UK and notes on microbial aspects of these industries*

Industry	%GNP	Microbial aspects
Building	18	Underground corrosion, moulds, dry and wet rot, septic sewage deterioration, air conditioning and water handling systems, coating deterioration
Food	3	Cooling water systems, sulfur stinkage
General engineering	8	Cutting oil deterioration, surface etching by moulds, lubricant breakdown
Government departments	4	Materials degradation in storage, fuel spoilage (mainly defence aspects)
Marine	21	Fouling of ship bottoms, fuel spoilage, filter blockages, pitting of piling and plate
Metal refining	1	Water treatment, surface etching
Oil and chemical	13	Internal and external pitting of vessels and pipelines, structural loading, plugging of reservoirs
Power	4	Cooling-water fouling, heat transfer loss
Transport	26	Fuel spoilage, filter bloackages
Water	2	Internal and external corrosion, pipe blockage, septic sewage

Note: From Anon, 1971.

have been estimated to be 0.5% GNP for the UK (Pritchard, 1981), though this evaluation includes corrosion costs; however, the bulk was identified as the energy penalty arising from the loss of heat-exchange capacity. As an illustration of the energy penalty of microfouling, films of 0.001–0.01 in. may reduce heat transfer by 10–50% (Haderlie, 1977). Second, utility costs have risen sharply over the last two decades, in particular energy and water costs. Third, the construction of modern plant and structures incorporates far less redundancy – modern plant is significantly more efficient. This arises from the combination of use of computer design techniques and improvement in the consistency of materials. Equipment can now be constructed with less material, heat-exchanger surfaces sized to closer tolerances, and equipment operated at higher temperatures and pressures. The result is an increased emphasis on materials performance. This emphasis is shown by the increase in the number of engineers involved in corrosion prevention.

Over the last 20 years the membership of corrosion associations has trebled and the number of publications dealing with corrosion has increased five-fold. Modern industry has largely designed out the 'simple' corrosion problems and not surprisingly, therefore, emphasis has moved to the minor, more complex corrosion aspects, which include microbial corrosion. As a field of study, microbial corrosion has seen a very significant upsurge in interest, annual publications increasing nearly ten-fold over the last two decades.

To put some financial perspective on the level of monitoring, the oil production industry spends around $12M per annum on testing for sulfate-reducing bacteria, comparing biocides in laboratory studies and on other relatively routine microbial tests. It is likely that the process industry, environmental and minor interest areas spend a similar sum on microbial monitoring. Though these sums ($20M–25M p.a.) are relatively minute in comparison to the amount spent on medical testing, the consequent amount spent on biocides, corrosion inhibitors, mechanical cleaning and environmental control programmes is massive.

Background

Microbial corrosion rarely occurs as an isolated phenomenon. Usually microbial processes are part of complex interactive processes that involve surface fouling with deposits and scales, local galvanic effects resulting from metallurgical variations in the metal surface, and differential aeration or concentration cells. When the plant or equipment is opened for inspection the conditions are markedly changed as the corrosion products oxidize in the presence of air or dry out. Until recently, engineers relied almost totally on periodic inspection for ensuring plant reliability. During these shutdowns there would be little or no time to do more than cursory analysis of the corrosion products; the emphasis would be on putting the plant back into service as soon as possible.

The increased complexity and cost of plant and the need to maintain a high return on investment means that there has been a change in emphasis away from inspection to monitoring. It is rare nowadays for plant to have an annual shutdown. Corrosion engineers increasingly rely on continuous or semicontinuous monitoring of the status of the plant from which to calculate trends in plant condition. From these trends they can schedule a refurbishment programme. This change in philosophy arose from the 'If it ain't broke, don't fix it' approach, applying the methods of preventative maintenance. The emphasis has thus changed to the measurement of on-stream parameters from which plant condition can be deduced. Modern microbial sampling and analysis are geared towards this monitoring approach.

Though some of the techniques have been 'borrowed' from the more advanced medical and food technology areas, there has been a rapid modification of these techniques to make them less sensitive to the skills of the operator. It is usually impracticable to rely on techniques requiring complex equipment or a high level of dexterity or skill; the industrial environment demands periodic repetitive but intensive testing under difficult conditions. The cost of providing this service by employment of specialists would be prohibitive; instead, the plant operatives must develop sufficient competence to allow them to provide the information required on a routine basis. Monitoring techniques that are successful are thus those providing consistent results quickly and reliably with minimum skill and equipment. The emphasis is necessarily on quantitative values that can be used to assess trends; purely qualitative information is often much less valuable.

The microorganisms that have been most studied are the sulfate-reducing bacteria (SRB). These organisms produce sulfide during growth and advertise their presence by simple testing. Other more discrete organisms have been less studied:

> sulfur-oxidizing bacteria, which cause concrete decay in sewers and damage to mining equipment;
>
> *Hormoconis resinae*, the fungus that degrades kerosene and causes filter blockage and metal damage in aircraft wing tanks and high performance surface ships;
>
> nitrite-oxidizing bacteria, which affect the corrosion inhibitors used in water circulation systems;
>
> oil-degrading organisms, which affect lubricants and cutting oils and some organic coatings (typically pseudomonads and *Aerobacter*);

slime-generating organisms, which affect heat exchange units;

iron-oxidizing bacteria, which cause blockage of water mains.

It should be noted that it is rarely necessary to identify these organisms at the species level. The corrosion engineer tends to regard them as groups of microorganisms that require specific treatments for control. If SRB are identified in a soil close to a pipeline then the engineer will adjust the protective coating and cathodic protection scheme to account for their presence. If similar organisms are found in the production fluids then the emphasis for control will be on the selection of an efficient biocide. Organisms that do not represent a threat to the operation of the plant or equipment are disregarded. Clearly this approach simplifies the requirements for the monitoring technique and also the skills needed to operate the technique.

Microbial consortia

Brief reference has been made to the complexity of fouling deposits on process plant equipment surfaces. Charaklis (1985) gave a neat classification of fouling phenomena:

1. Biological fouling.
2. Chemical reaction fouling.
3. Corrosion fouling.
4. Freezing fouling: deposit of low melting point materials on to cool surfaces.
5. Particulate fouling.
6. Sedimentation fouling: gravity settlement of material.
7. Precipitation fouling.
8. Scaling.

The combination of these fouling phenomena will be specific to a particular industry and process. For example, the oil industry suffers from types 1, 3, 4, 7 and 8 in oil production pipelines and from types 1, 3 and 8 in water injection systems. It is important that the microbe monitoring technique selected takes into account the alternative fouling processes.

Usually there is a range of microorganisms present that represents the most efficient balance of organisms for the particular plant conditions. The normal pattern observed is a limited range of organisms in a new plant – or in an older plant after a successful cleansing treatment. After a period the variety of organisms increases before declining to a limited variety of dominant organisms. The particular species and their balance will relate to the water quality, temperature, flow rate and biocide treatment regime. It is usual practice to change the biocide periodically to ensure that the regime does not allow the development of a consortia of bacteria resistant to the particular biocide.

The biofilm is often seen as active throughout its depth (Costerton & Geesey, 1985), though this is not borne out by analysis (Miller, 1982). Experience (King, 1980) also indicates that treatment of biofilms is expedited by the use of detergents, which strip the film from the metal surface, rather than by biocides, which merely treat the outer active surface. Indeed the new generation of biocides combines surface-active material with biocide.

Sampling

Whatever the monitoring technique used there remains a need to bolster the information using a conventional microbial enumeration. Most industrial microbial enumeration is done in the laboratory after sampling of the fluid streams, deposits or soils. Clearly the method of sampling is critical to the quality of the data derived from the analysis. Each industrial environment demands that a different sampling technique and guidance from specific industrial recommended practices should be sought (Miller, 1971; NACE, 1990).

Water streams are relatively simple to sample. Care must be taken when water is withdrawn through a side-tapping to allow the water to flow for long enough to ensure that the sample is not contaminated from atypical growths in the side-tapping line and valve. The use of clean sterile sampling containers is desirable. Where this is not possible the containers should be as clean as possible and rinsed thoroughly either with very hot water or with several changes of the water being sampled. The clean containers should be capped and the caps only removed prior to taking the sample; caps should then be replaced.

Oily water systems present problems as it is often difficult to obtain a sufficient volume of water. Repeat samples may need to be taken and the water decanted. It is useful to record the water cuts from these repeat samples so that the microbial numbers can be related back to the actual water content. In many cases an emulsion will be satisfactory but this assumption needs to be tested on a specific basis as some chemicals with biocidal properties are concentrated at the water/emulsion interface. It is extremely difficult to avoid external contamination during such a procedure and it is prudent to have the sample examined as soon as possible to minimize the effect of this contamination. Sampling solids can also represent considerable difficulties in minimizing external contamination. It is worth while trying a 'dry run' for new equipment to evaluate the contamination problems that may arise.

In some cases the level of microorganisms will be very low and some form of consolidation is needed. Filtration of large volumes of water through 0.45 μm pore membranes is suitable or large samples can be taken to the laboratory for centrifugation. NACE Standard TM-01-73 (NACE, 1992) gives details of membrane filtration methods. Clearly it is necessary to record the original volume of water sampled so that the microbial count can be related to the fluid streams.

For biofilm monitoring, special equipment can be used; it provides removable studs on which the biofilm has developed. This equipment is described below.

When a sample is taken a record should be made on the sample container or the container logged with the following information:

  date of sampling, time and location;

  temperature of the fluid stream sampled;

  pH of the fluid sampled;

  notes on the colour, turbidity, smell (especially of hydrogen sulfide), presence of slimes or deposits;

  notes on the chemical regime underway at the time of sampling, with particular reference to bioactive chemicals.

Overview of monitoring techniques

The use of growth media for plate counts and serial dilutions still represents the bulk of routine industrial microbial monitoring. The media used tend to be of limited specificity since the engineer requires only global figures. Some service companies do provide qualitative analysis of the microorganisms but this is rarely on a routine basis, is rarely exhaustive and is considered more as a sales ploy than as being necessary for deciding whether treatment is needed or for biocide selection.

The problem with the conventional culture techniques is the time needed to allow growth to detectable levels; up to 10 days may be required for low to medium populations of low activity organisms. Considerable effort has been expended on developing rapid analysis techniques that will provide quantitative information within hours if not minutes. This is the major area of development at present and the rapid techniques range from ATP analysis and radiorespirometry to enzyme analysis techniques and the use of polyclonal antibodies.

Microscopic examination is generally considered impracticable for general industrial usage, since the waters contain considerable debris. For specific types of algae and protozoa, however, the technique remains necessary (ASTM D1128). Recently the use of fluorescent tagging has revived microscopy as a rapid technique for general enumeration.

Since the late 1970s there has been an increased emphasis on the enumeration of microorganisms in biofilms on metal surfaces. The number of organisms in biofilms can be 10^2 to 10^4 times greater than in the water phase. It has always been common practice to provide small removable metal or plastic plates for the growth of microorganisms. These samples would be removed and stored in source water for transfer to the laboratory. For high pressure systems, insertion or side-stream equipment incorporating small removable studs is now common place. This type of equipment provides biofilm for periodic analysis, which gives a snapshot in time of the status of the microbial consortia, rather similar to weight loss coupons used for corrosion monitoring. The range of techniques to evaluate the biofilm on the studs is steadily increasing in sophistication and covers conventional culture techniques, ATP fluorescence and radiotracer techniques.

Continuous or semicontinuous monitoring is now being developed using electrochemical techniques. The problem is that these techniques give information on all the reactions occurring on the metal surface and there is no known method at present that can isolate the microbial contribution. The microbial component has to be deduced from the conventional fluid or biofilm monitoring. Monitoring techniques that are likely to be developed in the near future include light reflectance from the surfaces of fibre optics, electrochemical probes with self-cleaning surfaces incorporated, capacitance and electrochemical noise signal analysis.

Table 8.2. *Media for enumeration of heterotrophic bacteria*

Serial dilution

Beef extract	3.0 g
Peptone	5.0 g
Distilled water	1.0 litre

pH adjusted to 7 with NaOH prior to sterilization

Plate counts for low salinity waters

Beef extract	3.0 g
Tryptone	5.0 g
Dextrose	1.0 g
Agar	15.0 g
Distilled water	1.0 litre

pH adjusted to 7 with NaOH prior to sterilization

Plate counts for high salinity waters

Peptone	5.0 g
Yeast extract	1.0 g
Ferric citrate	0.1 g
Sodium chloride	19.5 g
Magnesium chloride	8.8 g
Sodium sulfate	3.3 g
Calcium chloride	1.8 g
Potassium chloride	0.6 g
Sodium bicarbonate	0.2 g
Agar	15.0 g
Distilled water	1.0 litre

pH adjusted to 8 with NaOH prior to sterilization

Monitoring using culture techniques

General heterotrophic bacteria are enumerated to provide a measure of the biological loading of the system. Clearly, heavily infested systems are likely to have more corrosion problems than systems with low counts. However, there is no agreed correlation between numbers and corrosion. Typical recipes for the growth media of these and similar organisms are given in Tables 8.2 to 8.4.

Table 8.3. *Basal medium for enumeration of oil-oxidizing bacteria*

Ammonium nitrate	2.5 g
Potassium chloride	0.3 g
Potassium dihydrogen phosphate	2.0 g
Magnesium sulfate (.7H$_2$O)	1.0 g
Calcium chloride (.6H$_2$O)	1.0 mg
Ferrous sulfate (.7H$_2$O)	2.0 mg
Zinc sulfate (.7H$_2$O)	2.0 mg
Manganese sulphate (.4H$_2$O)	1.5 mg
Sodium chloride	5.0 mg
Distilled water	1.0 litre

Salinity adjusted with sodium chloride to match source water

pH adjusted to 7 with NaOH before sterilization

Table 8.4. *Medium for enumeration of fermentative acid producers*

Beef extract	3.0 g
Yeast extract	3.0 g
Peptone	15.0 g
Ascorbic acid	0.1 g
Neutral red indicator	10.0 g
Distilled water	1.0 litre

Salinity adjusted with sodium chloride to match source water

pH adjusted to 7 with NaOH before sterilization

Enumeration of SRB is by serial dilution. The important requirement is to minimize the contact of the air with the medium. To this end the growth medium bottles comprise 9 ml of medium in a small glass phial fitted with a rubber septum. The water is injected into the phial with a hypodermic syringe. Suitable media are listed in Table 8.5. (Further details of the methods used are given in NACE, 1990.)

Table 8.5. *Media for enumeration of sulfate-reducing bacteria*

Modified API medium

Sodium sulfate	1.0 g
Sodium lactate (60–70% solution)	4.0 g
Yeast extract	1.0 g
Ascorbic acid	0.1 g
Magnesium sulfate (.7H$_2$O)	0.2 g
Potassium hydrogen phosphate	10.0 mg
Ferrous ammonium sulphate (.6H$_2$O)	0.2 g
Distilled water	1.0 litre

Salinity adjusted with sodium chloride or 70% source water, reducing the distilled water by this volume

pH adjusted to 7.3 with NaOH before sterilization

Modified Postgate medium

Potassium dihydrogen phosphate	0.5 g
Ammonium chloride	1.0 g
Sodium sulfate	1.0 g
Calcium chloride (.6H$_2$O)	0.1 g
Magnesium sulfate (.7H$_2$O)	2.0 g
Sodium lactate (60–70% solution)	5.0 g
Yeast extract	1.0 g
Sodium thioglycolate	0.1 g
Sodium ascorbate	0.1 g
Ferrous sulfate (.7H$_2$O)	0.5 g
Distilled water	1.0 litre

Salinity adjusted with sodium chloride

pH adjusted to 7.3 with NaOH before sterilization

Modified iron sulfite medium

Tryptone	10.0 g
Sodium sulfite	0.5 g
Iron citrate	0.5 g
Ferrous sulfate (.7H$_2$O)	0.5 g
Sodium lactate (60–70%)	3.5 g
Magnesium sulfate (.7H$_2$O)	2.0 g

Table 8.5 (*cont.*)

Agar	12.0 g
Distilled water	1.0 litre

pH adjusted to 7 with NaOH before sterilization

Akzo Chemie medium

Potassium hydrogen phosphate	0.5 g
Ammonium chloride	1.0 g
Sodium sulfate	1.75 g
Sodium lactate (60–70%)	2.5 g
Sodium thioglycolate	0.5 g
Ascorbic acid	0.1 g
Magnesium sulfate (.7H$_2$O)	1.5 g
Calcium chloride (.2H$_2$O)	0.1 g
Ferrous sulfate (.7H$_2$O)	20 drops
Yeast extract	1.0 g
Double distilled water	250 ml
Seawater	750 ml

pH adjusted to 7.2 with NaOH prior to sterilization

Torry Research Station medium

Potassium hydrogen phosphate	0.5 g
Ammonium chloride	1.0 g
Sodium sulfate	1.0 g
Calcium chloride (.2H$_2$O)	0.1 g
Magnesium sulfate (.7H$_2$O)	2.0 g
Sodium lactate (70%)	5.0 g
Yeast extract	1.0 g
Distilled water	1.0 g
For seawater testing add NaC1	2.5 g

After splitting into 200 ml portions, the following are added:

Sodium thioglycolate	0.02 g
Sodium ascorbate	0.02 g
Ferrous sulfate	0.1 g
Resazurin solution 0.1%	0.2 ml

pH adjusted to 7.8 with NaOH prior to sterilization

Postgate medium E

Potassium dihydrogen phosphate	0.5 g
Ammonium chloride	1.0 g
Calcium chloride (.2H$_2$O)	1.0 g
Magnesium chloride (.7H$_2$O)	2.0 g
Sodium lactate	3.5 g
Ferrous sulfate (.7H$_2$O)	0.5 g
Yeast extract	1.0 g
Thioglycolic acid	0.1 g*
Ascorbic acid	0.1 g
Tap water	1.0 litre

pH adjusted to 7.6 with NaOH prior to sterilization

* Sterilized by membrane filtration and added after the autoclaving

Note: API, American Petroleum Institute.

To enumerate biofilm samples on studs or coupons it is usual to solubilize the biofilm into sterile water or medium using some form of mild vibration or agitation. Ultrasonic agitation should not be used as the ultrasound can kill viable organisms on the studs and so reduce the bacterial count. The suspended biofilm is then treated as a water sample and plate or serial dilution counts made. Solids may be treated in the same manner.

Incubation of the inoculated growth medium should be at a temperature not too far removed from the source temperature. To accelerate the growth rate without distressing the organisms the temperature may be increased by 5 deg.C SRB vials should be stored in the dark.

Most growth media have a limited shelflife. Growth vials should be marked with the date when the medium was prepared; the usual shelflife is 1 month. The American Petroleum Institute (API) growth medium for SRB can have its sensitivity and shelflife extended by incorporating a small iron nail into the growth vials prior to sterilization and adding a small quantity of ammonium or sodium sulfite (100 p.p.m. max.) to the medium. These additions reduce the effect of oxygen on the medium; the oxygen enters the vial through the rubber septum (Farinha & King, 1980). It is usual to use triplicate vials for serial dilution enumeration of SRB. The number of bacteria can then be evaluated using Most Probable Number (MPN) tables.

Trend analysis

Biocide treatments to kill microorganisms in water systems may be applied continuously or batchwise. In the light of environmental concerns there is a trend to batch use of biocides. In this procedure a concentrated slug of biocide is introduced into the process or water stream and is carried around the plant or along a pipeline by the general flow. Though the biocide slug is diluted somewhat, the technique does allow special arrangements to be made for safe disposal of the treated water stream. The period between batch treatments should be determined by monitoring of either the number of bacteria or the corrosion rate. Because the corrosion rate results from several conjoint processes it is more common to use the microbial population as the determining factor for biocide treatment.

When using enumeration techniques for determining the population of microorganisms and by inference the level of corrosion in a system it is common practice to evaluate the seriousness of the problem by trend analysis. In its simplest form this involves plotting the population against time. No matter how much care is taken in deriving the values, there is a large scatter. Most engineers decide on a value at which they will initiate a treatment programme or at which they will review the need for a change in the biocide. A typical figure for SRB is 10^3 cells/ml. When the values have exceeded this critical level for two or three adjacent time periods then the treatment programmes will be initiated. An alternative analysis technique uses a rolling average based on the latest three values.

A more complex basis for decision may be the combination of population level and corrosion monitoring. In this case there is a need to evaluate the percentage contribution to the corrosion from the microorganisms. Clearly, if there is only a tenuous link the constant use of biocide would be wasteful. The most common technique used is the combination of biofilm and weight loss. Here a biofilm evaluation device is used either in a side-stream or directly into the main flow. The studs are removed from the device and the biofilm evaluated in the conventional manner by suspension of the biofilm in a sterile solution followed by plating and serial counting. The surfaces of the studs may be analysed; the analysis used will depend on the process thought likely to be occurring. For example, analysis for sulfide deposits if SRB attack is suspected or, for aircraft fuel fungal contamination studies, grain boundary etching of the aluminium alloy studs would be undertaken. Usually the studs have been preweighed and after cleaning may be reweighed, allowing a weight loss to be calculated. Since the main cost is the installation and removal of the studs, it is usual to maximize the information that can be obtained after their exposure.

Rapid enumeration techniques

These techniques have been developed and tested on SRB for use in the oil production industry. Their use for other organisms will undoubtedly require experimentation and development.

ATP photometry

The use of ATP assays relies on an assumption of a similar ATP level per unit cell carbon regardless of genus and physiological state of the cells. This may be reasonable in laboratory cultures but is dubious in the field. The SRB reduce sulfate to sulfide in a series of steps beginning with sulfate to sulfite using ATP:

$$SO_4^{2-} + ATP \; APS + PP_i$$
$$APS \rightarrow SO_3^{2-} + ADP$$

A measure of ATP availability in a culture is perhaps also a measure of the propensity for sulfate reduction. However, indirect work on hydrogenase-related sulfate reduction did not reveal a clear link: pH, temperature, salinity, soluble iron content, phase of growth when in batch culture, all affected the rate of sulfate reduction. Other difficulties experienced when ATP is used for SRB enumeration result from the biogenic sulfide, which interferes with luciferase function. The luciferase is the active ingredient for detection of ATP; in combination light is emitted and this can be related directly to ATP concentration. Since this reaction is also time dependent, there is a need for a very regimented sampling procedure (Littmann, 1977). In practical systems, the SRB count is below 10^3 cells/ml. For ATP assay the numbers must be increased by a consolidation technique, usually for convenience by membrane filtration; however, some adverse effects on ATP levels have been noted.

The extraction procedures for ATP can also cause inaccuracies: samples will often be oily and contain active precipitates and SRB are often adherent to the particulate matter. Boiling buffers and strong alkalis are not recommended for SRB extraction and internal ATP standards are usually used to correct for losses during extraction of 'dirty' samples. Most experience so far has been with firefly luciferase, which is sensitive to sulfide and some biocides.

Overall this is the longest-established, alternative and quick technique requiring limited skill and equipment. However, there are many factors that can affect the results; the procedure is complicated and interfering species need to be identified or avoided. Evaluating samples, though rapid, has to be done very quickly after sampling. The main disadvantage, however, is the lack of specificity for SRB. As a general tool for water quality testing the procedure is good, once tuned to the particular environment or circumstances. It does not assist when SRB-specific testing is required.

Radiorespirometry

Though an established technique in conventional microbiological laboratories, the industrial applications for corrosion and associated studies have only recently become available. There remain many obstacles, not least the irrational fear of radioactivity per se. Most publicized has been the [^{35}S]sulfate reduction procedure, used initially for solid samples and biofilms, but extended to plankton populations (Fig. 8.1).

The technique involves growth of SRB on [^{35}S]sulfate in tubes that can be tightly sealed and contain, hanging from the bung or seal, a piece of filter paper folded concertinawise and saturated in zinc acetate. After a defined period of incubation, usually 12–40 h, the culture is acidified to stop the growth reactions and release hydrogen sulfide, which is trapped in the filter paper wick. The wick is transferred to a liquid scintillation counter calibrated for ^{35}S detection (Hardy & Syrett, 1983; Rosser & Hamilton, 1983).

The technique has been used quite widely and correlations of the values with traditional MPN enumerations have been reported (Maxwell, 1987). Sadly there does not appear to be any clear relationship. The later tests suggest that this results from the production of sulfides that are not rapidly released by acidification. For specific systems the procedure can be quantified but the process is very sensitive to delays between sampling and incubation.

Table 8.6. *Sulfate-reducing bacteria (SRB) corrosion hazard/risk assessment*

	Population		
Activity	High	Medium	Low
Low	Some risk (5)	Some risk (3)	Low risk (1)
Medium	High risk (8)	Some risk (5)	Some risk (2)
High	Extreme risk (10)	High risk (8)	Nests of SRB (7)

Note: Hazard/risk is assessed on a 0–10 basis, 10 representing extreme risk of corrosion damage.

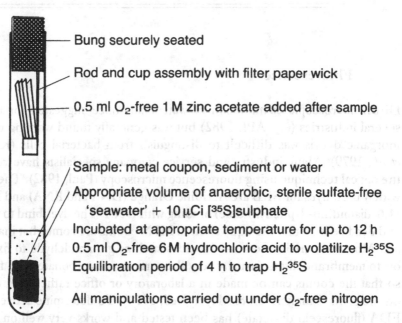

Bung securely seated

Rod and cup assembly with filter paper wick

0.5 ml O$_2$-free 1 M zinc acetate added after sample

Sample: metal coupon, sediment or water
Appropriate volume of anaerobic, sterile sulfate-free
'seawater' + 10 μCi [^{35}S]sulphate
Incubated at appropriate temperature for up to 12 h
0.5 ml O$_2$-free 6 M hydrochloric acid to volatilize H$_2$^{35}S
Equilibration period of 4 h to trap H$_2$^{35}S

All manipulations carried out under O$_2$-free nitrogen

Fig. 8.1 Apparatus for radiorespirometric detection of sulfate-reducing bacteria activity (after Maxwell & Hamilton, 1984).

The procedure was put forward as a means of quantifying the 'activity' of the SRB so that the engineering 'truth' table (see Table 8.6) related to biological corrosion hazard from SRB could be more closely assessed. The method does assist but is still too imprecise for general use; rate of blackening of conventional high iron SRB medium is still preferred (see Table 8.7).

Table 8.7. *Evaluation of numbers and activities of sulfate-reducing bacteria from conventional culturing by serial dilution*

Numbers/population evaluation	
Low	$<10^2$ cells/ml
Medium	10^2–10^4 cells/ml
High	$>10^4$ cells/ml
Activity evaluation	
Low	Blackening after 14 days
Medium	Blackening after 5 days but before 14 days
High	Blackening before 5 days

Fluorescence

Direct microscopic examination of waters was once suggested for use in several industries (e.g. API, 1982) but was generally found wanting in that inorganic debris was difficult to distinguish from bacterial cells (Kogure *et al.*, 1979). Many industry and service company specialists have revived the optical technique using fluorescence microscopy (Paul, 1982). The most widely used dyes for SRB are Acridine Orange (DNA and RNA) and DAPI (4,6-diamidino-2-phenylindole) binding with DNA. The dyes bind to viable and dead cells so that the equivalent to MPN counts are somewhat inaccurate. Most industrial testers use biocides such as glutaraldehyde to fix cells on to membrane filters (usually very flat surface polycarbonate pore filters) so that the counts can be made in a laboratory or office rather than *in situ* on the plant (Zimmerman & Meyer-Reil, 1974). To determine active cells, FDA (fluorescein diacetate) has been tested and works very well on water samples, though of course with all these optical methods all cells are counted, not SRB specifically.

Autoradiography has not yet been investigated, but would appear to be a promising technique using ^{35}S for SRB evaluation. In essence the bacteria are incubated with labelled material (usually intended to be incorporated into protein) then extracted on to membrane filters that are subsequently coated with photographic emulsion. The blackened silver spots can be counted.

Immunology

Immunological techniques would appear to offer a most suitable method for rapid *and* selective enumeration, even in complex environments. The main effort has been in the late 1980s in the USA and the UK, though research funding on this in the UK was unfortunately cut in the late 1970s. Both cases used specific antibodies (rabbit) stained with fluorescent dyes to produce SRB-specific fluorescence (Smith, 1982). To date, the resolution appears to be at the 3×10^3 cells/ml level, which implies for low population samples that there is a prior consolidation/extraction of SRB by filtration. The procedure developed for MTI uses rabbit antisera specific to SRB to bind with the SRB and later anti-immunoglobulin serum (sheep anti-rabbit) labelled with fluorescein thiocyanate (FTC; Pope & Zintell, 1988).

An alternative using the enzyme-linked immunosorbent assay (ELISA) has been developed and can detect down to 100 cells/ml (Bobowski, 1987; Gaylarde & Cook, 1987). This is a major step forward as it allows the usual industrial-sample low levels of SRB to be identified by filtration of reasonable volumes of water. It is very difficult to process much over 500 ml of typical industrial waters through bacterial quality filters; hence there is a lower limit to detection of cells/ml because of these practical limitations. In the ELISA, specific antigen is adsorbed on to a solid surface, the antiserum is added, incubated and washed. Specific SRB antiserum binds to SRB antigen and forms an antigen–antibody complex. An enzyme-labelled conjugate is added and attaches to the relevant anti-SRB serum. Enzyme substrate is added and incubated, followed by spectrophotometric measurement of the quantity of enzyme-hydrolysed substrate (usually arranged to be a colour change). Horseradish peroxidase has been used for the enzyme system.

APS reductase antibody

This is a similar technique to the ELISA method and has been developed by the DuPont Company (Odom *et al.*, 1987; Tatnall *et al.*, 1988). All SRB have a specific enzyme for the sulfate to sulfite reduction step, adenosine-*S*-phosphosulfate (APS) reductase. Antibodies are developed that are specific to this enzyme. The technique is straightforward. The SRB sample on a filter is cleaned of H_2S by rinsing then treated ultrasonically to disrupt the cells and release the APS reductase. A sample is taken and added to a tube containing a bead with antibody attached, and agitated. A colour-developing solution is added and the degree of coloration relates to the original population density of the SRB. The detection threshold appears to be 10^3 cells/ml.

Monoclonal antibody probes

The advantages of using monoclonal antibodies over polyclonal systems are the greater specificity and a more constant source of reactant. Lymphocytes or spleen cell antibodies are developed from hybrid myelomas from bone marrow, which are single lymphocyte producers, usually derived from mice. Some 77 monoclonal antibodies were produced in a particular test programme and from seven of these a broad-spectrum reagent for SRB was developed. The method has only recently begun to be field tested.

Gene probes

The possibility of using a DNA extract to identify and quantify SRB is attractive. The protein of interest would need to be both specific but general to SRB; cytochrome c_3 has been suggested. To date, these probes have been devised for organisms of medical interest but the biotechnological systems could easily be applied to industrial organisms such as SRB.

Hydrogenase test

This test has been developed by Caproco (Boivin, 1990). The SRB contain a hydrogenase that enables them to utilize hydrogen, evolved on metal and heavy metal sulfide surfaces, as an energy source. Consolidated samples from bulk filtration of water or solids are directly analysed. After digestion of the sample to lyse the cells and release the hydrogenase, the sample is placed in a hydrogen atmosphere and a reduced dye added that reacts with the hydrogenase. The quantity of hydrogenase is evaluated by the colour change of the dye, the basic assumption being that there is a direct relationship between SRB numbers and activity and colour intensity. SRB are, of course, not the only organisms that contain hydrogenase but in most industrial environments the results give values similar to conventional serial dilution evaluations.

Respirometry

The use of respirometry is not strictly a culture technique. When micro-organisms are active they consume oxygen or, if fermentative, produce gases (Wagner, 1986). SRB as resting cells consume hydrogen. When biocides are tested for time to kill, the level of testing can be very extensive and labour intensive. Farinha (1982) developed a respirometric method for evaluating the rate of biocidal action against SRB. The technique also gave some indication of the mode of operation of the biocide. For example quaternary ammonium compounds temporarily increased the rate of respiration as the cell membrane was degraded; glutaraldehyde caused a rapid fall in respirometric rate as the cell membrane became impermeable. The technique was found to be rapid and sensitive and, with semi-automatic equipment, required little labour.

Electrochemical methods of monitoring biofilms

General reviews on these techniques are available by Mansfeld & Little (1990) and Sussex et al. (1986).

Electrical resistance

Here a wire or thin tube or plate is exposed. As it corrodes, it becomes thinner and thus the electrical resistance increases. By measuring the change in resistance, the corrosion is measured. This is a widely used technique but has a drawback in that increased sensitivity means a thinner metal section and shorter life. Since biofilms usually cause pitting, the wires fail quickly and must be replaced. Equally any cause of thinning is measured, not only the biological aspect (Duquette & Ricker, 1986).

These probes have been used (Oganowski, 1985) to study the growth of SRB under marine fouling at different levels of cathodic protection (the probe can be polarized as an electrode). Such techniques are also being used for biological corrosion mechanisms at Harvard University (T. Ford, personal communication).

Linear polarization

Here, two metal electrodes are exposed and the potential (E) between them is fluctuated by up to 20 mV; the current response (i) is measured. At such low potential oscillations the relationship between E and i is linear, so a corrosion rate can be calculated. Such techniques have been widely used for microbiological studies where the corrosion rates with and without a biofilm/biological effect have been measured (Rosales, 1986; Videla *et al.*, 1987).

In the laboratory, this technique is cheap, rapid and reliable. It has been used to study SRB action on cast irons, copper–nickel alloys, C–Mn steels, and γ-stainless steels. In the field, where highly controlled conditions do not exist, such a technique does not give a characteristic signal related to biofilming alone.

Dynamic polarization

This is essentially the linear polarization method's 'big brother'. When the potential (E) on an electrode exceeds ±20 mV from its natural potential, then the current potential relationship is not linear but becomes logarithmic. The potential changes used are usually from ±500 mV to ±1000 mV. The technique does show the effects of biofilms (Gilbert *et al.*, 1987) but it also disturbs them or even destroys them such that a long period must elapse before the electrodes are refilmed as before.

Zero-resistance ammetry (ZRA)

Here two 'identical' electrodes are exposed, wired together through an electronic ammeter such that the measuring current is electronically compensated for and the electrodes are effectively short-circuited together. This technique was used in the earliest corrosion studies (done manually using null-detectors) and has blossomed again since the late 1970s with the advent of reliable microchip operational amplifiers. It has begun to be used for biofilm work (Little *et al.*, 1985; Wagner & Little, 1986). The findings (Gilbert *et al.*, 1987; Dexter *et al.*, 1989) that biofilms cause major interfacial alterations and potential differences on surfaces may be an indicator that such a technique, coupled to potential measurement, may be one of the most suitable methods of biofilm evaluation.

AC impedance/electrochemical impedance

Here the potential of one electrode with respect to another (or reference electrode) is oscillated sinusoidally (AC) but at an ever changing frequency from kHz to mHz. The current response is measured and its lead/lag calculated. The results can be presented as Bode plots (impedance versus frequency) or as Nyquist plots (imaginary versus real impedance). The shape and location on the axes of these plots gives valuable information as to the condition of the surface and hence the condition of the biofilm.

The technique requires expensive and complex equipment and is used presently only in the laboratory, for mechanistic studies (Merrique, 1978; Gilbert *et al.*, 1987; Moosavi, 1987; J. C. Danko, personal communication). Simpler forms of equipment are evolving and thus impedance techniques may be practicably applicable more widely in the near future.

Signal analysis techniques

Here, a sensitive recording voltmeter is used to monitor the natural fluctuations in the potential of an exposed electrode or in the current flowing through a ZRA system. A given pattern of fluctuations in the potential is characteristic of a surface process, e.g. film formation and breakdown. This technique was used by Iverson (1968; Iverson *et al.*, 1985) to determine SRB attack on buried pipelines. More recently, the signals have been captured on microcomputer and analysed by amplitude/frequency modelling. It appears that particular distribution patterns are related to particular events. To date, it is possible to determine SRB activity but only by a combination of noise signals and potential shift (King & Eden, 1988*a*).

Combined techniques

The signals received from the surface of our electrodes reflect the processes occurring thereon: corrosion, biofilm development, scaling, precipitation. To determine the extent of a particular process, e.g. biofilming, it is necessary to extract the relevant part of the signal. This clearly is not possible except under defined conditions. However, the engineer rarely needs absolute information. For example, if he or she knows there is a biofilm problem then monitoring of this is required until it becomes unacceptable, at which point a biocide treating programme will be initiated; now information is required on the efficiency of the treatment programme. This is possible using a set of electrochemical monitoring techniques but not by one monitoring procedure alone. The most useful combination appears at present to be potential plus potential noise and current noise through ZRA systems, or at least for SRB-laden biofilms (Cubicciotti & Licina, 1989). 'Simpler' biofilms may have a clearer fingerprint. Also worth considering is the option of using active (corrodible) and inert electrodes so that the biofilm component can be more easily identified from the combined signal.

Biofilm equipment

Understanding of the role of biofilms in corrosion has steadily improved. To a large extent this emphasis on biofilms has resulted from the occasional failure of conventional planktonic sampling to accurately reflect the behaviour of the biofilm and its control by biocides. A wide range of devices has been developed, all of which present multiple small studs to the fluids under test. One or multiple studs are removed periodically for analysis of the biofilm. More recently, electrically wired studs have been used; these allow the application of electrochemical techniques. However, as noted above the corrosion monitoring methods do not distinguish the contribution from the microbial corrosion mechanism.

The biofilm devices fall into three categories:

1. Insertion equipment, which fits directly into the operating pipework; typically this equipment is marketed by Caproco, Rohrbach-Cosasco and Petrolite, and fits through standard access fittings (Fig. 8.2).

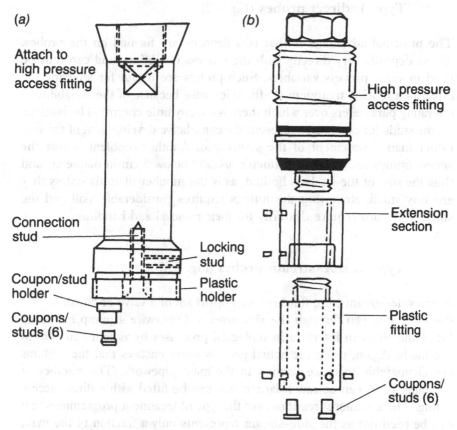

Fig. 8.2 (*a*) Caproco biofilm probe (from Caproco trade literature). (*b*) Petrolite bioprobe with Cosasco solid plug (from Rohrbach-Cosasco trade literature).

2. Side-stream apparatus linked into the process pipework; such instrumentation is custom built though some small-scale devices are commercially available such as the Robbins device (Fig. 8.3).
3. Laboratory recirculation rigs, which are used to simulate the conditions in the process plant.

Each method has advantages and disadvantages.

Type 1: direct probes (Fig. 8.2)

The principal advantage is that real deposits are formed on the probes. These deposits vary directly with the process conditions and can thus be used to study process variables. Such probes are useful for studying the effect of a biocide treatment. Difficulties arise because of the variability of operating parameters over which there is usually little control. The biofilms on the studs (or coupons) represent the cumulative development of the film rather than a statement of the status quo. Another problem is that the access fittings are of small diameter, usually below 5 cm in diameter, and thus the size of the studs is limited, as is the number of studs unless they are very small. Removing the fittings requires considerable skill and the small studs also require dexterity for their removal and handling.

Type 2: side-stream probes (Fig. 8.3)

In the side-streams, the fluid is taken upstream of a valve or choke so that the fluid is driven through the side-stream. Otherwise a pump has to be fitted and this can interfere in biological processes by violent agitation of the fluids. Again, using the actual process water ensures that the biofilms are comparable to those formed in the main pipework. The number of sampling studs can be much larger than can be fitted with a direct access fitting. There is more freedom over the type of treatment programmes that can be tried out as the side-stream represents only a fraction of the main flow. Often the side-stream flow is small enough for the fluid to be discharged. The principal disadvantage is that the system cannot model the main flow hydrodynamics or geometries. Great care has to be taken in the design and construction of the unit if it is to operate at high pressures. Usually quite a high level of skill is also required to operate the unit, though the advantage remains that if a mistake is made the unit can usually be isolated by positioning valves so that repairs can be made.

Increasingly frequently used for side-stream testing are small portable rigs that are transported by the service company to a client plant and hard-piped into the process pipework. For safety reasons these tend to operate on the low pressure areas only but the level of instrumentation is usually considerable. Such units measure biofilming, corrosion, scaling and allow testing of treatment chemicals (Sexsmith, 1984). Side-stream systems represent the best balance between reality and ease of experimentation. It

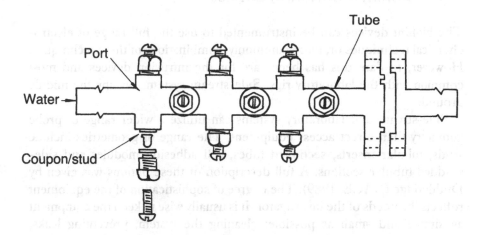

Fig. 8.3 Schematic diagram of ported tube type apparatus, e.g. Robbins device.

is likely that, as the more advanced corrosion monitoring techniques become established, and the equipment more reliable and robust, most plant monitoring will be by this form of system.

Type 3: laboratory rigs

Nearly all laboratory rigs are circulating rigs containing quite small volumes of simulated or actual process fluids. Such rigs can have instrumentation to a higher level of sophistication than units on site, though with the increasing flexibility of computer-led systems this advantage is reducing. Laboratory rigs allow full control of the operating parameters. The principal criticisms are that they are usually a poor reflection of reality and that the scale is generally small; hence geometry and hydrodynamics are unrealistic. The continued circulation of the same fluid is also unrealistic and great care is necessary to ensure that a bleed of fresh fluid is provided to avoid a rapid departure from an acceptable simulation.

Biofilm monitoring devices

The biofilm devices can be instrumented to use the full range of electro-chemical techniques or, more commonly, combinations of these techniques. However, to date this has been rare for the intrusion devices and most common with the laboratory rigs. Side-stream systems occupy the middle ground.

Side-stream and laboratory systems can utilize a wider range of probe geometry than direct access equipment. The range of geometries include studs, tubular inserts, sectioned tubes, cell adhesion modules and side-studded tubular sections. A full description of these options was given by Dudderidge (NACE, 1989). The degree of sophistication of the equipment reflects the needs of the investigator. It is usually wise to keep the equipment as simple and small as possible; cleaning the system, preventing leaks, contamination and air ingress, etc. can be very labour intensive.

A similar wide range of geometries is available for electrochemical probes. Most probes are either circular studs, such as probes fitted through insulating sleeves, or a sequence of metallic, insulating tubes bolted together to form a tube.

The development of the biofilm can be measured *in situ* if the flow can be adequately controlled. For each specific system the measured parameters have to be correlated with conventional enumeration. The two most common indirect parameters are the friction loss and the overall heat transfer coefficient. To measure the friction loss the flow rate has to be well controlled; as the biofilm increases in thickness so the friction increases. The biofilm grows until the waves induced in its surface by the flow cause sloughing off of the film. Heat transfer monitoring is more sensitive as the changes in heat transfer are significant for very small changes in biofilm thickness. A heated section is incorporated into the flow stream and the temperature downstream is measured. Accurate measurement of the flow rate and the heat input allow the thickness of the biofilm to be calculated from the overall heat transfer rate. The status of the biofilm is correlated to the corrosion rates obtained from the electrochemical monitoring equipment.

Supplementary analytical monitoring techniques

The cost of monitoring a microbial population is high in comparison to the costs of straightforward chemical analysis. Not surprisingly emphasis is placed on using chemical analysis whenever possible. It is necessary to ensure that sufficient testing has been done to allow sound correlations between chemical analysis and the perceived microbiological corrosion problems.

Water is essential for growth and for corrosion. The water may be in a discontinuous thin film. Microorganisms produce water during respiration and growth and corrosion products tend to hold the water to the metal surface. The corrosion problem once initiated thus becomes self-supporting. Even in 'dry' systems this form of corrosion is possible if the container walls are colder than the fluid, causing condensation. A suitable analysis technique is Karl–Fischer titration as given in ASTM D1744.

Oxygen levels determine the balance of species present in an environment but, as noted above, most corrosion processes occur in the presence of consortia of microorganisms and a complete range of conditions is likely to appertain within a mixed culture. Usually only bulk oxygen levels can be monitored; a suitable method is the Winkler titration, provided ferric ions are absent or in low concentration. Oxygen probes are also suitable if used *in situ* or great care is taken when sampling. The carbon source can also be altered by one member of the consortium into a food source for another organism. Several consortia have been identified that include the SRB: sulfate reduction coupled to sulfide oxidation in sulfureta, oil-degrading organisms and SRB, and iron-oxidizing bacteria and SRB. The SRB can metabolize a wide range of organic materials; indeed recent work has identified completely new SRB; these were comprehensively reviewed by King & Miller (1988). In nominally clean water streams it is often of value to evaluate the level of total organic carbon (TOC) present; this is often cyclic. TOC measurement requires sophisticated equipment; a suitable method is described in ASTM D2579.

Sulfate is, however, necessary for the SRB to flourish and cause corrosion problems. The level of sulfate required is difficult to define precisely, around 50–100 p.p.m. appears to be the minimum around which corrosion problems can become manifest though usually at these low levels there is a considerable time scale from initiation of a colony to the development of an active, localized corrosion environment. A suitable turbidometric method is described in ASTM 516. Alternatively commercial kits can be used such as the Hach HH/02251-00 or Merck 10019 (31521 2H). Minor nutrients are always present in sufficient quantities. Nitrogen can often be the limiting factor to growth; in such circumstances the addition of ammonium bisulfite as an oxygen scavenger or use of nitrite for corrosion inhibition can trigger significant microbial activity. Commercial kits are the most suitable for monitoring trace elements; suitable kits are available from Hach, Chemetrics, Merck and Lovibond.

Corrosion processes accelerate with increases in temperature as do the microbial processes; the corrosion rates can be extremely high. There are upper temperature limits to growth and if temperatures are maintained above the tolerance of the organisms then the biological corrosion processes will decrease over time. However, cyclical temperatures can lead to sustained corrosion rates as the organisms will recolonize the environment while the temperatures are moderate. Some of the recently discovered SRB are active over the temperature range 50–75 °C and these organisms have been identified as active and causing corrosion in oil field equipment. The same effects are observed with decreases in temperature when the biological processes are reduced, leading to a rapid decrease in corrosion rates; for example, microbiological corrosion of sheet steel piling in ports and harbours shows marked seasonality.

The pH tolerance of microorganisms varies widely. SRB are active over the pH range 6 to 9.5; sulfur-oxidizing bacteria (e.g. *Thiobacillus*) clearly tolerate considerably lower pH. Caution is needed when one is extrapolating from bulk measurements, however, as local environments in water streams may be suitable for microbial growth. The wide range of pH tolerance allows fairly crude pH monitoring procedures and indicator paper is usually adequate.

Sulfide is often taken as presumptive evidence of the activity of SRB in a water system. Sulfide monitoring using silver–silver sulfide electrodes has been used to determine the status of oil storage tank water bottoms; taking samples requires care to avoid air ingress into the sample. An alternative electrometric method is described in API RP 45.

Possible future techniques

To date, most attempts to develop a continuous low-skill monitoring technique for microbial corrosion have focused on a single method. These have been reasonably successful but tend to provide qualitative rather than quantitative information. The complexity of the processes occurring on the metal surface militates against such an approach. It is likely that a better approach would be to use several monitoring techniques and identify a 'fingerprint' characteristic of microbial corrosion. The availability of cheap computing power makes such an approach feasible. Some progress along this route has been made, using linear polarization techniques, by Kasahara & Kajiyama (1983). Work on a single metal probe gave conflicting patterns (King & Eden, 1988b) and a more suitable method would be to use pairs of active and inert probes or multiple monitoring techniques (King et al., 1985). The electrochemical noise techniques pioneered by Iverson (1968) appear to be the most suitable, coupled to linear polarization resistance.

Fibre optics offer an attractive method of continuously monitoring the development of a biofilm by light reflectance. The use of a single or selected wavelengths of light may allow some specificity in the measurement. Fibre optics terminating in chemical impregnated plugs that would give colour variations dependent on the rate of reaction at the plug would also appear to be an attractive method for monitoring under biofilms. Capacitance of thin films under self-cleaning surfaces (e.g. Teflon membrane) would also allow a continuous monitoring of the biofilm development. Whatever the continuous technique used, it remains clear that enumeration will always be needed to correlate the technique with actual microbial numbers and varieties.

References

Anon (1971). *Report of the Committee on Corrosion and Protection*. Chairman T. P. Hoare. HMSO, London.

American Petroleum Institute handbooks (in all cases the most recent revision/edition should be consulted).

API RP 38: *Recommended Practice for Biological Analysis of Subsurface Injection Waters*. API, Washington, DC.

API RP 45: *Recommended Practice for Analysis of Oilfield Waters*. API, Washington, DC.

American Society for Testing and Materials handbooks (in all cases the most recent revision/edition should be consulted).

ASTM 518: *Standard Technical Method for Testing Thermal Conductivity Detectors used in Gas Chromatography*. ASTM, Philadelphia.

ASTM D1744: *Standard Technical Method for Evaluation of Water in Liquid Petroleum Products by Karl Fischer Reagent*. ASTM, Philadelphia.

ASTM 2597: *Standard Technical Method for Analysis of Natural Gas–Liquid Mixtures by Gas Chromatography*. ASTM, Philadelphia.

Bobowski, S. (1987). Serological methods for SRB detection. In *Industrial Microbiology Testing*, ed. E. C. Hill & J. W. Hopton. Academic Press, London.

Boivin, J. (1990). The influence of enzyme systems on MIC. In *Corrosion 90*, Paper no. 128. NACE, Houston, TX.

Booth, G. H. (1964). Sulphur bacteria in relation to corrosion. *Journal of Applied Bacteriology*, 27, 174–81.

Brown, G. F. (1985). A simple electrical method for the rapid detection of brewery bacteria. *Laboratory Practice*, 34(10).

Characklis, W. G. (1985). Influence of microbial films on industrial processes. In *Proceedings of an Argentina–USA Workshop on Biodeterioration* (CONICET-NSF), ed. H. A. Videla, pp. 181–216. Aquatec Quimica S.A., Sao Paulo.

Costerton, J. W. & Geesey, G. G. (1985). The microbial ecology of surface colonization and of consequent corrosion. In *Biologically Induced Corrosion*, ed. S. C. Dexter, pp. 233–32. NACE, Houston, TX.

Cubicciotti, D. & Licina, G. J. (1989). Electrochemical aspects of MIC. In *Corrosion 89*, Paper no. 517. NACE, Houston, TX.

Dexter, S. C., Siebert, O. W., Duquette, D. J. & Videla, H. (1989). Use and limitations of electrochemical techniques for investigating microbiological corrosion. In *Corrosion 89*, Paper no. 616. NACE, Houston, TX.

Duquette, D. J. & Ricker, R. E. (1986). Electrochemical aspects of microbiologically induced corrosion. In *Biologically Induced Corrosion*, ed. S. C. Dexter, pp. 121–35. NACE, Houston, TX.

Farinha, M. (1982). Use of constant respirometry to evaluate the efficiency of biocides against the sulphate-reducing bacteria, M.Sc. dissertation, University of Salford.

Farinha, M. & King, R. A. (1980). Sensitivity of media for the enumeration of sulphate-reducing bacteria. Subsea Pipeline Project, UK Department of Energy, September, Paper no. 18.

Gaylarde, C. C. & Cooke, P. E. (1987). ELISA techniques for the detection of sulphate-reducing bacteria. In *Immunological Techniques in Microbiology*, ed. J. M. Grange, A. Fox & N. L. Morgan, Society for Applied Bacteriology Technical Series no. 24, pp. 231–44.

Gilbert, P., Attwood, P. A., David, T., Morgan, B. & Herbert, B. N. (1987). Biofilm associated corrosion. In *UK Corrosion 87*, 291–308. CCEJV.

Haderlie, E. C. (1977). *The Nature of Primary Organic Films in the Marine Environment and their Significance for Ocean Thermal Energy Conversion (OTEC) Heat Exchange Surfaces*. Report no. NPS-68Hc 77021 for ERDA OTEC Program, Naval Postgraduate School, Monterey, CA.

Hardy, J. A. & Syrett, K. R. (1983). A radiorespirometric method for evaluating inhibitors of sulphate-reducing bacteria. *European Journal of Applied Microbiology and Biotechnology*, 49, 17.

Iverson, W. P. (1968). The role of phosphorus and hydrogen sulphide in the anaerobic corrosion of iron and the possible detection of this corrosion by an electrochemical noise technique. *Journal of the Electrochemical Society*, 617, 49–51.

Iverson, W. P., Olson, G. J. & Heverley, L. F. (1985). The role of phosphorus and hydrogen sulfide in the anaerobic corrosion of iron and the possible detection of this corrosion by an electrochemical noise technique. In *Biologically Induced Corrosion*, ed. S. C. Dexter. NACE, Houston, TX.

Kasahara, K. & Kajiyama, F. (1983). Determination of underground corrosion rates from polarization resistance measurements. *Corrosion*, 39, 475–80.

King, R. A. (1980). Monitoring of microbiological activity and its relation to corrosion. In *Corrosion Monitoring in the Oil, Petrochemical and Process Industries*. IBC, London.

King, R. A. & Eden, R. (1988a). Evaluation of biofilms by advanced electrochemical monitoring. In *Biocorrosion*, ed. C. C. Gaylarde & L. H. G. Morton, pp. 134–49. Biodeterioration Society.

King, R. A. & Eden, R. (1988b). Biofilms. In *Microbiological Up-date for the Petroleum Industry*, ed. J. L. Shennan, pp. 35–46. API, Washington, DC.

King, R. A. & Miller, J. D. A. (1988). On the Sulphate-Reducing Bacteria and their Corrosive Activities. Plenary Paper. *Microbios '88*, Pretoria.

King, R. A., Skerry, B. S., Moore, D. C. A., Stott, J. F. D. & Dawson, J. L. (1985). Corrosion behaviour of ductile and grey iron pipes in environments containing sulphate-reducing bacteria. In *Biologically Induced Corrosion*, ed. S. C. Dexter, pp. 83–91. NACE, Houston, TX.

Kogure, K., Simudu, U. & Taga, N. (1979). A tentative direct microscopic method of counting living marine bacteria. *Canadian Journal of Microbiology*, 25, 415–17.

Little, B. J., Wagner, P. & Gerchakov, S. M. (1985). A quantitative investigation of mechanisms for microbial corrosion. In *Biologically Induced Corrosion*, ed. S. C. Dexter, pp. 209–14. NACE, Houston, TX.

Littmann, E. S. (1977). Use of ATP extraction in oil field waters. In *Oilfield Subsurface Injection of Water*, ASTM STP 641, ed. C. C. Wright, D. Cross, A. G. Ostroff & J. R. Stanford, pp. 79–88. ASTM, Philadelphia.

Mansfeld, F. & Little, B. (1990). The application of electrochemical techniques for the study of MIC – a critical review. In *Corrosion 90*, Paper no. 108. NACE, Houston, TX.

Maxwell, S. (1987). Monitoring sulphate reduction activity in the field using radiorespirometry. In *Biodeterioration – 7*, ed. D. R. Houghton, R. N. Smith & H. O. W. Eggins, pp. 411–17. Elsevier Applied Science, London.

Maxwell, S. & Hamilton, W. A. (1984). Activity of sulphate-reducing bacteria on metal surfaces in an oilfield situation. In *Proceedings of a Meeting of the Society for General Microbiology*, Warwick, Abstract.

Merrique, J. L. (1978). Corrosion monitoring in microbially contaminated systems. M.Sc. dissertation, University of Manchester, Institute for Science and Technology, Manchester.

Miller, J. D. A. (1971). *Microbial Aspects of Metallurgy*. Medical and Technical Publications, Aylesbury.

Miller, P. (1982). Biological fouling, film formation and destruction. Ph.D. thesis, University of Birmingham.

Moosavi, A. N. (1987). Application of novel electrochemical techniques in studies of biologically induced corrosion of reinforced concrete. Ph.D. thesis, University of Manchester Institute for Science and Technology, Manchester.

NACE (1987). *Review of Current Practices for Monitoring Bacterial Growth in*

Oilfield Systems, NACE-CCEJV Joint Document E1/1. NACE, Houston, TX.

NACE (1989). *Review of Non-Conventional and Supplementary Methods for the Detection of Sulphate-Reducing Bacteria in Oilfield Waters*, NACE-CCEJV Joint Document E1/4. NACE, Houston, TX.

NACE (1990). *Microbially Influenced Corrosion and Biofouling in Oilfield Equipment*, TPC-3; 1990 revision T-1D-26. NACE, Houston, TX.

NACE (1992). *Methods for Determining Water Quality for Subsurface Injection Using Membrane Filters*, NACE TM-01-73. NACE, Houston, TX.

Odom, J. M., Gawel, L. J. & Ng, T. K. (1987). Sulphate-reducing bacteria detection. Patent App. ICR 7780-USSN 946,547 DuPont Company.

Oganowski, C. H. (1985). Studies on the marine corrosion of cathodically protected steel by sulphate-reducing bacteria. M.Sc. dissertation, University of Manchester Institute for Science and Technology, Manchester.

Paul, J. H. (1982). Use of Hoechst Dyes 33258 and 33342 for enumeration of attached and planktonic bacteria. *Applied and Environmental Microbiology*, **43**, 934–44.

Payer, J. H., Dippold, D. G., Boyd, W. K., Berry, W. E., Brooman, E. W., Buhr, A. R. & Fisher, W. H. (1978). *Economic Effects of Metallic Corrosion in the United States*. A report to NBS by Batelle Columbus Laboratories, US Department of Commerce, Washington, DC.

Pope, D. H. & Zintel, T. P. (1988). Methods for the investigation of under-deposit microbiologically influenced corrosion. In *Corrosion 88*, Paper no. 249. NACE, Houston, TX.

Pritchard, A. M. (1981). Fouling: science or art? An investigation of fouling and antifouling measures in the British Isles. In *Fouling of Heat Transfer Equipment*, ed. R. Somerscales & K. Knudsen, p. 531. Hemisphere Publishing Corp., Washington, DC.

Rosales, B. M. (1986). Corrosion measurements for determining the quality of maintenance in jet fuel storage. In *Proceedings of an Argentina–USA Workshop on Biodeterioration* (CONICET-NSF), ed. H. A. Videla, pp. 135–43. Aquatec Quimica S.A., Sao Paulo.

Rosser, H. R. & Hamilton, W. A. (1983). Simple assay for accurate determination of ^{35}S-sulphate reduction activity. *Applied and Environmental Microbiology*, **45**, 1956–9.

Sexsmith, D. R. (1984). Corrosion monitoring in water cooling systems. In *Proceedings of the 2nd International Conference on Corrosion Monitoring and Inspection in the Oil, Petrochemical and Process Industries*. IBC, London.

Smith, A. D. (1982). Immunofluorescence of sulphate-reducing bacteria. *Archives of Microbiology*, **133**, 118–21.

Sussex, G. A. M., Hussain, K., Reid, C., Nabizadeh, H., Dawson, J. L. & King, R. A. (1986). Review of electrochemical monitoring techniques for studying corrosion of ferrous metals in soils. *Corrosion Australasia*, pp. 5–9.

Tatnall, R. E., Stanton, K. M. & Ebersole, R. C. (1988). Methods of testing for the presence of sulphate-reducing bacteria. In *Corrosion 88*, Paper no. 88. NACE, Houston, TX.

Videla, H. A., de Mele, M. F. & Brankevich, G. (1987). Microfouling of several metal surfaces in polluted seawater and its relation with corrosion. In *Corrosion 87*, Paper no. 365. NACE, Houston, TX.

Wagner, P. & Little, B. J. (1986). Application of a technique for the investigation of microbiologically induced corrosion. In *Corrosion 86*, Paper no. 121. NACE, Houston, TX.

Wakerley, D. S. (1979). Microbial corrosion in the U.K. industry: a preliminary survey of the problem. *Chemistry and Industry*, pp. 656–58.

Zimmerman, R. & Meyer-Reil, L. A. (1974). A new method for fluorescence of bacterial populations on membrane filters. *Kiel Meeresforschung*, 30, 24–7.

9

AC impedance spectroscopy in microbial corrosion

CÉSAR A. C. SEQUEIRA

Introduction

Although studies related to the corrosive effects of microorganisms have been carried out for something of the order of 90 years, it is only in recent times that the subject has gained widespread acceptance and recognition in relation to massive degradation.

This renaissance is in part related to the so-called 'energy crisis' and the substantial investment in off-shore structures, storage facilities and transmission lines associated with oil and gas production. Thus, the demands for return in investment, reliability and safety have justified extensive research and development in the areas of biofouling and anaerobic microbial corrosion. It would be wrong, however, to give the impression that biodeterioration problems relate only to the oil and gas industry. Conditions favourable to microbial growth can exist in a broad spectrum of industry and affect a variety of materials including concrete, cotton, wood, rubber and a variety of metals.

The number of technical symposia held in the last few years and the numbers of publications on the topic are adequate testimony to the increased awareness of the problem by those in industry who deal with the problem on a day-to-day basis. It has also become a 'scientifically valid' topic for research workers in several engineering and scientific areas. The result of much of this activity has been to 'turn the corner' from having to defend the idea that microbial corrosion is real, to being concerned with the mechanisms whereby it occurs, and how to treat and prevent it. The reader is referred to a number of publications dealing with case histories, methods of detection, treatment and prevention, and other aspects of microbial corrosion (e.g. Miller, 1971; Nielands, 1974; Postgate, 1979; Tiller, 1982; Hamilton, 1983; Stoecker, 1985; Hill *et al.*, 1987; Zehnder, 1987; Sequeira & Tiller, 1988, 1992), which prove the involvement of microorganisms in the corrosion processes.

As a result of this involvement, microorganisms contribute to corrosion by one or more of the following factors:

1. Direct influence on the rate of anodic or cathodic reaction.
2. Change of surface metal film resistance by metabolic production of aggressive species such as sulfuric or organic acids.
3. Creation of corrosive environment.
4. Establishment of a barrier by growth and multiplication so as to create electrochemical concentration cells on the metal surface.

In other words, microbial involvement does not involve a new corrosion mechanism but merely an acceleration of those already known to corrosion science, which are well recognized as being of electrochemical nature. Progress in understanding the mechanisms whereby microorganisms influence corrosion should therefore be made by electrochemical means, complemented by microbiological methods (e.g. cell-counting techniques, microscopic examination, determination of bacterial activity, immunological detection) and other approaches.

All electrochemical techniques are indirect methods based on Faraday's law, i.e. a correlation between the mass flux density and the electrical current density. The electrochemical methods are marked by the extremely high accuracy in measuring the electrical potential and the current density. Generally they also give instantaneous results. Therefore, they give information on the differential corrosion rate and are suitable for corrosion monitoring. Moreover, they are particularly useful and efficient in the study of corrosion mechanisms, which have been explained on the basis of reactions controlled by charge transfer, diffusion, and/or electrocrystallization, taking into account adsorbed reaction intermediates or products. This is a great advantage of electrochemical techniques, which is not exhibited by non-electrochemical measurements.

In many electrochemical techniques, a (clamped) DC potential is applied to the working electrode and the resultant current flowing in a circuit completed by a counter electrode is measured (see e.g. Bard & Faulkner, 1980; Bond, 1980; Kissinger & Heineman, 1984). Even in pulse voltammetric techniques, the measuring system is designed such that the potential difference between the working and reference electrodes, and also the size of the current ultimately measured, are constant for a greater or lesser period. However, the last 30 years or so have witnessed the increasing exploitation of sinusoidal exciting voltages in the study of electrode processes in aqueous media (see e.g. Breyer & Bauer, 1963; Schwan, 1966; Smith, 1966; Sluyters-Rehbach & Sluyters, 1970; Macdonald, 1977; Archer & Armstrong, 1980; Bard & Faulkner, 1980; Bond, 1980; Gabrielli, 1980; Buck, 1982; Macdonald & McKubre, 1982), an approach that possesses two advantages in particular:

1. The sinusoid offers convenient technical and mathematical features in such systems, together with an excellent signal : noise ratio predicated upon the use of a 'steady-state' analysis (see e.g. Creason *et al.*, 1973; Gabrielli & Keddam, 1974; Diamond & Machen, 1983; Marshall, 1983).
2. The frequency, as well as the voltage, of the exciting waveform may be altered, so that the technique may be used as a form of spectroscopy.

To put these another way, we may raise the idea, with which we are all familiar, that the frequency-dependent absorption of ultraviolet, visible and infrared light may be used in the analysis of microbiological (and other) systems. Yet light is only a form of electromagnetic radiation, albeit of a rather high frequency (10^{14} Hz or so), and there is thus no reason why the frequency-dependent absorption of electrical energy of lower frequencies might not be similarly exploited in microbial corrosion studies. In such cases, at least below 30 MHz or so, one requires electrodes to act as an interface between the exciting electrical field and the sample, so that, as in the 'pure' electrochemical case above, one may study the frequency-dependent, passive electrical properties of the system consisting of the electrodes plus the microorganism contaminant; in other words, one may study the frequency-dependent impedance or admittance of the metallic material/biological fluid system.

In the following, therefore, (a) I outline in very elementary terms what is meant by the concepts of electrical impedance and admittance, and (b) I discuss the application of such measurements in microbial corrosion.

My aim is predominantly to provide an introduction to a field which has been widely neglected by biologists and biophysicists, yet which underlies a great many present and future applications in studies of biodeterioration systems.

General AC theory

Let us consider a sinusoidally modulated voltage, of the form $V = V_m \sin \omega t$, where ω is the frequency in radians/s ($\omega = 2\pi f$, where f is the frequency in Hz), V_m is the maximum (peak-to-peak) voltage, and V the voltage at any given instant. If this voltage appears across the terminals of a passive circuit, device, or 'system', which may consist of pure electrical components or of a biological or chemical sample separating a pair of electrodes, the current flowing in the circuit (after any transients have died down) may be related to the voltage both by its magnitude and its phase, and is of the form $i = i_m \sin (\omega t + \theta)$. Thus, although the frequency and sinusoidal nature of the waveform are unchanged by interaction with the system (Fig. 9.1(a)), the characteristics of the system are reflected in the ratio V_m/i_m and by the value of θ.

Now systems may exhibit resistive, capacitive and inductive properties, properties which (by definition) may be distinguished from each other by their effects upon a sinusoidal voltage. Thus, for a pure resistor (R ohms), the current due to our exciting waveform ($V_m \sin \omega t$) is given by:

$$i = (V_m/R) \sin \omega t \tag{9.1}$$

For a pure capacitor (C farads):

$$i = \omega C \ V_m \sin [\omega t + (\pi/2)] \tag{9.2}$$

whilst for a pure (self) inductance of L henries:

$$i = (V_m/\omega L) \ \sin [\omega t - (\pi/2)] \tag{9.3}$$

Thus, for a pure resistor, there is no phase difference between V and i. In contrast, for a pure capacitor, the current leads the voltage by $\pi/2$ radians (90°), whilst for a pure inductor the current lags the voltage by the same amount. For systems with negligible inductances, we may therefore imagine intuitively (and correctly) that for a 'real' system, which possesses both resistive and capacitance properties (i.e. behaves as a leaky capacitor), θ takes a value between 0 and $\pi/2$, as illustrated in Fig. 9.1(b).

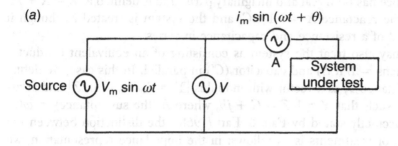

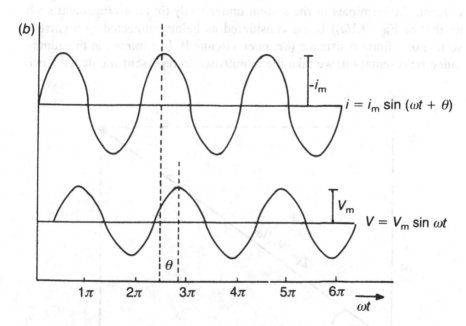

Fig. 9.1 (*a*) The impedimetric experiment, in which a small amplitude perturbation, in the form of a sinusoidal voltage, is applied to the system of interest. The sinusoidal voltage across the system may be measured using a (high impedance) AC vector voltmeter, V, whilst the sinusoidal current flowing in the circuit may be measured by means of an AC vector ammeter, A. (*b*) Phase relationships between voltage and current for a real system.

We may then define a vector quantity Z, the impedance, with modulus (magnitude) $|Z|$ and argument ('direction') θ, in a form analogous to that of a complex number $a + jb$ (where $j = \sqrt{-1}$) as in Fig. 9.2, where the modulus $|Z|$ of the impedance is equal to the ratio V_m/i_m. Thus, the impedance has both real and imaginary parts, and is defined as $Z = R + jX$, where the reactance $X = -1/\omega C$, and the system is treated as though it consisted of a resistance and capacitance in series.

We may also treat the system as consisting of an equivalent conductor (G siemens $= 1/R'S$) and capacitor (C') in parallel. In this case, we define an admittance Y, as a vector with modulus $|Y| = i_m/V_m = 1/|Z|$ and argument θ, such that $Y = 1/Z = G + jB$, where B (the susceptance) $= \omega C'$.

As succinctly stated by Falk & Fatt (1968), the distinction between the two sets of treatments is as follows: in the impedance representation, we take the impedance to represent the dependence of the voltage on the current, the terminals of the system under study (in an arrangement such as that of Fig. 9.1(a)) being considered as being connected to a current source of infinite resistance (i.e. open circuited). In contrast, in the admittance representation, we take the admittance to represent the dependence

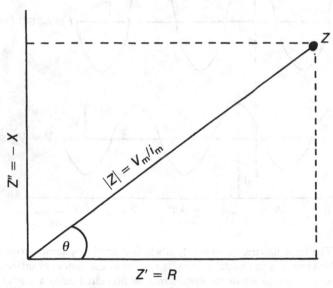

Fig. 9.2 Impedance as a complex quantity. There is a mathematical function known as Euler's identity, which states that $Ae^{\pm j\theta} = A\cos\theta \pm Aj\sin\theta$, where $j = \sqrt{-1}$. Thus, any complex quantity may be split up into its real (Z') and imaginary (Z'') part. The figure shows the manner in which this is done for the impedance function $Z = R + jX$. Simple geometrical considerations indicate (i) that $Z^2 = R^2 + X^2$, and (ii) that $R = |Z|\cos\theta$ and $X = -|Z|\sin\theta$. Thus R and X may be obtained from measurements of $|Z|$ and θ, and are known respectively as the 'in phase' and (90°) 'out-of-phase' components.

of the current on the voltage, the terminals being considered as being connected to a voltage source of zero resistance (short circuited).

For real circuits, then, the impedance $Z(\omega)$ or admittance $Y(\omega)$, and their component real and imaginary parts, are frequency-dependent quantities, the frequency dependence of which may be used to describe the actual equivalent electrical circuits. It should be noted that, by definition, the impedance and admittance are independent of the voltage across, and current flowing in, the system under study, and this 'linear property' should be taken into account when use is made of these representations.

In general, the most convenient means by which we can extract the magnitudes and topological relationship of the components constituting the equivalent circuit is by means of complex plane diagrams, a topic to which I now turn.

Impedance diagrams

For a variety of historical and other reasons, impedance (R/X) has dominated the electrochemical literature, although J. R. Macdonald and his colleagues (see e.g. Macdonald, 1980; Macdonald *et al.*, 1982) have stressed the utility of the three-dimensional perspective $R/X/\log f$ plot. Now the general aim in studies of purely electrochemical and, in many cases, of corrosion process impedances is to gain information about the mechanism of electrode processes, i.e. of processes occurring at the electrode–electrolyte interface. Thus, since such processes are obviously dependent upon the 'mean' potential of the working electrode, one should arrange to fix this potential at a known value, either by including both pairs of a redox couple of known $E\acute{o}$ in the medium (Faradaic impedance) or electronically. In the latter case in particular, it is usual to use a three-electrode system (Bard & Faulkner, 1980; Bond, 1980; Gabrielli, 1980). In such two- or three-electrode measurements, of course, one should either use identical electrodes or make the impedance of the working electrode very much greater than that of the counter-electrode.

The interpretation of electrochemical impedances is a vast, detailed, and complex field, and for the present purposes I want merely to give the simplest possible description of the salient ideas in corrosion research.

The electrical analogue of the corroding metal surface can be demonstrated and represented by a network consisting of resistors and capacitors – the equivalent circuit. Evaluation of the components of the equivalent circuit provides a characteristic measurement of the surface properties and an estimate of the corrosion resistance. The electrochemical reaction at the metal–solution interface is generally assumed to be very simple in nature and could be represented by the equivalent circuit shown in Fig. 9.3(a).

This circuit consists of the solution resistance R_0 between the surface and the reference electrode. The charge transfer resistance R_{ct} is in parallel with the double-layer capacitance C_{dl}. Another RC circuit is in series with R_{ct} and C_{dl} and contains the passive-film resistance R_{pf} and the passive-film capacitance C_{pf}. If the passive-film impedances (R_{pf} and C_{pf}) dominate the electrochemical reaction, then Fig. 9.3(a) can be simplified (Fig. 9.3(b)). Furthermore, if the electrode process takes into account the diffusion of charged species, another component known as the Warburg impedance will appear in the equivalent circuit. The surface interaction of the passive film with the aggressive environment can be analysed and represented by this simple model.

The measured impedance data can be displayed in the form of a Bode plot and/or a Nyquist plot, as shown schematically in Fig. 9.3(c) and (d), respectively. The Bode plot shows the frequency dependence of the absolute magnitudes of the impedance modulus and the phase angle. In the Bode diagram the measured impedance modulus will approach the value of the solution resistance R_0 at the high frequency end, and will approach the sum of the solution resistance, the charge transfer resistance and the passive-film resistance ($R_0 + R_{ct} + R_{pf}$) at the low frequency end. At these two frequency extremes the phase angle is found to be near $0°$ and this shows that the electrode properties can be represented by an ideal resistor whose response to an AC signal is nearly independent of the frequency. If the impedance data are displayed by the complex variables and separated into real and imaginary parts, a semicircle may be plotted in this complex plane plot; this is called a Nyquist plot. A detailed analysis of this type of equivalent circuit is outside the scope of this chapter and is described elsewhere (Randles, 1947; Hung et al., 1979; Macdonald et al., 1982).

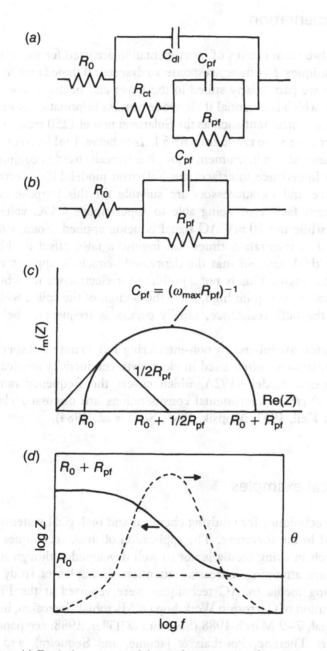

Fig. 9.3 (a) Equivalent circuit of the surface property of a passive metal and (b) its
simplified model. Impedance data can be displayed in the form of a Nyquist
plot (c) or a Bode plot (d).

Instrumentation

Experimentally, two main classes of instrumentation are used for measurement in AC techniques: frequency response analysers and impedance meters. The former are particularly suited to the lower end of the frequency regime, access to which is essential if electrode process information is to be obtained. A typical instrument such as the Solartron model 1250 frequency response analyser covers the range from 65.5 kHz to below 1 mHz. Because the input impedance of this instrument is low, it is typically used in conjunction with a high impedance interface; the Solartron model 1186 electrochemical interface and its successors are suitable for this purpose and have the additional facility of being able to superimpose a DC voltage on the test cell while the 10 mV AC signal is being applied. Some early interfaces have slow integration times that impose a false offset on high frequency (>10 kHz) data, so that the depressed semicircle appears not to go through the origin. This is not a problem for electrolytes for which bulk resistance values are quite high, since the bottom of the spike, which corresponds to the bulk resistance, usually occurs at frequencies below 10 kHz.

Impedance meters are inherently non-interfering and do not need special interfaces. An instrument often used in electrolyte conductivity studies is the Hewlett-Packard model 4192A, which covers the frequency range 5 Hz–13 MHz. Further experimental considerations are discussed elsewhere (Harris & Kell, 1983; Mopsik, 1984; Steel *et al.*, 1984).

Practical examples

The use of AC techniques for studying chemical and biological systems is well documented in the literature. The application of these techniques to corrosion research in living media is not so well developed, although it is clear that they are attracting increasing attention. Examples of study of corrosion in living media by AC techniques were reported at the First European Federation of Corrosion Workshop on Microbial Corrosion, held in Sintra, Portugal, 7–9 March 1988 (Sequeira & Tiller, 1988; see papers by Guezennec & Therene, Pourbaix & Jacome, and Sequeira), and at the International Congress on Microbially Influenced Corrosion, held in Knoxville, Tennessee, USA, 7–12 October 1990 (Dowling *et al.*, 1988; see

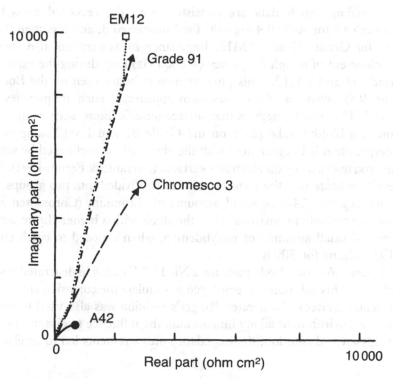

Fig. 9.4 Nyquist plots obtained with the steel electrodes exposed to *Desulfovibrio vulgaris* batch cultures for 500 h. The symbols represent 10 mHz (from Ferrante & Feron, 1991).

papers by Deshmukh *et al.*, Ferrante & Feron, Feron, Ignatiadis *et al.*, Jones & Walch, Kasahara & Kajiyama, Kearns & Deverell, Little & Wagner, and Mansfeld). Below, I draw attention to the use of AC techniques, presenting some examples of their application.

The influence of chromium and molybdenum as alloying elements on the corrosion behaviour of ferritic steels (containing 0–9%Cr and 0–2%Mo) in batch cultures of *Desulfovibrio vulgaris* was investigated by Ferrante & Feron (1991) by biological and electrochemical techniques, including impedance diagrams. Impedance data obtained after 500 h are given in Fig. 9.4 as Nyquist plots and indicate a great similarity in the behaviours of EM12 (9%Cr, 2–10%Mo) and Grade 91 (9.5%Cr, 10.5%Mo), which have a high charge transfer resistance. The steels containing less chromium-like Chromesco 3 (2.25%Cr, 0.9–1.1%Mo) exhibit a lower resistance, which is particularly small for A42 (0%Cr, 0%Mo), indicating that the electrode is corroding. Such data are consistent with the recorded mass losses: 1.8 mg/cm² for A42, 0.4 mg/cm² for Chromesco 3, and less than 0.1 mg/cm² for Grade 91 and EM12. Impedance measurements also show the development of a high frequency (≈ 2000 Hz) loop during the exposure of Grade 91 and EM12. This phenomenon is better seen on the Bode plot (Fig. 9.5), where a phase maximum appears at such frequencies (bold arrow). This result suggests that surface modifications, such as the formation of a biofilm, take place on the Grade 91 and EM12 samples. This interpretation is in agreement with the observations performed by scanning electron microscopy on electrode surfaces (Ferrante & Feron, 1991). These results indicate that the tested steels can be divided into two groups: those containing no (A42) or small amounts of chromium (Chromesco 3) and more susceptible to corrosion than the steels with a higher chromium content and small amounts of molybdenum, when exposed to batch cultures of *D. vulgaris* for 500 h.

Figure 9.6 shows Bode plots for a Ni–15%Cr alloy in deaerated Ringer's solution. This solution was employed to simulate the corrosion environment in dental crevices. An aerated Ringer's solution was also used to simulate the oral environment taking into account the influence of dissolved oxygen. In this aerated solution, the impedance measurements led to similar Bode

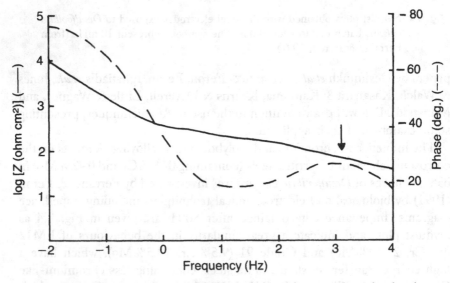

Fig. 9.5 Bode plot obtained with a EM12 steel electrode exposed to a batch culture of *Desulfovibrio vulgaris* for 500 h (from Ferrante & Feron, 1991).

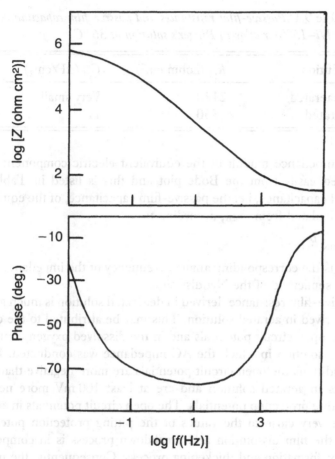

Fig. 9.6 Bode plots for a Ni–15%Cr alloy in deaerated Ringer's solution at 36 °C.

curves (L. F. F. T. T. G. Rodrigues & C. A. C. Sequeira, unpublished data).

This study indicated that the alloy/electrolyte corrosion process could be characterized by the simple equivalent circuit model shown in Fig. 9.3. Only one maximum value of the phase lag was observed for the alloy. This result indicated that the impedance of the passive film is much greater and overshadows that of the double-layer equivalent RC circuit. Therefore, the equivalent circuit with two RC circuits in series can be simplified to eliminate the double-layer RC circuit, as shown in Fig. 9.3(b), since the influence of the double-layer components is relatively small. Accordingly, the

Table 9.1. *Passive-film resistances and passive-film capacitances of the Ni–15% Cr alloy in Ringer's solution at 36 °C*

Solution	R_{pf} (kohm cm²)	C_{pf} ($\mu F/cm_2$)
Deaerated	2120	Very small
Aerated	350	11

respective impedance moduli of the equivalent electric component could be calculated easily from the Bode plot and this is listed in Table 9.1. The parallel capacitance, i.e. the passive-film capacitance, of the equivalent circuit is calculated from ω_{max}, according to

$$C_{pf} = 1/\omega_{max} R_{pf} \tag{9.4}$$

where ω_{max} is the corresponding angular frequency of the impedance at the apex of the semicircle of the Nyquist plot.

The passive-film resistance derived in deaerated solution is much greater than that derived in aerated solution. This may be attributed to the differences in the open circuit potentials and in the dissolved oxygen content of the Ringer's solution in which the AC impedance was conducted. In deaerated conditions the open circuit potentials are more negative than their counterparts in aerated solution and are at least 100 mV more negative than the pitting protection potentials. The open circuit potentials in aerated solution are very close to the values of the pitting protection potentials. Therefore, the film dissolution and breakdown process is in competition with the film formation and thickening process. Consequently, the passive film that is formed despite the film dissolution process in aerated Ringer's solution is less compact and thinner than the passive film formed in deaerated solution at more negative potentials. Therefore, the passive-film resistance is reduced.

The passive-film capacitances were also calculated. However, the centre of the semicircular Nyquist plots in the complex plane were found to fall below the real axis. One explanation for this effect is that the uneven current distribution caused by a porous surface layer or a highly roughened surface can facilitate this depression. The occurrence of the depressed semicircle could cause an error in the calculation if equation (9.4) is applied directly. The parallel capacitances calculated were, therefore, estimated values calculated using equation (9.4). It is frequently assumed that the reciprocal value of the passive-film capacitance is linearly proportional to the thickness of the passive film on the metal surface, regardless of other influential factors. Hence, the passive-film thickness of the Ni–15%Cr alloy is greatest for the lowest capacitance and highest resistance values. Since the passive-film thickening process is more difficult in the aerated solution, the susceptibility to localized corrosion is also greatly increased in aerated solutions.

The role of sulfate-reducing bacteria (SRB) in the localized corrosion of ductile iron has also been studied in our laboratory by means of AC impedance measurements. Apart from obtaining results expected for simple equivalent circuits such as that shown in Fig. 9.3(*a*), we observed, in the case when SRB did not grow, inductive semicircle types of impedance locus throughout the entire test period, indicating the adsorption of iron sulfate on to the electrode surface as a corrosion product (Fig. 9.7; L. F. F. T. T. G. Rodrigues & C. A. C. Sequeira, unpublished data).

The occurrence of the inductive loop has created an additional problem with respect to its significance and relationship to the polarization resistance, R_p, which is defined as:

$$R_p = \lim_{\omega \to 0} Z'_{E_{corr}} \tag{9.5}$$

where $Z'_{E_{corr}}$ is the real component of the electrode impedance at the free corrosion potential. Epelboin & Keddam (1970), on the basis of experimental results for iron in sulfuric acid containing propargyl alcohol and a non-uniform corrosion model, found it necessary to define the charge transfer resistance as:

$$R_{ct} = \lim_{\omega \to \infty} Z'_{E_{corr}} \tag{9.6}$$

and claimed a better agreement of weight loss data with R_{ct} than with R_p.

Lorenz & Mansfeld (1981) stated that, in relatively simple corrosion systems exhibiting continuous polarization curves under steady state polarization conditions, electrochemical DC and AC data agree well with non-electrochemical corrosion rate measurements. In the case of linear systems, the corrosion current density is unequivocally correlated to the polarization resistance measured at the corrosion potential using DC techniques according to the Stern–Geary technique or using the expression of the absolute impedance measured by the AC impedance technique. The question arises then as to whether AC impedance measurements in non-linear systems giving 'system responses' instead of 'real impedance data' can be used for the evaluation of kinetic parameters. This open problem requires further work, hence wrong interpretations may occur at present in AC impedance data analysis.

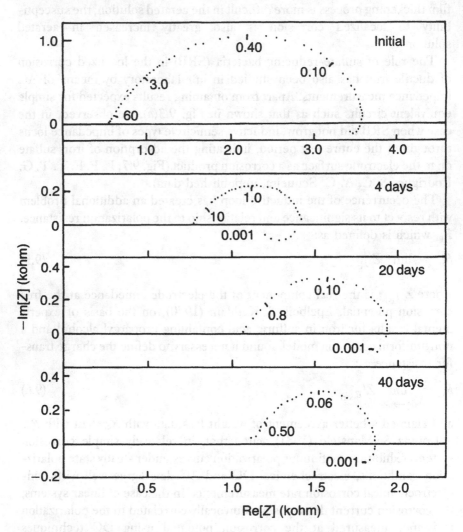

Fig. 9.7 AC impedance loca for ductile iron subject to localized corrosion under conditions where sulfate-reducing bacteria are inactive.

Conclusion

From the above discussion, the conclusion may be reached that AC impedance spectroscopy methods are very useful in microbial corrosion practice. However, it has to be emphasized that no method is universally applicable and that the methods should be selected by taking into account the different aspects of the problem of concern. Moreover, there are novel techniques such as electron spectrochemical analysis (ESCA), Auger spectroscopy, strain electrometry, ellipsometry, transmission and scanning electron microscopy (TEM and SEM), low energy electron diffraction (LEED), reflection electron diffraction (RED), and ion microprobe mass spectrometry, which, depending on the circumstances, can act as a powerful adjunct to AC impedance techniques, giving much greater information on the corrosion processes.

The author is grateful to the Ministry of Industry and Technology, as well as to JNICT, Lisbon, Portugal, for financial assistance (PEDIP – Measure F, Action Type T2L19, Project C/P-F15). He also expresses his affectionate thanks to his wife, Maria Elisa, who accomplished tasks such as the compiling of the literature, and drawing of the figures.

References

Archer, W. I. & Armstrong, R. D. (1980). The application of A.C. impedance methods to solid electrolytes. In *Electrochemistry*, ed. H. R. Thirsk, vol. 7, pp. 157–202, Specialist Periodical Reports. The Chemical Society, London.

Bard, A. J. & Faulkner, L. R. (1980). *Electrochemical Methods*. John Wiley & Sons, Chichester.

Bond, A. M. (1980). *Modern Polarographic Methods in Analytical Chemistry*. Marcel Dekker, New York.

Breyer, B. & Bauer, H. (1963). *Alternating Current Polarography and Tensammetry*. Wiley-Interscience, New York.

Buck, R. P. (1982). The impedance method applied to the investigation of ion-selective electrodes. *Ion-Selective Electrode Review*, 4, 3–74.

Creason, S. C., Hayes, J. W. & Smith, D. E. (1973). Fourier transform faradaic admittance measurements. III. Comparison of measurement efficiency for various test signal wave forms. *Journal of Electroanalytical Chemistry and Interfacial Electrochemistry*, 47, 9–46.

Diamond, J. M. & Machen, T. E. (1983). Impedance analysis in epithelia and the problem of gastric acid secretion. *Journal of Membrane Biology*, 72, 17–41.

Dowling, G., Mittelman, M. & Danko, J. (eds.) (1991). *Microbially Influenced Corrosion and Biodeterioration*. University of Tennessee, Knoxville, TN.

Epelboin, I. & Keddam, M. (1970). Faradaic impedances: diffusion impedance and reaction impedance. *Journal of the Electrochemical Society*, 117, 1052–6.

Falk, G. & Fatt, P. (1968). Passive electrical properties of rod outer segments. *Journal of Physiology*, 198, 627–46.

Ferrante, V. & Feron, D. (1991). Microbially influenced corrosion of steels containing molybdenum and chromium: a biological and electrochemical study. In *Microbially Influenced Corrosion and Biodeterioration*, ed. G. Dowling, M. Mittelman & J. Danko, pp. 355–65. University of Tennessee, Knoxville, TN.

Gabrielli, C. (1980). *Identification of Electrochemical Processes by Frequency Response Analysis*. Solartron Electronic Group, Farnborough.

Gabrielli, C. & Keddam, M. (1974). Progrès récent dans la mesure des impédances electrochemiques en régime sinusoidal. *Electrochimica Acta*, 19, 355–62.

Hamilton, W. A. (1983). The sulphate reducing bacteria: their physiology and consequent ecology. In *Microbial Corrosion Conference*, pp. 1–5. NPL Teddington, The Metals Society, London.

Harris, C. M. & Kell, D. B. (1983). The radio-frequency dielectric properties of yeast cell measured with a rapid, automated, frequency-domain dielectric spectrometer. *Bioelectrochemistry and Bioenergetics*, 11, 15–28.

Hill, E. C., Shennan, J. L. & Walkins, R. J. (eds.) (1987). *Microbial Problems in the Offshore Oil Industry*. John Wiley and Sons, Chichester.

Hung, B. N., Beard, R. B., Brownstein, M., Dubin, S. E., Niazy, N. & Miller, A. J. (1979). Correlation of linear A.C. polarization impedance studies with tissue ingrowth for porous stimulating electrodes. In *Electrical Properties of Bone and Cartilage*, ed. C. T. Brighton, J. Black & S. R. Pollack, pp. 249–66. Grune and Stratton, New York.

Kissinger, P. T. & Heineman, W. R. (eds.) (1984). *Laboratory Techniques in Electroanalytical Chemistry*. Marcel Dekker, New York.

Lorenz, W. J. & Mansfeld, F. (1981). Determination of corrosion rates by electrochemical DC and AC methods. *Corrosion Science*, 21, 647–72.

Macdonald, D. D. (1977). *Transient Techniques in Electrochemistry*. Plenum Press, New York.

Macdonald, D. D. & McKubre, M. C. H. (1982). Impedance measurements in electrochemical systems. In *Modern Aspects of Electrochemistry*, ed. J. O'M. Bockris & B. E. Conway, vol. 4, pp. 61–150. Plenum Press, New York.

Macdonald, J. R. (1980). Interface effects in the electrical response of non-metallic conducting solids and liquids. *IEEE Transactions, Electrical Insulation*, EI-15, 65–82.

Macdonald, J. R., Schronman, J. & Lehnen, A. P. (1982). The applicability and power of complex non-linear least squares for the analysis of impedance and admittance data. *Journal of Electroanalytical Chemistry*, 131, 77–95.

Marshall, A. G. (1983). Transform techniques in chemistry. In *Physical Methods in Modern Chemical Analysis*, ed. T. Kuwana, vol. 3, pp. 57–135. Academic Press, New York.

Miller, J. D. A. (ed.) (1971). *Microbial Aspects of Metallurgy*. Medical and Technical Publishing Co. Ltd, Aylesbury.

Mopsik, F. (1984). Precision time-domain dielectric spectrometer. *Reviews of Scientific Instruments*, 55, 79–87.

Nielands, J. B. (ed.) (1974). *Microbial Iron Metabolism*. Academic Press, New York.

Postgate, J. (1979). *The Sulphate Reducing Bacteria*. Cambridge University Press, Cambridge.

Randles, J. E. B. (1947). Kinetics of rapid electrode reactions. *Discussions of the Faraday Society*, 1, 11–19.

Schwan, H. P. (1966). Alternating current electrode polarisation. *Biophysik*, 3, 181–201.

Sequeira, C. A. C. & Tiller, A. K. (eds.) (1988). *Microbial Corrosion*, vol. I. Elsevier Science Publishers, London and New York.

Sequeira, C. A. C. & Tiller, A. K. (eds.) (1992). *Microbial Corrosion*. EFC Publications no. 8. The Institute of Materials, London.

Sluyters-Rehbach, M. & Sluyters, J. H. (1970). Sine wave methods for the study of electrode processes. In *Electroanalytical Chemistry*, ed. A. J. Bard, vol. 4, pp. 1–128. Marcel Dekker, New York.

Smith, D. E. (1966). A.C. polarography and related techniques; theory and practice. In *Electroanalytical Chemistry*, ed. A. J. Bard, vol. 1, pp. 1–155. Edward Arnold, London.

Steel, M., Sheppard, R. J. & Grant, E. H. (1984). A precision method for measuring the complex permittivity of solid tissue in the frequency domain between 2 and 18 GHz. *Journal of Physics*, E. *Scientific Instruments*, 17, 29–34.

Stoecker, J. (1985). Overview of industrial biological corrosion: Past, present and future. In *Biologically Induced Corrosion*, ed. S. C. Dexter, pp. 56–71. NACE, Houston, TX.

Tiller, A. K. (1982). Aspects of microbial corrosion. In *Corrosion Processes*, ed. R. N. Parkins, pp. 115–59. Applied Science Publishers, London.

Zehnder, A. J. B. (ed.) (1987). *Biology of Anaerobic Microorganisms*. John Wiley & Sons, Chichester.

10

Design, selection and use of biocides

CHRISTINE C. GAYLARDE

Introduction

The prevention of microbially induced corrosion is an economically important and, in addition, an achievable goal. To some extent the use of corrosion-resistant materials may satisfy this aim, but it is not always practicable or economic, and toxic chemicals aimed at destroying or inhibiting the corrosion-causing microorganisms are commonly used. These biocides take many forms and can be employed in many ways. The wide variety of microorganisms whose activity or presence may promote corrosion has been described in the preceding chapters and there is a similar diversity of remedial treatments aimed at eliminating or inhibiting these organisms.

In industry, the prevention of microbiological problems is better than cure. The correct use of machinery, regular cleaning cycles and normal hygienic precautions can help to avoid the need for remedial treatment, but it is impossible to avoid entirely contamination by fungal and bacterial spores and vegetative cells. The removal of such microbial contamination, once established, can be a difficult and expensive process. The economic importance of biocides used to control microbial growth is obvious. There is a multi-million pound industry devoted to their evaluation, production and marketing.

New biocides or novel formulations of established antimicrobials continue to be produced, but it is only in recent years that the search for new products has become systematic, with development chemists liaising with microbiologists to produce substances likely to have the desired properties. This chapter is a review of the latest developments in the world of industrial biocides used to control corrosion-related problems.

Methods used in biocide treatment

Most industrial firms are sufficiently aware of the economic and environmental costs of biocide treatment that, before resorting to this action, they will have considered alternatives such as clean-up of the systems and inspection of plant for points of ingress of contamination, with subsequent plant modification. However, when control of the problem is not possible by physical methods, then treatment with an appropriate biocide may be indicated. Before such treatment is initiated, it is necessary to consider the following:

1. If the source of the contamination can be pinpointed prior to treatment, then the chemical can be effectively used locally. The recent introduction of biofilm testing has made the detection of localized infections possible. In a case study in an oil production plant in central Alberta, presenting severe corrosion problems, biofilm monitoring pinpointed the causative organisms in the treaters and recycling oil tank. Further testing of water sources entering this system showed that the contamination originated from a nearby gas plant water tank. Biocide treatment was thus restricted to the affected areas, and costly and unnecessary treatment of the entire system avoided (Boivin *et al.*, 1990).

2. Although the type and source of corrosive organisms may be detected, biocide may be unable to gain access to the cells. For example, dead spaces in pipelines can lead to the build-up of thick biofilms that can protect the cells within them from chemicals in the environment (Costerton, 1984). Since the recognition of these problems, biocide companies have begun to produce new formulations of products aimed at removing biofilms or aiding the penetration of biocide through biofilms.

3. When physical prevention of microbial corrosion has been shown to be impractical, then biocide treatment must be considered as the only possible strategy. Such treatments are not curative and microbial contamination will recur. It will, therefore, be essential to monitor the system carefully if biocide is not to be wastefully

used. Continuous treatment with a biocide, in addition to being often environmentally unacceptable, is not economic, and regular testing, with the introduction of chemical treatment when indicated, is the best policy (Nunes, 1982; Sanders, 1988).

Biocide application

Where there is prior recognition of the possibility of microbial corrosion problems, biocides can be incorporated into surface coatings on pipes and other structures. This can be a highly effective form of protection, but the presence of defects, or 'holidays', in the coatings will lead to increased electrochemical attack at these unprotected sites, resulting in localized rapid perforation of the metal rather than slow, more generalized, corrosion. The integrity of the protective coating is therefore important, but some protection against microbial corrosion may be afforded to uncoated areas for a while by biocide leaching out of surrounding protective films. Surface coatings are particularly useful in the fight against corrosion associated with fouling organisms, although in this case it is often the non-corrosive effects, such as increased drag on boats, which are considered the main problem.

Where incorporation of the biocide into a surface coating is not feasible in closed systems, systemic dosage is the alternative. Continuous treatment with biocides is not recommended. Apart from the expense, this regime runs the risk of encouraging the development of resistant forms of micro-organisms, with the potential for eventual massive failure. Systematic discontinuous treatment should be the method of choice if at all possible. Such shock, or slug, treatment will maintain adequate control if the microbial loading is not too high.

Biocides may be used both to gain and to maintain microbiological control. In order to establish control over a fouled system, thorough cleaning (in so far as it is possible) and the use of a biofilm-penetrating biocide are essential. It is foolish to add chemicals to a fouled system indiscriminately. This will result only in temporary (if any) improvement and in wasted expenditure.

Once control has been established, a common practice is to add high concentrations of biocide regularly but infrequently, without any regard for the levels of microbial contamination. This type of treatment often works, as high concentrations of biocide rapidly kill those cells present and reduce the possibility of resistant forms arising, and is thus preferable to continuous low level treatment. The prevention of microbial resistance is further aided by alternating use of different biocides or by using two biocides in combination. In the latter case, the use of subinhibitory concentrations of each of the products may be possible. A microbial population reduced and, perhaps, weakened by one biocide may be readily eliminated by the second. This corresponds to the so-called 'Hurdles Concept' (Scott, 1989), which applies to the use of subinhibitory concentrations of chemicals in combination. Where combined treatment is intended, it is important to ensure that the chemicals are not antagonistic in action and this can be shown by microbiological testing.

Biocide testing and monitoring of treatment

The effectiveness of a biocide against planktonic populations does not necessarily predict its performance against sessile cells (Ruseska *et al.*, 1982; Gaylarde & Johnston, 1983; Costerton & Lashen, 1984; Lunden & Stastny, 1985; Videla *et al.*, 1991). Thus traditional biocide assays, measuring activity against a suspension of organisms in pure culture, may have little relevance to the actual situation. It is important that testing of biocides prior to use in the field, whether for the development of a novel compound or for the selection of the optimum product from a range of available compounds, should take this fact into account. The use of biofilm monitors in biocide testing is now almost standard (see King, Chapter 8), especially in the petroleum extraction and some water treatment industries and it is not the intention of this review to cover these methods. It is, however, important to note the disadvantages of the traditional Minimum Inhibitory Concentration test, which is still in use in many laboratories (Piddock, 1990). This method of testing antimicrobial substances (termed the 'MIC test' long before this acronym was adopted by microbial corrosion scientists) has been the standard technique for many years. Its drawbacks are associated with the difficulties of extrapolation of results to the real environment:

1. Chemicals are tested only for their ability to inhibit growth and not for their potential to kill microorganisms.
2. The biocide is not tested under 'in-use' conditions, but merely in the presence of a growth medium and under optimum growth conditions for the organism. It is not possible to alter any of these conditions outside those required for good growth.

3. The activity against sessile organisms is not determined.
4. Since tests are performed using a young, highly active inoculum, the ability of the biocide to act against old cells, which may be more resistant, is not considered.
5. In the traditional form of the test, only batch cultures are used. It has recently been recognized that microorganisms in batch culture may be more sensitive to inhibitors than those in continuous cultures. Chow & Russell (1990) demonstrated the increased resistance of *Streptococcus bovis* cells in continuous culture to the ionophores lasaloic acid and monensin, and Haack *et al.* (1988) previously noted the lack of correlation between results of biocide assays against sessile bacteria in static and flowing systems.

The disadvantages noted above may be overcome by using a form of the 'time-kill' test. This was the preferred method prior to the adoption of the MIC. Kronig & Paul, in 1897, used a time-kill test to compare the biocidal activity of a wide range of compounds. They introduced the concept of 'exponential death', which is still recognized as being approximately true. Cells in a chosen state and environment are treated with varying concentrations of biocide. After set time intervals, portions are removed and the numbers of living cells determined using any suitable method. The incorporation of this technique with a flow-through system in which biofilms may also be assayed for their viable cell content should fulfil most requirements for a test for biocides to be used intermittently and, indeed, this type of design has been much in use recently (Eager *et al.*, 1986; Kinniment & Wimpenny, 1990; Kramer, 1991). When low dose continuous biocide treatment is adopted, the MIC test is more analogous to the field situation and therefore may be a more reliable guide.

Even if a standard test method should be adopted by biocide manufacturers, it is important that this can be adapted to give a more realistic prediction of the results of using a biocide in the field and this is obviously in the interests of the user. The American Society for Testing and Materials (ASTM) has prepared a set of guidelines for use by industrial firms wishing to test biocides or other chemicals for their ability to prevent or treat biofilms. ASTM Committee E35.15 on antimicrobial agents has considered a wide variety of techniques that have been used to prepare and measure biofilms, and interested firms can choose those most appropriate for their situations.

A biocide and treatment regime having been selected, it is important to monitor the results in order to know whether the treatment has been effective and equally important to continue monitoring in order to detect when treatment needs to be reinstated. Monitoring may be performed by simple enumeration techniques on samples taken from the system, using traditional microbiological methods (growth techniques) or the more recently introduced tests such as radiorespirometry for sulfate-reducing bacteria (SRB), ATP measurements or even the enzyme-linked immunosorbent assay (ELISA). Reviews of these methods are given by King (Chapter 9, this volume) and Gaylarde (1990).

Monitoring should be performed immediately before and after slug treatment and at regular intervals during lengthier treatments. After the completion of dosing, examination of the results of the monitoring tests will indicate the degree of success. It should not be expected that all cells will be killed by the biocide, although this may occur. It is essential, however, that a substantial reduction in numbers be produced. A count of $10^7–10^8$ cells/ml should fall after slug treatment to below $10^3–10^4$ cells/ml. Sometimes a rise in numbers due to the removal of cells from a biofilm into the sampling (planktonic) phase occurs (Gaylarde & Videla, 1992). This should be followed by a fall in planktonic numbers as the biocide exerts its effect on these cells and some of the specially designed biocides mentioned later below are aimed at exactly this 'remove and kill' effect.

Modes of action of biocides

The major means whereby biocides exert their effects are described below, but of course many compounds have an unknown mode of action and a number of biocides act on more than one cellular target.

Enzyme poisons and protein denaturants

These chemicals may be able to act against specific groups of microorganisms and hence may be more environmentally acceptable than some other biocides. However, most enzyme inhibitors that have found wide application in industry have as their sites of action enzymes that are common to many organisms, including macroorganisms. The cytochromes, for example, are commonly affected. A good example of this group is the bisthiocyanates, which are effective against all organisms reliant on iron-containing cytochromes, both anaerobes and aerobes. These chemicals are particularly useful, because of their hydrophobic nature, for incorporating into certain surface coatings such as paints and bitumens. Salts of heavy metals such as copper and tin may also act as enzyme poisons at low concentrations. The isothiazolones, currently a much used group of biocides, react with thiol groups in proteins and have been said to affect membrane structure (Collier *et al.*, 1990). The aldehydes, such as formaldehyde and formaldehyde adducts (e.g. hexamethylenetriamine), act not only on proteins but also on lipopolysaccharides in the bacterial cell envelope (Cloete *et al.*, 1992). A formaldehyde-releasing biocide has recently been shown to be highly effective in laboratory tests against a biofilm of *Pseudomonas fluorescens* (Menezes *et al.*, 1994).

Oxidizing agents

Kronig & Paul (1897) listed oxidants, amongst the many other compounds that they tested, in the following order of decreasing biocidal activity: HNO_3, CrO_7, chloric acid, Cl_2, $H_2S_2O_8$, MnO_4. This group of biocides is still, perhaps, the most widely used. Chlorine is a good antimicrobial compound for use in the water industry, where it has found application for many years (Kawata, 1980), but it has obvious disadvantages in situations where readily oxidizable metal is present. In addition, chlorine has been shown to react, under certain conditions, with compounds that contain ammonia. This can result in the formation of carcinogenic trichloromethanes (Cocnet *et al.*, 1986). For this reason, chlorine dioxide is beginning to replace the use of chlorine gas. Chlorine acts by combining with proteins and is particularly active at low pH, since the active forms are hypochlorous acid, $HClO$, and molecular chlorine. At pH 9 or above it is not an effective biocide and bromine might be preferred. Figure 10.1 shows the effect of pH on the concentrations of the molecular species of bromine and on the killing time. As chlorine is more reactive than bromine, the corresponding equilibrium constants are greater and the curves show a general shift to the left. For use against metal-corroding organisms, one of the chlorine compounds, such as the chloramides or chloramines, may also be used. Chloramines are active at high pH, and at pH 10 some have higher activity than free chlorine itself. However, in general the chlorine compounds are

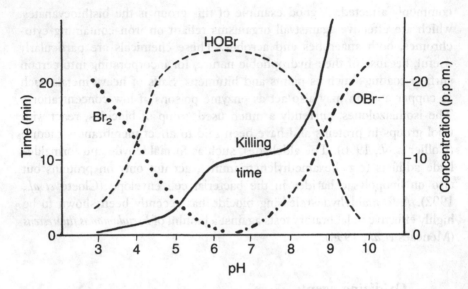

Fig. 10.1 Graph showing variation in concentrations of ionic species and killing time
with pH for bromine. (Modified from Wyss & Stockton, 1947.)

less active than chlorine both as corrosive and as biocidal agents. They may
also be more expensive and less easily inactivated in the environment, the
latter feature having advantages for certain users as well as disadvantages
for the natural population.

Surfactive agents

These compounds act upon microbial and other cell surfaces causing leakage and eventual lysis. They are amphipathic molecules with a hydrophilic
and a hydrophobic portion that can insert into the lipid-containing membranes of cells and may be either anionic or cationic, depending on the
nature of the hydrophilic portion.

Quaternary ammonium compounds (the 'quats') have been widely used
to inhibit microbial growth for many years. Their antimicrobial activity
varies with the length of the organic side-chain. Molecules with a side-chain
of less than eight carbon atoms have little activity. Biocidal activity increases
with lengthening side-chain to give optimal activity at C_{16}–C_{18}. Thereafter,
molar specific activity decreases slowly. These are fairly active biocides,

stable over a wide range of pH and causing relatively little harm to the environment. They are normally used at high concentrations to ensure effectiveness and at such concentrations foaming can be a problem. An excellent article on the modes of action of biocides has been produced by Denyer (1990).

Why are new biocides necessary?

The failure of a biocide treatment can have several causes, but in at least a number of cases products with the required properties are unavailable. Biocide manufacturers with the research underlying their industry continue to be active in the development of new products. However, the rapid changes taking place in the user industries and the adaptation of the problem-causing microorganisms make the need for new biocides ever more urgent.

Deficiencies of biocides in current or recent use

A number of failures of biocide treatment are due to an incorrect choice of biocide, which could have been prevented by better knowledge and understanding on the part of the user; for instance, the selection of a biocide that is inactivated by another chemical in the system or is unable to penetrate a biofilm. In other cases, the failure of treatment could have been predicted only by biocide testing against samples from the site, indicating the presence of resistant microorganisms. Some case histories demonstrating the above points were described by Gaylarde & Latorre (1992).

Interactions with other chemicals in the system

There are two major problems encountered: inactivation of the biocide and biocide-induced enhancement of corrosion. An example of the latter is the removal of bacterial competitors from a biocide-treated environment, allowing the growth of algae that secrete glycolic acid, reducing the chromate corrosion inhibitor. Hence the long-term effect can be an increase in corrosion because of the removal of the corrosion inhibitor rather than because of the direct corrosive effect of the microorganisms. This problem can also occur with the dithiocarbamate biocides if they are used with chromate-protected metals. High concentrations of quats and substituted guanidines will precipitate chromate, thus reducing the levels of both corrosion inhibitor and biocide and rendering both treatments useless. The replacement of chromate as a corrosion inhibitor in many countries has reduced these problems, although it has introduced others which are mentioned later.

Chromate itself has antimicrobial activity, but polyphosphate corrosion inhibitors may actually promote growth. Hence, biocides will be required more frequently in such systems. This is true also for environments that are rich in nutrients, or for those materials from which nutrients can leach. An example of the latter is creosoted wood. In high concentrations, the phenolics present in creosote are toxic to microorganisms; at a low leach rate the levels will be subinhibitory. At these concentrations, certain microorganisms, such as the *Pseudomonas* spp. and the 'jet fuel' fungus, *Hormoconis resinae*, can utilize the compounds as nutrients causing increased corrosion rates. When biocides are added to an already contaminated system, their efficacy can be very different from that in a similar environment containing the same number of newly added microorganisms. In some way, the growth of organisms affects the environment such that the biocides are less effective. This has been noted for example in the metal-working fluid environment (Rossmoore & Rossmoore, 1991). A number of biocides were shown to be less effective in 'used', as opposed to fresh, cutting oil. The metabolic cell product responsible for this change was not identified, but the well-known inactivating effect of proteins on many biocides suggests that these macromolecules may be involved.

Inability to penetrate biofilms
In heavily fouled environments, where a biofilm has already formed on the metal surface, many biocides are ineffective. Indeed, a thick biofilm is not required to enhance the resistance of the cells; even biofilms of bacteria at 10^7 cells/cm^2 can show higher resistance than the same, unattached, cells (Holah *et al.*, 1990). Unexpectedly, the biocides regarded as acting as surfactive agents (quats, amphoterics and biguanides) are not necessarily more effective on surfaces. In the work quoted above, the most effective chemicals against planktonic bacteria were peracids, amphoterics and quats, whilst only the peracids, along with iodophores, showed good activity against sessile organisms. Mrozek (1982) has also demonstrated the supremacy of peracids over quats in the treatment of surface contamination. However, Jones *et al.* (1991) found that yeast cells dried on to stainless steel surfaces were more sensitive to membrane-active biocides such as alcohols and quats

than were planktonic cells, but that the sensitivity of surface-attached cells to oxidizing biocides such as peracetic acid was similar to that of cells in suspension. Hence, surfactive agents may act well at surfaces, whilst being inefficient within a biofilm.

Even when added prior to biofilm formation, biocides may not always be able to prevent the formation of the biofilm. Chlorine and chlorine dioxide were found to be unable to prevent the deposition of a manganese-containing biofilm in certain areas of a water distribution system because of the relatively low concentrations of biocides reaching these areas (Sly et al., 1990). Chlorination was also shown to be ineffective in killing sessile cells in oil field water injection systems (Whittingham & Hardy, 1985). The lack of efficacy of biocides against sessile organisms, well documented in the past few years, is probably due to the inability of the chemicals to penetrate the biofilm, in addition to physiological differences between sessile and planktonic cells (Brown & Gilbert, 1993). A number of workers have shown that biocide sensitivity can be altered up to 1000-fold by changes in nutrients and growth rate (Gilbert & Brown, 1978, 1980; Wright & Gilbert, 1987a,b). Although Brown et al. (1990) emphasize the need for cautious interpretation of results of antibiotic assays against sessile cells, Evans et al. (1990) have shown that newly formed cells, whether sessile or planktonic, show the highest sensitivity to certain inhibitors and Page & Gaylarde (1990) demonstrated the increased resistance of older cells of Legionella micdadei to the biocide 2-bromo-2-nitro-1,3-propanediol, which could have been associated with an altered outer membrane protein. The increased resistance of biofilmed cells is, it seems, likely to be caused by their situation, protected within deposits and slimes, and by the possibly increased age and reduced growth rate of the cells and their altered surface structures. Another possible explanation for failures of biocides in fouling situations is removal of biocide by the biofilm matrix. Cationic biocides, such as biguanides and quats, adsorb to the surface of extracellular polymeric materials in the biofilm but may not be absorbed into the bulk biofilm and hence do not reach the microbial cells embedded within and beneath it. Gaylarde & Gaylarde (1992), using a model biofilm system, showed that the kinetics of uptake of even a simple biocide into a polysaccharide biofilm is complex and it is difficult to predict active concentrations within the film.

The isothiazolones are excellent biofilm penetrants, but they have the disadvantages of being inhibited by hydrogen sulfide and being incompatible with some corrosion inhibitors. Glutaraldehyde, a well-tried and long-used biocide, is also relatively cheap. It shows good activity against sessile organisms and has been demonstrated to control biofilms in a laboratory simulation of a circulating metal-working-fluid system (Kramer, 1991) and to accelerate the removal of cells from the biofilm (Eager *et al.*, 1986; van der Wende, 1990). However, it is by no means completely effective against bacteria within biofilms (Gaylarde & Johnston, 1984; Videla *et al.*, 1991) and its efficacy as a sporocide has also recently been called into question (Power & Russell, 1990). Formaldehyde has been shown to be effective to some extent against *Pseudomonas aeruginosa* in a biofilm (Kinniment & Wimpenny, 1990), but, as with glutaraldehyde, the great disadvantage of this chemical is its toxicity to non-target organisms. It should be used only in closed systems and its subsequent discharge into the environment be carefully controlled.

A further, and by no means minor, problem associated with biofilm treatment has recently been recognized. The use of subinhibitory levels of biocide can cause stress to some microbial cells, such that they increase their production of extracellular polysaccharide (slime) and thereby enhance biofilm thickness (Dunne, 1990). Furthermore, it has been demonstrated that biofilm formation is more effectively prevented by a single large dose of biocide than by several smaller applications (Hassan & Oh, 1989).

Resistant microorganisms

Biocides may be degraded by chemical and physical factors, such as pH and heat, or by biological effects, such as enzymic activity, or by adsorption to surfaces. These factors can result in the failure of biocide treatment. However, even when no such inactivation occurs, failure may still result from the presence, or arrival, of 'resistant' microorganisms.

Microorganisms are probably the most adaptable group of living things. Problems of their resistance, or adaptation, to antibiotics are well documented and in many instances the molecular basis of this resistance is known. Anecdotal accounts of failures of biocide treatments are legion (e.g. see Gaylarde & Latorre, 1992), but there has been no truly systematic and thorough study of this phenomenon. The development of biocide resistance by mutation is still questioned by some people. However, Sharma, in 1984, reported a biguanide-resistant mutant of *Desulfovibrio desulfuricans* that had a decreased permeability to the biocide, and Sanders (1988) reported the presence of biocide-resistant SRB in an oil field, although the cellular changes conferring resistance were not investigated. In a much earlier study, a strain of the Gram-negative bacterium *Serratia marcescens* was found to have developed resistance to a particular quat by elaborating a lipid-containing outer membrane that was not disrupted by the chemical (Chaplin, 1952). Many resistant bacteria are found to have a high lipid content in the cell envelopes and this seems to be a common form of resistance. A recent study has surveyed the resistance of a number of environmental isolates to various commercial products and concluded that inducible resistance to at least the isothiazolones and some quats is rare, although a number of organisms show constitutive resistance (Brözel & Cloete, 1991). Larson & Ventullo (1991) were able to produce resistant microbial populations in the laboratory and in the field by exposure to chronic surfactant treatment.

Some claims of resistance are, in fact, due to the inactivation of the biocide by a second, truly resistant, microorganism. Bronopol (2-bromo-2-nitropropane-1,3-diol), long used as a pharmaceutical preservative, has been shown to be inactivated by a highly resistant form of the fungus *Fusarium solani* (Thomas & Moss, 1990). Inactivation of the biocide resulted in 'preserved' antacid becoming contaminated with various species of bacteria, none of which was resistant to the chemical.

The relatively non-specific action of biocides means that major changes will have to take place within a microbial cell in order for a biocide to become ineffective. However, there is no doubt that microorganisms are capable of such changes without serious effect on their viability and hence true biocide resistance is possible.

Changes in industrial practices

The ways in which alterations in industrial processes can result in the need for different biocides can be demonstrated by examining two areas – industrial cooling water and the pulp and paper industry.

The treatment of industrial cooling waters has changed dramatically over the last 20 years or so because of increased environmental awareness. The chromate- and zinc-based corrosion inhibitors previously favoured are now almost universally discouraged, and phosphate- or organic-based substances, more active at high than low pH, have been substituted (Lamot, 1988). At the same time, the use of sulfuric acid for scale control has been replaced by more specific inhibitors such as polycarboxylates. The resulting increase in the pH of the water has reduced the efficiency of the chlorine biocides previously used and made it difficult to find an acceptable substitute. Dithiocarbamates, a possible alternative, can cause effluent problems

(Sequeira *et al.*, 1988). Both for these reasons, and because of the increasing use of recycled water, many cooling water systems are having more contamination problems than before and better biocides are required.

Similar changes have occurred in the pulp and paper industry and have also resulted in increased pH values in systems requiring treatment. Once more, increased contamination and biofilm (slime) formation have been the result and this has led to more problems with anaerobic bacteria (Lamot, 1988). Again, therefore, new biocides are required.

Impact of environmental issues

The breakdown of biocides by living organisms reduces the active life of the chemical and, although this can be a disadvantage for the user, such biodegradability ensures the non-persistence of the toxic chemical in the environment. In 1984 alone, 500 tons of biocides were discharged into the North Sea as a result of offshore oil production operations (Bedborough & Blackman, 1987). The introduction of legal controls over the discharge of hazardous materials in recent years has affected the biocide production industry to no small extent (Halleux, 1990), in addition to posing problems of disposal to biocide users (Haggett & Morchat, 1991). Both in the USA and Europe, 'chemical blacklists' have been published by governmental bodies. In 1990, these lists contained 114 (Environmental Protection Agency) and 118 (European Community) organic compounds respectively, considered to be of major environmental concern, and many more are currently being tested for possible addition to the list (Valls *et al.*, 1990). In addition to the commonly recognized toxic hazards of biocides, other effects such as the role of chlorine compounds on ozone decomposition in the upper atmosphere also warrant regulation. Although not all countries have introduced tight controls and enforcement is often inadequate even when regulations exist, it is now recognized by most biocide manufacturers that their products must be rigorously tested for environmental impact if they are to succeed in today's market.

Toxicity of biocides

Before a new biocide can be sold, its toxicity to a variety of higher organisms must be determined. The extent of this toxicity testing considerably increases the cost of launching a new formulation. Animal toxicity is usually assessed as the LD50 (lethal dose 50%), the concentration of chemical which, administered by the stated route (intradermally, by inhalation, etc.), will kill half of the animals tested in a given time. For example, the oral LD50 for rats is 40 mg/kg for acrolein, 190 mg/kg for tributyltin oxide (TBTO), 200 mg/kg for pentachlorophenol, and around 2000 mg/kg for the quats. Toxicity to fish is also an important parameter, especially where the biocide is likely to be released into rivers or seas. Thus an application to register a new compound in the UK or USA will include information on the LD50 or LC50 (lethal concentration 50%) values for a variety of aquatic animals. Data required might include the oral LD50 for mallards and dietary LC50s for quail, rainbow trout and bluegill sunfish, in addition to a value for the toxic effects on daphnia.

Although the concentration of biocide that is lethal to a variety of animals is obviously an important parameter, the LD50 may be misleading, since non-lethal, but nevertheless harmful, effects can occur at much lower concentrations. The ED50 (effective dose 50%) gives a measure of the ability of a chemical to cause specified symptoms, such as paralysis, and this measurement may be more important than the LD50. In recent years, these traditional tests are gradually being superseded by the 'rising dose toxicity profile', in which the highest non-lethal and the lowest lethal doses are quoted (W. G. Guthrie, personal communication) and it is well recognized that such factors as accumulation in tissues under chronic dosage and ability to cause skin sensitization (not a lethal effect) are also important parameters that must be tested.

Unfortunately, all these types of test necessarily involve the use of living animals. No *in vitro* toxicity test has yet been accepted by governmental bodies for biocide registration purposes. A considerable amount of work is currently in progress to develop acceptable *in vitro* tests. The Ames test, which uses mutagenesis in *Salmonella* as a measure of carcinogenicity, is well recognized, but cytotoxicity testing using animal cell cultures has not been shown to correlate sufficiently well with animal tests to satisfy the authorities. New tests under development include the chorioallantoic membrane test in fertilized hens' eggs and the use of human epidermal cell cultures. Both of these can indicate inflammatory activity and may be able to replace the Draize test in rabbits (Goldberg & Frazier, 1989).

Reducing the environmental impact of biocides
Toxicity testing is, of course, essential, as are the control regulations laid down by governments, both over marketing and over disposal of biocides after use. That governmental regulations can be effective is shown by the

declining levels of DDT in Europeans since the introduction of controls (Jensen, 1983; Greve & van Zoonen, 1990). However, new laws are not always so rapidly effective. The use of other organochlorine products has also been considerably reduced over many years and yet levels of these compounds in human tissues do not appear to have declined over the last 20 years or so (Greve & van Zoonen, 1990). The organochlorines, of course, are particularly persistent substances.

The recent introduction into the cooling-water biocide market of the extremely short-lived compound ozone (a highly active oxidizing agent) is an example of how environmental issues may affect the choice of chemical agent. Ozone is at the moment a relatively expensive option, but it may have sufficient advantages, especially from the environmental regulation viewpoint, to attain a prominent position in the market (Gaylarde & Latorre, 1992; Gaylarde & Videla, 1992).

In addition to legally enforceable regulations, education of the biocide user is important. Nichols (1988) suggests that education of boat-owners could reduce the release of biocide into harbour waters by at least one-third. The dissemination of information might readily be undertaken by biocide producers and distributors and those who are not already involved in such educational activities should be encouraged to become so.

An area of intense research at the present time is the biodegradation of xenobiotic materials (those resistant to biological attack). If a biocide is particularly persistent in the environment, then the development of some system that would degrade the chemical prior to release would be a great advantage. Although not strictly within the scope of this chapter, it is important to note that research to this end is in progress in a number of establishments. Two recent, and rather novel, ideas will be mentioned. These suggestions include the use of biological products, rather than whole organisms, as degradative systems.

Nicell et al. (1991) reported the removal of phenolics from wastewaters using the enzyme horseradish peroxidase. After oxidation by enzymic action, aggregation occurs (non-enzymically) and the insoluble products are readily removed from the water.

Sublette et al. (1990) have used a different system to degrade persistent compounds. The 'biomimetic agent' haematin (a porphyrin) is able to catalyse the oxidation or reduction of a variety of organic compounds. Sublette and his co-workers were able to oxidize chlorinated phenols (using t-butyl-hydroperoxide) and reduce nitrotoluenes (using dithiothreitol) sufficiently quickly and efficiently to make this process worthy of further research. The success of such strategies, of course, will depend on the diminution of toxic hazard in the treated waste or on the ease of removal of the products from the waste if toxic properties are not eliminated.

Recent introductions and research in the field of biocides

The newer biocides on the market today are mostly electrophilically active. They react with nucleophilic groups, such as those on proteins; the nucleophilic groups in the active centres of enzymes are often extremely susceptible to such reagents. Hence, these biocides inhibit or kill living organisms efficiently. In addition they have the advantage of being non-persistent in the environment because they are rapidly inactivated. An example of this class of compound is the isothiazolones, which react with nucleophilic substances as mentioned above (Paulus, 1991). This mode of action makes the isothiazolones efficient biocides with relatively good environmental acceptability. However, their reactivity with –SH groups leads to some problems in areas of SRB activity, where they may be inactivated much too rapidly by biogenic H_2S to be fully effective.

New compounds and new uses for existing compounds

It is rare to find completely new compounds being developed as biocides today. This is, at least partially, due to the cost of such programmes, which is becoming prohibitive (Lloyd, 1990). However, some new active substances have been registered recently.

2-Bromo-2-nitropropane-1-ol is such a new biocidal product (Elsmore & Guthrie, 1990). This compound has been shown to be effective as both a bactericide and a fungicide and, being highly soluble in organic solvents, could be an interesting option for in-can paint preservation. A demonstrated MIC of 6–12 µg/ml for algae suggests its possible use in antifoulants.

Although a new product, this chemical is related to biocides already in use. In this way, it resembles the development of a new formaldehyde-releasing agent. This group of biocides has been in use for many years, but still new compounds, with slightly differing structures, continue to be synthesized (Paulus, 1988). The new phosphonium biocides, however, represent a new group of active agents, albeit that they are basically quats in which the ammonium ion has been replaced by a phosphonium ion. Three phosphonium biocides are listed by Lloyd (1990), the best studied being tetrakis-hydroxyphosphonium sulfate (THPS). This compound is said to have a more favourable environmental profile than many other biocides whilst still being very effective. Page & Gaylarde (1990) showed that it was particularly useful for the treatment of *Pseudomonas* contamination and its activity against SRB has also been demonstrated (P. E. Cook & C. C. Gaylarde, unpublished data; Lloyd, 1990). Akihiko *et al.* (1993) showed that polymers of phosphonium salts were twice as active as the corresponding quaternary ammonium salt polymers against *Escherichia coli* and *Staphylococcus aureus*, once more indicating the potential of these agents.

The search for new active compounds can involve a rational approach such as that used by Vincentini *et al.* (1989). They investigated purine-like structures for the development of new fungicides and had some degree of success. Where specific organisms are the target, it may be possible to look for inhibitors of pathways peculiar to this group. An example is the potential use of inhibitors of the polyamine biosynthetic pathway to control bacteria with growth requirements for polyamines. Midorikawa *et al.* (1991) demonstrated the restricted activity of methylglyoxal bis(guanylhydrazone) analogues against some Gram-negative bacteria. The most sensitive organism was *Aeromonas sobria*, against which methylglyoxal bis(butylamidinohydrazone) had an MIC of 50 μmol/l.

An alternative strategy is to determine the molecular structures responsible for antimicrobial activity of known biocides and use this knowledge in the synthesis of new compounds. Massolini *et al.* (1989) have found that the fungitoxic activity of phenylpyridyl ketoxime derivatives depends on both lipophilic and steric factors (for instance, variations in benzene ring substituents and the position of the pyridine nitrogen atom with respect to the free oxime group). Novel compounds can now be prepared in accordance with this knowledge.

Yet a further possibility is to study the substances produced by biological control agents. A number of organisms are known that inhibit other microorganisms but from which the substance responsible for this inhibition has not been isolated. Rogers (1989) has identified a novel pyridone compound, produced by *Trichoderma harzianum*, that could be a useful fungicide. There are also a number of well-studied antibiotic substances unsuitable for veterinary or human therapy that might be reconsidered for industrial use.

A group of biocides with a mode of action not previously mentioned includes the azole derivatives, triazoles and imidazoles. These substances prevent the biosynthesis of ergosterol, an important membrane constituent in fungi, by inhibiting the demethylation of the intermediate compound lanosterol (Paulus, 1991). Ergosterol is not an important constituent of bacteria and hence these compounds are useful only in situations where fungal contamination is the problem. Nevertheless, they can be efficient biocides in such cases. One advantage is that the development of specific resistance to these demethylation inhibitors (DMIs) is normally slow. The resistance mechanism is not certain, but could be due to active efflux (quoted by Koller & Wubben, 1989). There is no evidence that resistance is due to decreased lipid content of the microorganisms. The differential sensitivity of two strains of *Cladosporium cucumerianum* was found to have no correlation with their lipid compositions (Carter *et al.*, 1989).

Much work is being carried out on the development of compounds that can prevent fouling (and often associated corrosion) of metal structures in contact with seawater. An interesting report of the isolation of a natural compound, derived from eucalyptus, which has antifouling properties was given by Yamashita *et al.* (1989). Acylated rhaponticin, a stilbene glycoside, was shown to be active against the blue mussel, *Mytilus edulis*.

A large number of biocides have been used in metal-working fluids. The huge range of possible contaminants in this situation has led to the requirement for broad spectrum biocides. Constant reinoculation in the workshop environment results in new populations of organisms being present over the course of time, even when a biocide is continuously used ('resistance'), and so product switching is commonplace. In an environment so closely associated with human workers, the toxic properties of biocides become more apparent and skin absorption and sensitization are real hazards. Following exposure to anionic detergents at pH 9.2–9.4, a mild, clinically insignificant, irritant dermatitis will commonly occur, and even severe reactions may occasionally be encountered. These skin changes will lead to increased skin permeability and any toxic effect of the biocide (or other constituents of the alkaline metal-working fluid) will be therefore enhanced. Hence, metal-working fluids present biocide manufacturers with a real challenge. Sandin *et al.* (1992) suggested that one solution might be to find biocides more active at high than at low pH, since the pH of metal-working fluids (9.4) differs from that of the human skin (about 5). They have demonstrated (Sandin *et al.*, 1991) that butylethanolamine and dimethylaminomethylpropanol, used as corrosion inhibitors, can control microbial contamination in cutting oils under machine workshop conditions. In a survey of alkanolamines aimed at finding the compound most useful as a biocide at high pH, and which had relatively low activity at the lower pH of human skin (Sandin *et al.*, 1992), octylmonoethanolamine was shown to have a minimum bactericidal concentration of 0.4 mM (equal to 69 p.p.m.) at pH 9.2. It may be, indeed, that this is a useful biocide, but it is unlikely that this strategy will be effective in reducing toxic skin effects. The skin is very poorly buffered and, in contact with a fluid of pH 9.2–9.4, will rapidly equilibrate to this level. Furthermore, the variation of biocidal activity with pH does not necessarily correlate with its skin-sensitizing potential.

Problems over the last few decades with bacterial contamination in metal-working fluids have led to the development of the new synthetic cutting oils. These are more resistant to bacterial growth, but, unfortunately, have turned out to be susceptible to fungal infections. Here, then, a new field has opened for the use of antifungal agents. There is a wide variety of antifungals known (many from work in the agricultural field) and these may now find new application. The fungicide diiodomethyl-*p*-tolylsulfone is currently being tested for activity in metal-working fluids (Pohlman, 1990) and many others remain to be tested.

Improved formulation of biocides

Apart from new uses for old products, another way of bringing novel biocides to the market today within a reasonably short time span and with relatively low expenditure is to improve the formulation. This may include adding a surfactive agent to improve biofilm penetration, manipulation to improve the survival of the active biocide in the environment without potentiating its hazardous effects, or mixing two different biocidal products. The mixing of two different active agents to produce a novel biocide formulation is not new. Paulus & Genth, in 1983, commented on the advantages of combinations of phenol derivatives with formaldehyde-releasing agents, benzimidazolylmethylcarbamate or thiazolylbenzimidazole. The mixtures have broad spectrum activity together with chemical stability and low toxicity (Paulus & Genth, 1983). However, these formulations were devised simply by using an empirical approach. Currently, a more rational approach is being brought to the design of new formulations.

Surfactive agents may be added to antimicrobial chemicals in order to increase the ability of these agents to reach the target cells, which may be hidden within thick biofilms (Lapin-Scott & Costerton, 1989). Even before the importance of sessile organisms in biocorrosion was realized, such bio-cide formulations were in use to help to overcome slime and corrosion product deposition. However, empirical data have shown that surfactant addition does not necessarily improve biocide activity (Falk & Bayer, 1989). Surfactants, as well as other complexing agents, may also be used to solubil-ize otherwise non-water-soluble products. Benzothiazole, for instance, may be used in an aqueous environment by this means (Katayama Chemical Works Co. Ltd, Japanese Patent application, 1989).

The problems associated with the use of chlorine as a biocide, mentioned in the Introduction to this chapter, have been overcome to some extent by using new bromine compounds. The bromamines have the advantages of being relatively non-persistent in the environment, and thus more environ-mentally acceptable (Ginn et al., 1989), and of having good activity in nitrogen-containing environments (Conley et al., 1987). Other bromine compounds that have been suggested for use include bromine chloride (Sanger & Connell, 1990), a bromosulfamate (Smyk et al., 1989) and dialkylphosphonodibromo-acetates and -acetonitriles (Direktor & Effenberger, 1991). Fellers et al. (1988) discussed the relative advantages of bromine over chlorine treatment in cooling-water systems and considered that, in addition to the advantages already mentioned, bromine treatments are to be preferred because of the lower corrosion rates, reduced require-ments for mechanical cleaning and lower overall costs.

A relatively new biocide, which incorporates both bromine and chlorine activity, is 1-bromo-3-chloro-5,5-dimethylhydantoin (BCDMH). This was first introduced into cooling-water systems in 1980 and has gained in popu-larity since then. The compound is generally more active than chlorine, especially in modern cooling-water environments, but is, apparently, inef-fective against *Legionella pneumophila* (Fliermans & Harvey, 1984). Zhang & Matson (1989), noting that the activity of BCDMH is intermediate between that of chlorine and that of bromine, suggested a more effective and cheaper biocide might be produced by using an organic chlorine-releasing compound and sodium bromide, thus providing separate sources of the two halogens.

Prolonged survival of a chemical under in-use conditions may be achieved by a number of means without necessarily increasing the ecotoxicity of the product. An innovative idea in this area has been developed by Kurita Water Industries Ltd, who have converted isothiazolones to their clathrates by reaction with bisphenols (Sekikawa et al., 1989). The resultant compounds give a sustained release of active biocide. Controlled release formulations, such as microencapsulation (Tadros, 1989), have been investigated for the improvement of the active life of a biocide. Prasad *et al.* (1990) showed that chemical complexation with metals (cobalt or copper) could increase the working and shelf life of some organophosphorus compounds.

Development of synergistic formulations

The cost of developing and bringing on to the market a completely new biocide means that many industrial companies are now showing great interest in developing biocides composed of two or more recognized products with synergistic activity. The 'Hurdles Concept' (Scott, 1989), mentioned on p. 330, can be extended to include more than two biocides or to incorporate other inhibitory stages. For example, adverse physical conditions, such as raised or lowered temperatures, may provide a further hurdle for the microbial cells to overcome. The incorporation of materials that are not, in themselves, biocidal, but have an adverse effect on cell metabolism or integrity, is another application of this concept. Ethylenediaminetetra-acetic acid (EDTA), for instance, has been shown to affect the composition and physical integrity of the outer membrane of the SRB species *Desulfovibrio vulgaris* (Bradley *et al.*, 1984) and has bacteristatic activity against *Staphylococcus aureus* (Kraniak & Shelef, 1988). The weakening of bacterial cell envelopes by this chemical would render the cells more susceptible to attack by biocides acting on internal cell metabolic processes. Hill (1990) also suggested this possibility, in addition to proposing the examination of enzymes as aids to biocide permeation. He described the use by Freis (1984) of an enzyme hydrolysing the polymer laevan to promote slimicide activity in paper mills and suggested that enzymes such as lipases and lysozyme might be tested for their ability to enhance biocide uptake through bacterial cell envelopes. The use of model membrane systems would facilitate such investigations. Barker *et al.* (1984) used Millipore filters impregnated with isopropylmyristate to study membrane transport, and their results indicate that hydroxybutylamines and hydroxypropylamines could facilitate uptake of anionic compounds.

Another approach to the problem is to identify the deficiencies in the biocide in use and try to correct these with a second product. An example of this is a new biocide for use in metal-working fluids. Bromonitropropanediol (BNPD), the initial product, controlled bacterial, but not fungal, contamination in synthetic metal-working fluids. After several available antifungal biocides with acceptable toxicity profiles had been tested, 2-(thiocyanome-thylthio)benzthiazole (TCMTB) was chosen for the production of an effective commercial product based on a mixture of the two compounds (Parr, 1990).

ICI UK has patented combinations of isothiazolones and a disulfide compound that have been shown to be highly effective in cooling water, paper mills and as a paint additive (1987). The isothiazolones may also be potentiated by copper salts. Cu(II), as disodium copper citrate, as copper sulfate, or as copper nitrate can increase the activity of 5-chloro-2-methyl-4-isothiazolin-3-one (Riha et $al.$, 1992). It is thought that the Cu(II) cation has two actions: (a) to protect isothiazolone from nucleophilic attack in an aqueous environment and hence prolong its active life, and (b) to enhance the antibacterial activity of isolthiazolone by an unknown mechanism. Whatever the mode of action, the mixture has been shown to be active in the metal-working fluid environment. Copper also appears to act synergistically with formaldehyde and formaldehyde adducts (Rossmoore, 1990). Disodium copper citrate and copper sulfate were both found to potentiate the activity of formaldehyde, but only if added together with, or before, the aldehyde. This suggests that copper acts by removing glutathione (Sondossi et $al.$, 1990), which is required for one type of formaldehyde resistance in microorganisms. Hence the interaction is not between the two chemicals themselves and this should be regarded as an example of quasi-synergism.

Yet another synergistic combination with copper is zinc pyrithione as an antifouling additive in marine paints (Ruggerio & Farmer, 1991). This formulation could replace the more commonly used Cu(II) oxide or tributyl-tin oxide. The quasi-synergistic effect of zinc and copper could be due to the occurrence of organisms with differential sensitivities to the two substances. The diatoms $Amphora$ $coffeaeformis$ and $A.$ $hyalina$ show such differential sensitivity, the former being more resistant to copper but more sensitive to zinc than the latter (French & Evans, 1988).

In conjunction with chlorine treatment, copper is found to compare favourably with conventional electrolytic copper dosing, chlorine dosing, or copper and aluminium dosing in the control of biofouling in closed seawater systems (Williams & Knox-Holmes, 1989). The combination was at least as effective in reducing fouling inside steel pipes and on titanium heat-exchanger surfaces as conventional hypochlorite treatment at levels of chlorine between five and ten times less than that usually used and at six times lower copper levels than those used to control macrofouling.

Although the use of copper as a protectant in aqueous systems is not new, the above examples show that a little imagination may produce yet more applications for this inorganic and fairly safe chemical. Recently, the metal itself has been tested as a protectant for cooling-water systems in submarines. Lewis & Smith (1990) showed that electrostatically released copper at 0.1 mg/l could protect these systems from hydroid (tubeworm) settlement.

It is important to remember, when attempting to compare novel formulations with traditional biocides, that laboratory testing may produce results far different from those encountered in the field. Singer (1990) quoted the case of two sanitizers that gave opposing results in laboratory versus field trials designed to select the most effective agent.

Treatments that could replace biocides

An alternative use of electrochemistry in control of biofilms has been demonstrated by Nakamura et al. (1989). They were able to kill sessile *Vibrio alginolyticus* by the application through a basal plane pyrolytic graphite electrode of 0.8 V (SCE) for 10 min. They suggested that cell death was caused by the electrochemical oxidation of intracellular coenzyme A.

Blenkinsopp et al. (1992) and Boivin et al. (1992) have demonstrated that the application of a low voltage electrical field can enhance the effectiveness of biocides against sessile bacteria. If this technique is proved to be efficacious, then it may permit the use of lower doses of biocides in a system, thus reducing both costs and the environmental hazard.

In the marine area, improved surface coatings with low fouling potential reduce the need for biocides. An interesting innovation for the production of non-toxic antifouling coatings has been suggested by Nanishi et al. (1989). They produced coating films with separated hydrophilic/hydrophobic and hydrophobic/hydrophobic phase structures using silicone resins, liquid paraffins and non-ionic silicone surfactants. Both laboratory studies and initial immersion tests in Shimizu Bay, Japan, indicated that adsorption of proteins and biofouling were lower for the more hydrophobic structures. Another piece of work from Japan indicates that it may be possible to use ultraviolet irradiation to reduce marine fouling (Yamashita, 1990).

Finally, a brief mention must be given to the possibility of replacing the chemical biocides with biological control agents. The use of harmless microorganisms to combat microbially induced problems is something that has long been a goal of microbiologists and ecologists. Several pieces of work suggest that this might be possible for fouling and metal corrosion. Thomas & Allsopp (1983) demonstrated a significant reduction in fouling of glass surfaces by the marine alga *Enteromorpha* when slides were previously colonized with a marine pseudomonad, indicating a possible use for this bacterium as a biological anti-fouling agent. Gaylarde & Johnston (1982) showed that the bacterium *Vibrio anguillarum*, isolated from estuarine waters, could reduce corrosion of mild steel coupons, while more recently it has been suggested that the production of H_2S by SRB may be controlled by the introduction of a sulfide-resistant strain of *Thiobacillus denitrificans* (Sublette *et al.*, 1989). Another biocontrol option is the use of bacterial viruses, the bacteriophages, to kill troublesome microorganisms. The Fuji Spinning Co. Ltd, in Japan, has considered the use of bacteriophages immobilized on chitosan as a new form of biocide (Yabe *et al.*, 1987). Immobilization extends the lifetime of the viruses and leaves only the problem of selecting bacteriophages with suitable specificity for the organisms to be attacked. The great specificity of bacteriophages for their host species means that this could be an onerous undertaking.

Biological control of environmental problems is an attractive option for the operator, since living organisms, being self-replicating, can be used in low and infrequent doses. However, in most cases the unpredictability of the material limits this option. In spite of much research in this area in a number of different industries over the years, relatively few biocontrol programmes exist. It seems that in the foreseeable future, biocides will continue to be employed in the fight against biocorrosion.

Concluding remarks: the future

We have begun to approach the development of new biocides rationally, but we still have a long way to go. The established empirical methods for biocide development will continue to be important. However, the path to be followed in the future must increasingly be knowledge-led. Ideally, the microbiologist will take his or her understanding of microbial cell structure and physiology to a developmental chemist and together they will determine potential inhibitory structures. A knowledge of comparative biochemistry will be essential, since the systems to be attacked must be unique to micro-organisms. In addition, the physicochemical characteristics of the products will be selected to ensure efficient biofilm penetration. Suggested outline schemes for the rational development of biocides are shown in Fig. 10.2.

The introduction of new active agents will be complemented by the development of improved formulations including synergistic mixtures, complexes and novel release systems. Together with efficient and appropriate testing systems, this will ensure the user industries of the opportunity to control microbial corrosion effectively.

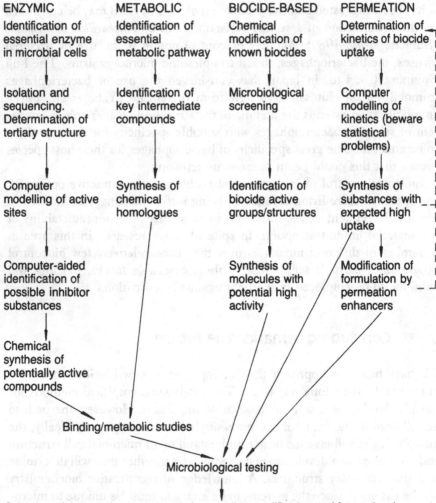

Fig. 10.2 Possible approaches to the development of 'designer' biocides.

I thank my husband, Peter, for his considerable help in the preparation of this chapter. In addition, my thanks go to my colleague, Bob Thomas, in Porto Alegre, for his helpful comments on the manuscript.

References

Akihiko, K., Tomiki, I. & Takeshi, E. (1993). Novel cationic biocides: synthesis and antibacterial activity of polymeric phosphonium salts. *Journal of Polymer Science. Part A: Polymer Chemistry*, 31, 335–43.

Barker, N., Hadgraft, J. & Wotton, P. K. (1984). Facilitated transport across liquid/liquid interfaces and its relevance to drug diffusion across biological membranes. *Faraday Discussions of the Chemical Society*, 77, 97–104.

Bedborough, D. R. & Blackman, R. A. (1987). A survey of inputs to the North Sea resulting from oil and gas development. *Proceedings of the Royal Society, London*, 316, 495–509.

Blenkinsopp, S. A., Anderson, C. P., Khoury, A. E. & Costerton, J. W. (1992). Electrical enhancement of biocide action for improved biofouling and biocorrosion control. *American Chemical Society Division of Fuel Chemistry*, 37, 1540–4.

Boivin, J. W., Shapka, R., Khoury, A. E., Blenkinsopp, S. A. & Costerton, J. W. (1992). An old and a new method of control for biofilm bacteria. In *Corrosion 92*, Paper no. 171. NACE, Houston, TX.

Boivin, J., Laishley, E. J., Bryant, R. & Costerton, J. W. (1990). The influence of enzyme systems on MIC. In *Corrosion 90*, Paper no. 128. NACE, Houston, TX.

Bradley, G., Gaylarde, C. & Johnston, J. (1984). A specific interaction between ferrous ions and lipopolysaccharide in *D. vulgaris*. *Journal of General Microbiology*, 130, 441–4.

Brown, M. R. W., Allison, D. G. & Gilbert, P. (1990). Resistance of bacterial biofilms to antibiotics: a growth-related effect? *Journal of Antimicrobial Chemotherapy*, 22, 777–83.

Brown, M. R. W. & Gilbert, P. (1993). Sensitivity of biofilms to antimicrobial agents. *Journal of Applied Bacteriology*, 74, 87S–97S.

Brözel, V. S. & Cloete, T. E. (1991). Fingerprinting of commonly available water treatment bactericides in South Africa. *Water, SA*, 17, 57–66.

Carter, G. A., Kendall, S. J., Burdan, R. S., James, C. S. & Clark, T. (1989). The lipid composition of 2 isolates of *Cladosporium cucumerinum* do not explain their differences in sensitivity to fungicides which inhibit sterol biosynthesis. *Pesticide Science*, 26, 181–92.

Chaplin, C. E. (1952). Bacterial resistance to quaternary ammonium disinfectants. *Journal of Bacteriology*, 63, 453–8.

Chow, J. M. & Russell, J. B. (1990). Effect of ionophores and pH on growth of *Streptococcus bovis* in batch and continuous culture. *Applied and Environmental Microbiology*, 56, 1588–93.

Cloete, T. E., Brözel, V. S. & von Holy, A. (1992). Practical aspects of biofouling control in industrial water systems. *International Biodeterioration*, 29, 299–341.

Cocnet, L., Courtois, Y. & Mallevialle, J. (1986). Mutagenic activity of disinfection by-products. *Environmental Health Perspective*, 69, 165–75.

Collier, P. J., Ramsey, A., Waigh, R. D., Douglas, K. T., Austen, P. & Gilbert, P. (1990). Chemical reactivity of some isothiazolone biocides. *Journal of Applied Bacteriology*, 69, 578–84.

Conley, J. C., Puzig, E. H. & Alleman, J. E. (1987). Bromine chemistry, an alternative to dechlorination in cooling water and wastewater disinfection. In *Proceedings of the 48th Annual Meeting, International Water Conference*, Pittsburgh, 2–4 November, Paper no. 42. Engineers Society of Western Pennsylvania, Pittsburgh.

Costerton, J. W. (1984). The formation of biocide-resistant biofilms in industrial, natural and medical systems. *Developments in Industrial Microbiology*, 25, 363–72.

Costerton, J. W. & Lashen, E. S. (1984). Influence of biofilm. Efficacy of biocides on corrosion-causing bacteria. *Materials Performance*, 23, 34–7.

Denyer, S. P. (1990). Mechanisms of action of biocides. *International Biodeterioration*, 26, 89–100.

Direktor, D. & Effenberger, R. (1991). Dialkylphosphonodibromoacetates and -acetonitriles active against organisms isolated from cooling water in a fertilizer plant. *Journal of Chemical Technology and Biotechnology*, 51, 253–62.

Dunne, W. M. Jr (1990). Effects of subinhibitory concentrations of vancomycin or cefamandole on biofilm production by coagulase-negative staphylococci. *Antimicrobial Agents and Chemotherapy*, 34, 390–3.

Eager, R. G., Theis, A. B., Turakhia, M. H. & Characklis, W. G. (1986). Glutaraldehyde: impact on corrosion causing biofilms. In *Corrosion 86*, Paper no. 125. NACE, Houston, TX.

Evans, D. J., Brown, M. R. W., Alison, D. G. & Gilbert, P. (1990). Susceptibility of bacterial biofilms to tobramycin: role of specific growth rate and phase in the division cycle. *Journal of Antimicrobial Chemotheraphy*, 25, 585–91.

Falk, R. H. & Bayer, D. E. (1989). Structure–activity–residue relationships of alkylphenol polyoxyethylene non-ionic surfactants and MSMA. *Pesticide Science*, 27, 243–51.

Fellers, B. D., Flock, E. L. & Conley, J. C. (1988). Bromine replaces chlorine in cooling-water treatment. *Power*, 132, 15–20.

Fliermans, C. B. & Harvey, R. S. (1984). Effectiveness of 1-bromo-3-chloro-5,5-dimethylhydantoin against *Legionella pneumophila* in a cooling tower. *Applied and Environmental Microbiology*, 47, 1307–10.

Freis, R. E. (1984). The effect of a specific enzyme on biocide use. *Journal of the Technical Association of the Pulp and Paper Industry*, 67, 100–2.

French, M. S. & Evans, L. V. (1988). The effects of copper and zinc on growth of the fouling diatoms *Amphora* and *Amphiprora*. *Biofouling*, 1, 3–18.

Gaylarde, C. C. (1990). Advances in detection of microbiologically induced corrosion. *International Biodeterioration*, 26, 11–22.

Gaylarde, C. C. & Johnston, J. M. (1982). The effect of *Vibrio anguillarum* on anaerobic metal corrosion induced by *Desulfovibrio vulgaris*. *International Biodeterioration Bulletin*, **18**, 111–16.

Gaylarde, C. C. & Johnston, J. M. (1983). The effect of some environmental factors on biocide sensitivity in *Desulfovibrio*: implications for biocide testing. In *Microbial Corrosion*, pp. 91–7. The Metals Society, London.

Gaylarde, C. C. & Johnston, J. M. (1984). Some recommendations for sulphate-reducing bacteria biocide tests. *Journal of Oil and Colour Chemists Association*, **12**, 305–9.

Gaylarde, C. C. & Latorre, W. (1992). Microbiological problems in cooling water systems. *Biodeterioration Abstracts*, **6**, 329–37.

Gaylarde, C. C. & Videla, H. A. (1992). Biocide action on metal biofilms. In *Proceedings of the PanAmerican Congress on Corrosion and Protection*, Mar del Plata, pp. 371–8. NACE, Houston, TX.

Gaylarde, P. M. & Gaylarde, C. C. (1992). The kinetics of biocide uptake in a model biofilm. *International Biodeterioration and Biodegradation*, **29**, 273–83.

Gilbert, P. & Brown, M. R. W. (1978). Influence of growth rate and nutrient limitation on the gross cellular composition of *Pseudomonas aeruginosa* and its resistance to 3- and 4-chlorophenol. *Journal of Bacteriology*, **133**, 1066–72.

Gilbert, P. & Brown, M. R. W. (1980). Cell-wall mediated changes in the sensitivity of *Bacillus megaterium* to chlorhexidine and 2-phenoxyethanol, associated with growth rate and nutrient limitation. *Journal of Applied Bacteriology*, **48**, 223–30.

Ginn, S. T., Conley, J. C., Sargent, R. H. & Fellers, B. D. (1989). Bromine biocides in alkaline and high demand cooling waters. In *Corrosion 89*, Paper no. 157. NACE, Houston, TX.

Goldberg, A. M. & Frazier, J. M. (1989). Alternatives to animals in toxicity testing. *Scientific American*, **261**, 24–30.

Greve, P. A. & van Zoonen, P. (1990). Organochlorine pesticides and PCBs in tissues from Dutch citizens (1968–1986). *International Journal of Environmental and Analytical Chemistry*, **38**, 265–77.

Guthrie, W. G. & Elsmore, R. (1990). A broad spectrum biocide combination. New developments in industrial biocides. *Speciality Chemicals*, **10**, 345–6.

Haack, T. K., Lashen, E. S. & Greenley, D. E. (1988). The evaluation of biocide efficacy against sessile microorganisms. *Developments in Industrial Microbiology*, **29**, 247–53.

Haggett, R. D. & Morchat, R. M. (1991). Microbial contamination: biocide treatment in naval distillate fuel. *International Biodeterioration and Biodegradation*, **29**, 78–99.

Halleux, P. (1990). Regulatory demands for biocides today and in the 1990s. *International Biodeterioration*, **26**, 251–8.

Hassan, R. S. & Oh, I. C. P. (1989). Effect of sodium hypochlorite (Chlorox) and its mode of application on biofilm development. *Biofouling*, **4**, 353–61.

Hill, E. C. (1990). Biocides for the future. *International Biodeterioration*, **26**, 281–5.

Holah, J. T., Higgs, C., Robinson, S., Worthington, D. & Spenceley, H. (1990). A conductance-based surface disinfection test for food hygiene. *Letters in Applied Microbiology*, **11**, 255–9.

Jensen, A. A. (1983). Chemical contaminants in human milk. *Residue Reviews*, **89**, 1–129.

Jones, M. V., Johnson, M. D. & Herd, T. M. (1991). Sensitivity of yeast vegetative cells and ascospores to biocides and environmental stress. *Letters in Applied Microbiology*, **12**, 254–7.

Kawata, K. (1980). Mode of bacterial inactivation by chlorine dioxide. *Water Research*, **14**, 635–41.

Kinniment, S. & Wimpenny, J. W. T. (1990). Biofilms and biocides. *International Biodeterioration*, **26**, 181–94.

Koller, W. & Wubben, J. P. (1989). Variable resistance factors of fungicides acting as sterol demethylation inhibitors. *Pesticides Science*, **26**, 133–45.

Kramer, J. F. (1991). Glutaraldehyde is effective in controlling biofilms in laboratory simulation of metal-working circulating system. In *Proceedings of the 8th International Symposium on Biodeterioration and Biodegradation*, Windsor, Ontario, August 1990, pp. 463–4.

Kraniak, J. M. & Shelef, L. A. (1988). Effect of ethylenediaminetetraacetic acid (EDTA) and metal ions on growth of *Staphylococcus aureus* 196E in culture medium. *Journal of Food Science*, **53**, 910–13.

Kronig, B. & Paul, T. (1897). Die chemischen Grundlegen der Lehre von der Giftwirkung und Desinfektion. *Zeitschrift für Hygiene*, **25**, 1–49.

Lamot, J. E. (1988). Role of biocides in controlling microbial corrosion. In *Microbial Corrosion I*, ed. C. A. C. Sequeira & A. K. Tiller, vol. I, pp. 224–34. Elsevier Applied Science, London and New York.

Lapin-Scott, H. M. & Costerton, J. W. (1989). Bacterial films and surface biofouling. *Biofouling*, **1**, 323–42.

Larson, R. J. & Ventullo, R. M. (1991). Acclimation and biodegradation response of natural microbial communities to surfactants. In *Proceedings of the 8th International Symposium on Biodeterioration and Biodegradation*, Windsor, Ontario, August 1990, pp. 373–4.

Lewis, J. A. & Smith, B. S. (1990). Hydroides settlement in Sydney Harbour (Australia) and its control in seawater cooling systems. In *Abstracts of the 8th International Symposium on Biodeterioration and Biodegradation*, Windsor, Ontario, August 1990.

Lloyd, G. (1990). The development of 'safer' compounds for biocidal use. *International Biodeterioration*, **26**, 245–50.

Lunden, K. C. & Stastny, T. M. (1985). Sulfate reducing bacteria in oil and gas production. In *Corrosion 85*, Paper no. 296. NACE, Houston, TX.

Massolini, G., Kitsos, M., Gandini, C. & Cacciolanza, G. (1989). Fungicidal activity of phenylpyridylketoximes and their O-acetyl derivatives. *Pesticide Science*, **26**, 209–14.

Menezes, T. M., Band, D. E. & Gaylarde, C. C. (1994). Biofilm and biocide assessment using epifluorescence microscopy. In *Proceedings of the 9th International Biodeterioration and Biodegradation Symposium*, Leeds, England, 5–10 September, in press.

Midorikawa, Y., Hibasami, H., Gasaluck, P., Yoshimura, H., Masiyi, A., Nakashima, K. & Imai, M. (1991). Evaluation of the antimicrobial activity of methylglyoxal bis(guanylhydrazone) analogues, the inhibitors for polyamine biosynthetic pathway. *Journal of Applied Bacteriology*, **70**, 291–3.

Mrozek, H. (1982). Development trends with disinfection in the food industry. *Deutsche Molkerei-Zeitung*, **12**, 348–52.

Nakamura, N., Kitajima, Y. & Matsunaga, T. (1989). Electrochemical sterilisation of marine microorganisms. In *Program of the 1st International Marine Biotechnology Conference*, p. 53.

Nanishi, Y., Yonehara, Y. & Kishihara, M. (1989). Influence of structural and thermodynamic properties of phase-separated films on adsorption of proteins and marine fouling. In *Program of the 1st International Marine Biotechnology Conference*, p. 50.

Nicell, J., Siddique, M., Bewtra, J., St. Pierre, C., Biswas, N. & Taylor, K. (1991). Enzyme catalyzed removal of aromatic compounds from aqueous solution. In *Proceedings of the 8th International Symposium on Biodeterioration and Biodegradation*, Windsor, Ontario, August 1990, pp. 518–19.

Nichols, J. A. (1988). Antifouling paints: use on boats in San Diego Bay and a way to minimize adverse effects. *Environmental Management*, **12**, 243–7.

Nunes, N. V. (1982). Bactérias indutoras da corrosão. *Boletim Técnico da Petrobras*, **25**, 147–51.

Page, S. & Gaylarde, C. (1990). Biocide activity against *Legionella* and *Pseudomonas*. *International Biodeterioration*, **26**, 139–48.

Parr, J. A. (1990). Industrial biocide formulation – the way forward. *International Biodeterioration*, **26**, 237–44.

Paulus, W. (1988). Developments in microbicides for the protection of materials. In *Biodeterioration 7*, ed. D. R. Houghton, R. N. Smith & H. O. W. Eggins, pp. 1–19. Elsevier Applied Science, London and New York.

Paulus, W. (1991). Microbiocides for the protection of materials – yesterday, today, tomorrow. In *Proceedings of the 8th International Symposium on Biodeterioration and Biodegradation*, Windsor, Ontario, August 1990, ed. H. W. Rossmoore, pp. 35–52. Elsevier, London.

Paulus, W. & Genth, H. (1983). Microbiocidal phenolic compounds – a critical examination. In *Biodeterioration 5*, ed. T. A. Oxley & S. Barry, pp. 701–12. John Wiley & Sons, Chichester.

Piddock, L. J. V. (1990). Techniques used for the determination of antimicrobial resistance and sensitivity to bacteria. *Journal of Applied Bacteriology*, **68**, 307–18.

Pohlman, J. (1990). Fungicidal efficacy of a diiodomethyl-*p*-tolylsulfone emulsion in metal working fluids. In *Abstracts of the 8th International Symposium on Biodeterioration and Biodegradation*, Windsor, Ontario, August 1990.

Power, E. G. M. & Russell, A. D. (1990). Glutaraldehyde – new aspects. *Letters in Applied Microbiology*, **11**, 231–2.

Prasad, B. P., Kantam, M. L., Choudary, B. M., Sukumar, K. & Satyanarayana, K. (1990). New pesticide metal complexes for controlled release. *Pesticide Science*, **28**, 157–65.

Riha, V. F., Sondossi, M. & Rossmoore, H. W. (1990). The potentiation of industrial biocide activity with Cu^{2+}. II. Synergistic effects with

5-chloro-2-methyl-2-isothiazolin-3-one. *International Biodeterioration*, **26**, 303–13.

Rogers, P. B. (1989). Potential of biocontrol organisms as a source of antifungal compounds for agrochemical and pharmaceutical product development. *Pesticide Science*, **27**, 155–64.

Rossmoore, H. W. (1990). The interaction of formaldehyde, isothiazolone and copper. *International Biodeterioration*, **26**, 225–36.

Rossmoore, H. W. & Rossmoore, L. A. (1991). Effect of microbial growth products on biocide activity in metalworking fluids. *International Biodeterioration*, **27**, 145–56.

Ruggerio, M. A. & Farmer, D. A. (1991). Preliminary evaluation of the efficacy of zinc pyrithrone as a microbiocide in antifouling marine coatings. In *Proceedings of the 8th International Symposium on Biodeterioration and Biodegradation*, Windsor, Ontario, August 1990, pp. 476–7.

Ruseska, I., Robbins, J., Costerton, J. W. & Lashen, E. S. (1982). Biocide testing against corrosion causing oil-field bacteria helps control plugging. *Oil and Gas Journal*, **80**, 253–8.

Sanders, P. F. (1988). Control of biocorrosion using laboratory and field assessments. *International Biodeterioration*, **24**, 239–46.

Sandin, M., Allenmark, S. & Edebo, L. (1992). The role of alkyl chain length on the antibacterial activity of alkyl ethanolamines. *Biomedical Letters*, **47**, 85–92.

Sandin, M., Mattsby-Baltzer, I. & Edebo, L. (1991). Control of microbial growth in water-based metal-working fluids. *International Biodeterioration*, **27**, 61–74.

Sanger, E. & Connell, G. F. (1990). Successful bromine/chlorine use in cooling water treatment. In *Official Proceedings of the 51st International Water Conference*, pp. 308–14. Engineers Society of Western Pennsylvania, Pittsburgh.

Scott, V. N. (1989). Interaction of factors to control microbial spoilage of refrigerated foods. *Journal of Food Protection*, **52**, 431–5.

Sekikawa, A., Sugi, H. & Takahashi, R. (1989). European Patent Application EP362,262, 2 August 1989.

Sequeira, C. A. C., Carrasquinho, M. P. N. A. & Cebola, C. M. (1988). Control of microbial corrosion in cooling water systems by the use of biocides. In *Microbial Corrosion I*, ed. C. A. C. Sequeira & A. K. Tiller, vol. I, pp. 240–55. Elsevier Applied Science, London and New York.

Sharma, A. P. (1984). Biological aspects of the control of sulphate-reducing bacteria. Ph.D. thesis, Heriot-Watt University, Edinburgh.

Singer, M. (1990). The role of antimicrobial agents in swimming pools. *International Biodeterioration*, **26**, 159–68.

Sly, L. I., Hodgkinson, M. C. & Arunpairojana, V. (1990). Deposition of manganese in a drinking water distribution system. *Applied and Environmental Microbiology*, **56**, 628–39.

Smyk, E. B., Smyrniotis, L. R. & Wiatr, C. L. (1989). Method for inhibiting corrosion in cooling systems and compositions therefor containing a nitrite corrosion inhibitor and bromosulfamate. US Patent US4,992,209, 1989.

Sondossi, M., Riha, V. F. & Rossmoore, H. W. (1990). The potentiation of industrial biocide activity with Cu^{2+}. I. Synergistic effect of Cu^{2+} with formaldehyde and formaldehyde-releasing biocides. *International Biodeterioration*, 26, 51–61.

Sublette, K. L., Hasan, S., Cho, P. & Pak, D. (1990). Porphyrin catalyzed degradation of phenols and nitro-substituted toluenes. In *Abstracts of the 8th International Symposium on Biodeterioration and Biodegradation*, Windsor, Ontario, August 1990.

Sublette, K. L., Woolsey, M. E., Manning, F. S., Montgomery, A. D. & McInerney, M. J. (1989). Microbial control of hydrogen sulfide production by sulfate reducing bacteria. USA Patent Application, 1989.

Tadros, Th. F. (1989). Colloidal aspects of pesticidal and pharmaceutical formulations – an overview. *Pesticide Science*, 26, 51–77.

Thomas, J. L. & Moss, M. O. (1990). The loss of biological activity of the preservative Bronopol associated with *Fusarium solani*. *International Biodeterioration*, 26, 327–35.

Thomas, R. W. S. P. & Allsopp, D. (1983). The effects of certain periphytic marine bacteria upon the settlement and growth of *Enteromorpha*, a fouling alga. In *Biodeterioration 5*, ed. T. A. Oxley & S. Barry, pp. 348–57. John Wiley & Sons, Ltd, Chichester.

Valls, M., Bayona, J. M. & Albaiges, J. (1990). Broad spectrum analysis of ionic and non-ionic contaminants in urban wastewaters and coastal receiving aquatic systems. *International Journal of Environmental and Analytical Chemistry*, 39, 329–48.

van der Wende, E. (1990). Biocide action on biofilms. *IPA Bulletin*, 5, 6–8.

Videla, H. A., Sautu, A. E., Gomez de Saravia, S. G., Guiamet, P. S., de Mele, M. F. L., Gaylarde, C. C. & Beech, I. B. (1991). Impact of glutaraldehyde on biofouling and MIC of different steels. A laboratory assessment. *Corrosion 91*, Paper no. 105. NACE, Houston, TX.

Vincentini, C. B., Poli, T., Veronese, A. C., Brandolini, V., Manfrini, M., Guarneri, M. & Giori, P. (1989). Synthesis and in vitro anti-fungal activity of 6-trifluoromethylpyrazolo(3,4-D)pyrimidin-4(5H)-thiones. *Pesticide Science*, 27, 77–83.

Whittingham, K. P. & Hardy, J. A. (1985). Microbial corrosion control in water injection systems. In *U.K. Corrosion 85*, pp. 271–80. Institution of Corrosion Science and Technology, Birmingham.

Williams, E. E. & Knox-Holmes, B. (1989). Marine biofouling solutions for closed seawater systems. *Sea Technology*, 30, 17–18.

Wright, N. E. & Gilbert, P. (1987a). Influence of specific growth rate and nutrient limitation upon the sensitivity of *Escherichia coli* towards chlorhexidine diacetate. *Journal of Applied Bacteriology*, 62, 309–14.

Wright, N. E. & Gilbert, P. (1987b). Antimicrobial activity of n-alkyltrimethylammonium bromides: influence of specific growth rate and nutrient limitation. *Journal of Pharmacy and Pharmacology*, 39, 685–90.

Wyss, O. & Stockton, J. R. (1947). Germicidal action of bromine. *Archives in Biochemistry*, 12, 267–71.

Yabe, H., Ito, Y., Seo, H., Minamide, J., Negoro, M. & Kamiyoshi, H. (1987).

Bacteriophages immobilised on chitosan substrate as bacteriocides. Japanese Patent Application No. 87/197,165, 6 August 1987.

Yamashita, N., Etoh, H., Sakata, K., Ina, H. & Ina, K. (1989). New acylated rhaponticin isolated from *Eucalyptus rubida* as a repellent against the blue mussel *Mytilus edulis*. *Agricultural and Biological Chemistry*, **53**, 2827–9.

Yamishita, K. (1990). Influence of ultra-violet irradiation on the larvae of barnacles. In *Abstracts of the 8th International Symposium on Biodeterioration and Biodegradation*, Windsor, Ontario, August 1990.

Zhang, Z. & Matson, J. V. (1989). Organic halogen stabilisers. Mechanisms and disinfection efficiencies. In *Proceedings of the Cooling Tower Institute 1989 Annual Meeting*, New Orleans, 23–25 January, Paper no. T89-05. Cooling Tower Institute, Houston, TX.

Index